American Public Health Association

VITAL AND HEALTH STATISTICS MONOGRAPHS

Mental Disorders / Suicide

Mental Disorders / Suicide

MORTON KRAMER, EARL S. POLLACK,
RICHARD W. REDICK, AND BEN Z. LOCKE

HARVARD UNIVERSITY PRESS
Cambridge, Massachusetts
1972

Library of Congress Catalog Number 74-186673
SBN 674-56735-8
Printed in the United States of America

Preface

So that prospective readers of this monograph will not be misled by its title, *Mental Disorders/Suicide*, the authors wish to disabuse them immediately of any notion that this volume is presenting the results of a study of the relationship of mental disorders to suicide. The title of this volume arose from the fact that the organizing committee of this series decided that mental disorders and suicide are two important public health problems, and that statistical data on both should be included in the same volume. Ideally, these data should conform to the basic purposes of all of the monographs in the series: (1) to present detailed morbidity and mortality rates for major problems of disease and disability for the United States and its various subdivisions utilizing the 1960 census data as denominators for the rates; (2) to present trends of these rates; (3) to use these data and other relevant information to determine the health status of the population as of 1960 and, where time series are available, changes that have occurred up to that point; and (4) to establish baselines against which to measure further change.

It is not possible to meet these objectives for the mental disorders because the types of annual morbidity statistics required to do so do not exist for the United States, or for any other country of the world. For reasons reviewed in Chapter 1, no health agency has developed a mechanism for the systematic collection of morbidity data on the mental disorders which can be used to provide reliable, current estimates of their incidence and prevalence (American Public Health Association, 1962). Indeed, the only systematic morbidity statistics on the mental disorders that are reasonably compatible with the above stated purposes are those dealing with the mentally ill who are admitted to mental hospitals and certain other types of psychiatric facilities. Thus, the chapters of this monograph dealing with mental disorders will, for the most part, describe variations in the patterns of use of such services. Admittedly, these are medical care rather than true morbidity statistics and, as such, they have many limitations for epidemiologic purposes. However, data on the number of "patients under care" and rates and ratios derived from them have served many useful purposes in the past for epidemiologic as well as for administrative studies and will continue to do so in the future. Indeed, such statistics have become increasingly important as a result of the intensified national effort to provide improved systems for delivery of mental health and related services and to evaluate their effectiveness.

The situation with respect to statistics on suicide is different from that for mental disorders in one respect and quite similar in others. The National Death Registration system provides systematic information for all deaths that occur in the United States on underlying and associated causes of death and the demographic characteristics of the deceased. Thus, it is possible to establish systematic mortality rates for suicide that conform to the basic purposes of the monograph. However, there are many problems related to the reporting of suicide as a cause of death. In addition, because of the absence of systematic national statistics on attempted suicides, it is impossible to present a complete statistical picture of the suicide problem which includes rates not only on the characteristics of the persons who are successful suicides but also on the persons who attempt such an act. This problem is much the same as that which exists in relation to the mental disorders. Although systematic data are available on the characteristics of persons who use certain types of psychiatric services, morbidity data are not available on the distribution of mental disorders in the general population. Thus, it is not possible to relate the rates at which people enter into psychiatric care to the rates of incidence and prevalence of mental disorders in the general population.

Chapter 1 expands on these basic problems and concepts. The data presented in this monograph on the institutionalized mentally ill are first admission and resident patient rates of state and county mental hospitals by age, sex, and diagnosis for the United States and its various subdivisions for the years 1959-61 and trends in these rates for the period 1940-67. These data form the basis for a first approximation to a descriptive epidemiology of mental disorders. Chapter 2 presents a description of the national program for collection of such data, definitions of "first admission" and "resident patient" and the rates computed from these data, the statistical classification of mental disorders used in this monograph, and a discussion of problems related to the accuracy of psychiatric diagnosis and consistency with which diagnostic terms are used by psychiatrists. Chapter 3 depicts overall trends in the patterns of use of state and county mental hospitals during the period 1946-66 and presents detailed rates of first admission and resident patients by age, sex, and diagnosis for the United States, its regions, and the individual states. Chapter 4 illustrates the patterns of use of the universe of psychiatric facilities consisting of the mental hospitals (state, county, private, and Veterans Administration), outpatient clinics, and psychiatric inpatient services of the general hospitals for the United States for 1966, the first year for which such a complete picture of psychiatric care in the U.S. was available.

Unfortunately, the National Reporting Program did not collect data on the demographic characteristics of the patients under care of psychiatric facilities by race, place of residence, occupation, income, and marital status. However, the National Institute of Mental Health collaborated with various states in the analysis of data such as those which were collected through the statistical systems in their state mental hospital programs as well as through special studies designed to obtain data on the relationship of living arrangements to patterns of psychiatric care. Chapter 5 presents data on the changes in first admission rates to the mental hospitals in the state of Ohio for the period 1949-51 and 1959-61 and in the patterns of use of all psychiatric facilities for years 1959-61 specific for selected diagnoses and a range of demographic variables. Chapter 6 presents first admission rates to the universe of psychiatric facilities (defined as above) in the states of Maryland and Lousiana during 1960 specific for age, sex, diagnosis, living arrangements, and selected socioeconomic variables.

Chapter 7 is concerned with death rates from suicide specific for age, sex, method of suicide, and several other variables for the years 1959-61 and trends in these rates for the period 1900-1965.

The authors wish to express their deep appreciation to current and former members of the staff of the Biometry Branch of the National Institute of Mental Health for their many contributions which helped to produce this volume. Special mention must be given to some of them individually for their key roles: Dr. Anita Bahn and Mr. Carl Taube, who provided much of the national data used in this volume; Mrs. Henrietta Duvall, who organized the tabulations of national data and supervised much of the detailed computational work; and Mrs. Dorothy Goldklang, who researched the literature and prepared a substantial part of the initial draft of the chapter on suicide. Miss Sarah Turner, of the Center for Epidemiologic Studies, NIMH, provided valuable assistance in organizing the Ohio material in Chapter 5. Our thanks also go to Mrs. Linda Woolson, Miss Patricia

Weidlein, and Mrs. Ruby Kaster of the Biometry Branch, NIMH, for their typing of numerous drafts of text and tables. Finally, we wish to express our appreciation to the mental health authorities of the various states whose cooperation over the years in the data collection activities of the Biometry Branch of the National Institute of Mental Health has made possible much of the patient data presented in this volume.

Morton Kramer
Earl S. Pollack
Richard W. Redick
Ben Z. Locke

Contents

Tables

Appendix Tables

Figures

Foreword

Rapid advances in medical and allied sciences. changing patterns in medical care and public health programs, an increasingly health-conscious public, and the rising concern of voluntary agencies and government at all levels in meeting the health needs of the people necessitate constant evaluation of the country's health status. Such an evaluation, which is required not only for an appraisal of the current situation but also to refine present goals and to gauge our progress toward them, depends largely upon a study of vital and health statistics records.

Opportunity to study mortality in depth emerges when a national census furnishes the requisite population data for the computation of death rates in demographic and geographic detail. Prior to the 1960 census of population there had been no comprehensive analysis of this kind. It therefore seemed appropriate to build up for intensive study a substantial body of death statistics for a three-year period centered around that census year.

A detailed examination of the country's health status must go beyond an examination of mortality statistics. Many conditions such as arthritis, rheumatism, and mental diseases are much more important as causes of morbidity than of mortality. Also, an examination of health status should not be based solely upon current findings, but should take into account trends and whatever pertinent evidence has been assembled through local surveys and from clinical experience.

The proposal for such an evaluation, to consist of a series of monographs, was made to the Statistics Section of the American Public Health Association in October 1958 by Mortimer Spiegelman, and a Committee on Vital and Health Statistics Monographs was authorized, with Mr. Spiegelman as Chairman, a position he held until his death on March 25, 1969. The members of this Committee and of the Editorial Advisory Subcommittee created later are:

Committee on Vital and Health Statistics Monographs

Carl L. Erhardt, D.Sc., Chairman
Paul M. Densen, D.Sc.
Robert D. Grove, Ph.D.
William H. Stewart, M.D.
(Withdrew June 1964)
Conrad Taeuber, Ph.D.

The early history of this undertaking is described in a paper presented at the 1962 Annual Conference of the Milbank Memorial Fund.[1] The Committee on Vital and Health Statistics Monographs selected the topics to be included in the series and also suggested candidates for authorship. The frame of reference was extended by the Committee to include other topics in vital and health statistics than mortality and morbidity, namely fertility, marriage, and divorce. Conferences were held with authors to establish general guidelines for the preparation of the manuscripts.

Support for this undertaking in its preliminary stages was received from the Rockefeller Foundation, the Milbank Memorial Fund, and the Health Information Foundation. Major support for the required tabulations, for writing and editorial work, and for the related research of the monograph authors was provided by the United States Public Health Service (Research Grant CH 00075, formerly GM 08262). Acknowledgment should also be made to the Metropolitan Life Insurance Company for the facilities and time that were made available to Mr. Spiegelman before his retirement in December 1966 after which he devoted his major time to administering the undertaking and to serving as general editor. Without his abiding concern over each monograph in the series and his close work with the authors, the completion of the series might

[1] Mortimer Spiegelman, "The Organization of the Vital and Health Statistics Monograph Program," *Emerging Techniques in Population Research (Proceedings of the 1962 Annual Conference of the Milbank Memorial Fund;* New York: Milbank Memorial Fund, 1963), p. 230. See also Mortimer Spiegelman, "The Demographic Viewpoint in the Vital and Health Statistics Monographs Project of the American Public Health Association," *Demography,* vol. 3, No. 2 (1966), p. 574.

have been in grave doubt. The published volumes will be a fitting memorial to Mr. Spiegelman even though his name does not appear as an author.

The New York City Department of Health allowed Dr. Carl L. Erhardt to allocate part of his time to administrative details for the series from April to December 1969, when he retired to assume a more active role. The National Center for Health Statistics, under the supervision of Dr. Grove and Miss Alice M. Hetzel, undertook the sizable tasks of planning and carrying out the extensive mortality tabulations for the 1959-1961 period. Dr. Taeuber arranged for the cooperation of the Bureau of the Census at all stages of the project in many ways, principally by furnishing the required population data used in computing death rates and by undertaking a large number of varied special tabulations. As the sponsor of the project, the American Public Health Association furnished assistance through Dr. Thomas R. Hood, its Deputy Executive Director.

Because of the great variety of topics selected for monograph treatment, authors were given an essentially free hand to develop their manuscripts as they desired. Accordingly, the authors of the individual monographs bear the full responsibility for their manuscripts, and their opinions and statements do not necessarily represent the viewpoints of the American Public Health Association or of the agencies with which they may be affiliated.

James R. Kimmey, M.D.
Executive Director
American Public Health Association

Notes on Tables and Figures

1. Regarding 1959-61 mortality data:
   a. Deaths relate to those occurring in the United States (including Alaska and Hawaii);
   b. Deaths are classified by place of residence (if pertinent);
   c. Fetal deaths are excluded;
   d. Deaths of unknown age, marital status, nativity, or other characteristics have not been distributed into the known categories, but are included in their totals;
   e. Deaths are classified by cause according to the Seventh Revision of the International Statistical Classification of Diseases, Injuries, and Causes of Death (Geneva: World Health Organization, 1957);
   f. All death rates are average annual rates per 100,000 population in the category specified as recorded in the United States census of April 1, 1960;
   g. Age-adjusted rates were computed by the direct method using the age distribution of the total United States population in the census of April 1, 1940, as a standard.[1]
2. Symbols used in tables of data:
   --- Data not available;
   ••• Category not applicable;
   – Quantity zero;
   0.0 Quantity more than zero but less than 0.05;
   * Figure does not meet the standard of reliability or precision:
      a) Rate or ratio based on less than 20 deaths;
      b) Percentage or median based on less than 100 deaths;
      c) Age-adjusted rate computed from age-specific rates where more than half of the rates were based on frequencies of less than 20 deaths.
3. Geographic classification:[2]
   a. Standard Metropolitan Statistical Areas (SMSA's): except in the New England states, "an SMSA is a county or a group of contiguous counties which contains at least one city of 50,000 inhabitants or more or 'twin cities' with a combined population of at least 50,000 in the 1960 census. In addition, contiguous counties are included in an SMSA if, according to specified criteria, they are (a) essentially metropolitan in character and (b) socially and economically integrated with the central city or cities." In New England, the Division of Vital Statistics of the National Center for

[1]M. Spiegelman and H. H. Marks, "Empirical Testing of Standards for the Age Adjustment of Death Rates by the Direct Method," *Human Biology*, 38 (1966) 280.

[2]National Center for Health Statistics, *Vital Statistics of the United States*, 1960, Vol. II – Mortality, Part A, Section 7, p. 8.

Health Statistics uses, instead of the definition just cited, Metropolitan State Economic Areas (MSEA's) established by the Bureau of the Census, which are made up of county units.

b. Metropolitan and nonmetropolitan: "Counties which are included in SMSA's or, in New England, MSEA's are called metropolitan counties; all other counties are classified as nonmetropolitan."

c. Metropolitan counties may be separated into those containing at least one central city of 50,000 inhabitants or more or twin cities as specified previously, and into metropolitan counties without a central city.

4. Sources:

In addition to any sources specified in the figures, text tables, and appendix tables, the deaths and death rates for the period 1959-61 are derived from special tabulations made at the National Center for Health Statistics, Public Health Service, U.S. Department of Health, Education, and Welfare, for the American Public Health Association.

5. Population denominators and rates:

The general population denominators used for computation of rates in Chapters 1, 3, and 4 were the resident civilian population as obtained from the Bureau of the Census. For the rates in the remaining chapters the published total population figures, excluding armed forces overseas, were used.

6. Standard population for morbidity rates:

The total United States population in the Census of April 1, 1950, was used as a standard for adjustment of rates in Chapter 3, unless otherwise noted. The total United States population in the Census of April 1, 1960, was used as a standard for adjustment of rates in Chapter 6.

Mental Disorders / Suicide

1 / Basic Problems and Concepts

The development of annual morbidity rates for the mental disorders is a problem that has defied satisfactory solution. Standardized basic instruments required to develop such data are not available: case-finding techniques for detecting persons in the general population with mental disorders; differential diagnostic techniques for assigning each case to a specific diagnostic group with a high degree of reliability, and methods for establishing dates of onset and termination of specific disorders. Until such instruments become available and procedures and programs are developed for their application to population groups, it is difficult to see how systematic morbidity statistics on the mental disorders can be collected. As Frost (1927) states in his classic paper on epidemiology: "since description of the distribution of any disease in a population obviously requires that the disease must be recognized when it occurs, the development of epidemiology must follow and be limited by that of clinical diagnosis and of the rather complex machinery required for the systematic collection of morbidity and mortality statistics."

PREVALENCE SURVEYS

A considerable number of community surveys have been carried out in various parts of the world to determine the prevalence of mental disorders. Lin and Standley (1962) reviewed the surveys carried out before 1960. More recently, Shepherd et al. (1966), have also reviewed this literature, highlighting the contributions made by the British investigators, particularly through determination of psychiatric morbidity rates in surveys of general practices. The prevalence rates reported in these various surveys do not lend themselves to precise comparisons because of differences in their underlying purposes. Each survey used different definitions of a case of mental disorder, case-finding techniques, diagnostic categories, and data analysis methods. Despite the lack of comparability, each study emphasizes that sizeable proportions of population groups in different parts of the world suffer from mental disorders.

Data from five surveys carried out in the U.S. during the past 30 years may be used to illustrate these points:

(a) Of the total population of an urban area, 60 per 1,000 were on the active rolls of mental hospitals and a large number of other health, welfare, social, educational, and correctional agencies that provided services to persons with mental disorders during 1938, the year of the survey (Lemkau et al., 1941).

(b) At least 70 per 1,000 of the population of a rural county were found to be mentally ill as of a given day and would have been referred to a mental health clinic had one existed in the county (Roth and Luton, 1943).

(c) At least 100 per 1,000 of the noninstitutional population, all ages, of a major urban area were found to have a serious mental disorder as of a given date (Pasamanick et al., 1957).

(d) Of the noninstitutional population, 240 per 1,000, aged 20-59 years, of a large metropolitan area were seriously impaired by mental disorder (Srole, et al., 1962).

(e) Of the population of another metropolitan area, 8 per 1,000 were known to be under the care of a private psychiatrist, a psychiatric clinic, or a mental hospital during a six-month period (Hollingshead and Redlich, 1958).

STATISTICS ON THE USE OF PSYCHIATRIC FACILITIES

In the absence of more precise statistics on the incidence and prevalence of the mental disorders, statistics on the patterns of use of psychiatric facilities, particularly mental hospitals, have been used as a first approximation to a descriptive epidemiology of mental disorders. As MacMahon (1967) has pointed out, such statistics provide an operational measure of manifest disability resulting from such disturbances at one or more of the following levels:

1. The persons affected use mental hospitals.
2. They are under psychiatric care either in or out of a mental hospital.
3. They exhibit symptoms or signs such that they would be judged by psychiatric experts as being disabled by mental illness.

He further states that such data are useful in epidemiologic studies: "There is considerable disagreement among psychiatrists as to the conceptual organization of a classification of mental illness, the distribution of individual patients within any single classificatory scheme, and even as to the utility of attempting any classification of this group of illnesses. Nevertheless, certain terms representing broad subgroups of mental illness are widely used clinically. In that these subgroups of illnesses have different patterns of distribution in the population, they seem to have utility in epidemiologic studies and, potentially, for implementation of preventive measures." These patterns of distribution have been derived by applying epidemiologic concepts to analysis of data on the annual numbers of persons admitted to psychiatric facilities and the numbers resident in them as of a given day. Two basic indexes. modeled after the incidence and prevalence rates for a disease, have been used in these analyses. To illustrate, assume that: (1) a mental hospital is designated to serve exclusively all the residents of a given subdivision of a state (catchment area); (2) each patient admitted to that hospital is classified as a "first admission" or a "readmission"; and (3) a census is taken of all patients resident in that hospital as of a given date.

By using the annual number of first admissions to the hospital as the numerator and the population of the catchment area as the denominator, a first admission rate is obtained. This rate, specified for a given mental disorder, is related to, and, under certain limited conditions, may be identical to the incidence rate for that disorder (Kramer, et al., 1961). By using the resident patient count on a given day as a numerator, and the catchment area population (as of the same date) as a denominator, a resident patient rate is obtained. This rate bears the same type of relationship to an admission rate as the prevalence rate for a disease bears to an incidence rate (Kramer, 1957; MacMahon, Pugh, and Ipsen 1960); that is, prevalence of a specific disease is a function of its incidence and duration (i.e., interval between onset, recovery, or death), and the number of resident patients for a specific mental disorder is a function of the number of admissions and their durations of stay following admission. A hypothetical model illustrates this point in Appendix A.

As illustrated in this model, the resident patient population consists of the survivors of groups of patients admitted over many years. The number in each residual group on a given date, therefore, depends on the initial size of the group at time of admission and its subsequent rate of depletion through release or death. Thus, a group of a given size which is depleted relatively quickly makes a smaller contribution to the resident population than another group of the same size which is depleted more slowly. Under certain conditions, a small group can make a greater contribution to the resident population than a larger group. For example, the large group of aged patients with diseases of the senium experience very high mortality rates both in the first few months following admission and in their subsequent hospital experience. Patients in this diagnostic category, therefore, constitute a much smaller proportion of residents than of first admissions. On the other hand, schizophrenics are essentially in the age group 15-54 years at time of admission, remain longer, are readmitted more often, and have a relatively low mortality rate. Therefore, a large number of schizophrenic patients have accumulated, and they represent a considerably higher proportion of residents than of first admissions (Kramer et al., 1956).

Limitations of statistics on psychiatric facility utilization

The limitations of the first admission and resident patient rates as measures of incidence and prevalence should be noted. First admission rates are a result of the incidence of mental disorders and a series of socioeconomic, attitudinal, administrative, and related nosocomial factors that determine the number of persons who are eventually admitted to mental hospitals (Svendsen, 1952; American Public Health Association, 1962). These include availability of mental hospital beds, availability and uses of other community resources for diagnosis and treatment of mental disorders, and public attitudes toward hospitalization. Thus, differences in rates for a specific disorder from time to time and place to place may be influenced as much or more by such factors as by the incidence of mental disorders.

Under certain limited conditions a first admission rate may be a satisfactory measure of the incidence rate for a specific disorder, as, for example, when the characteristics of a disease are such that essentially all persons who develop it are admitted to a hospital. Chronic brain syndrome with central nervous system syphilis is such a disorder (Kramer, 1957; Group for Advancement of Psychiatry, 1961). First admission rates may also be used to provide measures of relative difference in incidence of a specific disorder among members of different demographic subgroups. There are two situations when this might be true: (1) if the ratio of the number of persons becoming hospitalized per year to the number developing the disorder per year is constant between groups, so that the ratio of the first admission rate in Group A to the corresponding rate in Group B is a true measure of relative morbidity risk, and (2) the incidence among persons in Group A is so much greater than that among persons in Group B that regardless of the differences in the ratio of the number of persons hospitalized to the number becoming ill, the difference in first admission rates would still be in the same direction as the true difference in incidence. To amplify these statements, a theoretical formulation of the relationship of the incidence rate to a first admission rate is given in Appendix B.

The resident patient rate also has distinct limitations as a measure of the prevalence of mental disorders. These rates are a function of the rates of first admission, readmission, release, and death operating in these hospitals. The level of the resident patient rate is, therefore, determined by the same factors that affect the admission rates, plus the characteristics of the communities from which these patients are drawn and to which they return, the presence or absence of other facilities for the care and treatment of the mentally ill, the official and unofficial policies of the hospital which affect the admission or release of patients, the staffing patterns and treatment programs, the degree of improvement expected of the patients by the hospital staff before their return to the community, and the attitudes of the patients' family and the community toward the mentally ill and the mental hospital (Belknap, 1956; Brown et al., 1966; Dunham and Weinberg, 1960; Greenblatt et al., 1955, Rawnsley et al., 1962).

Use of first admission and resident patient rates

Despite their limitations for epidemiologic purposes, first admission and resident patient data from mental hospitals and other types of psychiatric services have served many important uses. First admission rates may be used to identify subgroups of the population which are affected by major problems of disability associated with the mental disorders. The very fact of admission to a mental hospital may, in itself, be defined as an index of the occurrence of a serious disability. Thus, studies of first admission rates specific for such variables as age, sex, color, and marital status can provide useful data for planning and developing programs for the control of mental disorders and for planning research. They delineate population groups in which high rates of disability exist and indicate groups which should be singled out for special attention in planning of community mental health services. They also suggest important variables to be considered in the search for causes and effects of mental disorders per se and of hospitalization. Studies of trends of first admission rates specific for age and sex are also very useful in demonstrating changes in the patterns of use of mental hospitals by the communities they serve. With respect to resident populations of mental hospitals, distributions of these populations by age, sex, diagnosis, and length of stay are basic in measuring long-term disability associated with mental disorders and serve as a starting point for many programs designed to reduce chronicity in the mental hospital (Kramer, 1968; Patton, 1958). Historical series of distributions by length of stay are useful in showing whether the number of patients in each of the length of stay categories is rising or falling (Richman, 1966; Richman and Kennedy, 1965).

Recently attempts have been made to extend the concepts of admission to a mental hospital to encompass admission to a universe of psychiatric facilities, which include the mental hospital, outpatient psychiatric clinics, inpatient psychiatric services of general hospitals, and related psychiatric services. Psychiatric case registers have been established in several places in the United States and other countries which collect, collate, and link records on patients admitted to and separated from such a defined universe of psychiatric facilities that serve the residents of the defined catchment area (Bahn et al., 1966; Gardner et al., 1963; Baldwin et al., 1965; Wing et al., 1967; Juel Nielsen et al., 1961; Krupinski and Stoller, 1962). This device makes it possible to determine first admission rates to such a universe. Practical uses of data on first admissions and on resident patients are similar to those described for first admissions and resident patient rates for mental hospitals. The advantage of the register approach is that it permits the development of statistics on an individual person basis rather than an event basis and makes it possible to study the fate of patients over various patterns of facility use. However, data on patterns of use of psychiatric facilities are still a type of medical care data and provide information only on that segment of the universe of mentally ill persons who come in contact with the universe of facilities that report to the register. Admissions to and separations from a specific type of facility are determined by a variety of administrative, attitudinal, socioeconomic, and related factors. Consequently, variations in the rates of usage of the universe of psychiatric facilities or of one of its specific elements are a function of these selective factors as well as of the level of incidence and prevalence of mental disorders of the population groups from which patients are drawn.

The data presented in Chapters 3 to 6 on first admission and resident patient rates to mental hospitals in the United States illustrate uses mentioned above and provide baselines against which to measure change in size and composition of these facilities during the 1970s.

MORTALITY STATISTICS AND MENTAL DISORDERS

Although mortality statistics are an important source of basic data on the distribution of many diseases, they are not a useful source of information on the distribution of mental disorders. National and state data on underlying causes of death provide a very unsatisfactory picture both of the mortality of persons with mental disorders and of the extent of the problems of mental disorders. To illustrate, Table 1.1 presents for the United States the number of

Table 1.1 Annual deaths and crude death rates per 100,000 population in which the underlying cause of death is a mental disorder listed in Section V of the International Classification of Diseases, Seventh Revision (Nos. 300-326): United States, 1950, 1960, and 1967

Cause of death and ICD code (7th Revision)	Number of deaths			Crude rate per 100,000		
	1950	1960	1967	1950	1960	1967
Total (300-326)	4,868	4,487	5,663	3.2	2.5	2.9
Psychoses (300-309)	2,231	1,496	1,853	1.5	0.8	0.9
Schizophrenic disorders (300)	349	161	106	0.2	0.1	0.1
Manic depressive reactions (301)	159	42	17	0.1	0.0	0.0
Senile psychosis (304)	1,053	396	211	0.7	0.2	0.1
Alcoholic psychosis (307)	255	438	599	0.2	0.2	0.3
Other (302, 303, 305-6, 308-9)	361	459	920	0.2	0.3	0.5
Psychoneurotic disorders (310-318)	54	81	96	0.0	0.0	0.0
Disorders of character, behavior and intelligence (320-326)	2,583	2,910	3,714	1.7	1.6	1.9
Alcoholism (322)	2,267	2,235	2,982	1.5	1.2	1.5
Mental deficiency (325)	252	483	526	0.2	0.3	0.3
Other (320-1, 323-4, 326)	64	192	206	0.0	0.1	0.1

Source: Vital Statistics of the United States, Vol. II, Mortality, Part B for 1950, 1960, 1967.

deaths and crude death rates per 100,000 population for 1950, 1960, and 1967 in which a mental disorder was reported as the underlying cause of death. The total numbers of such deaths were 4,868 in 1950, 4,487 in 1960, and 5,663 in 1967.*

Although only a relatively small number of deaths was reported in which a mental disorder was stated to be an underlying cause of death, such disorders were reported more frequently as a contributory cause of death. A study of the National Center for Health Statistics (1965) on multiple causes of death in the United States demonstrated that in 1955 mental disorder was coded as the underlying cause of death 3,574 times, only 9 percent of the 39,660 times they were coded as either an underlying or a contributory cause of death.

MORTALITY OF THE MENTALLY ILL

A large number of deaths occur among persons known to have had a history of mental illness or to be under treatment in an institution for the mentally ill. Thus, in 1967, 39,600 deaths – about 2 percent of all the deaths in the United States – occurred among 801,000 patients under care during that year in the state and county mental hospitals of the nation.** This corresponds to an annual crude rate of 90 deaths for every 1,000 of the average daily number of patients in these institutions.

A variety of studies have demonstrated that the age-specific mortality rates among the hospitalized mentally ill as well as among those under care of outpatient clinics, private psychiatrists, and psychiatric units of general hospitals are considerably in excess of those in the corresponding age groups of the general population. In 1930 the age-adjusted mortality rate from all causes for both sexes in age groups 15 years and over in the mental hospitals of New York State was 78.4 per 1,000 resident patients, about four times the mortality rate of 20 per 1,000 for the general population of New

---

*Source: Vital Statistics of the United States, vol. II, *Mortality*. Part B for 1950; 1960; 1967.

**This estimate is based on the number of patient care episodes to state and county mental hospitals in 1967, i.e., the number of persons under care as of January 1, plus all of the admission actions during the year.

York State in the same age range (Malzberg, 1934). By 1962, the respective rates had decreased by about one third – to 51.4 for the mental hosptial population and 13.4 per 1,000 for the general population – so that the ratio still remained four to one (Kramer, 1968). A recent study has demonstrated that the population of persons (all ages) reported to a psychiatric case register by public and private inpatient and outpatient facilities in Monroe County, New York, during the period 1960-66 had experienced a mortality rate, adjusted for age, that was 2.5 to 3.0 times that of the general population (Babigian and Odoroff, 1969). It is not always clear as to the manner in which mental disorders or institutionalization for them play a role either as a contributory or an underlying cause of death. However, the underlying cause of death tabulation reported from the national mortality statistics in Table 1.1 certainly under-represents the role of mental disorders in mortality.

SUICIDE

Suicides accounted for 21,325 or 1.2 percent of all deaths in the United States in 1967, corresponding to an annual death rate of 10.8 per 100,000 population. The death certificate provides relatively little information about the medical or psychiatric conditions of the deceased. The multiple cause of death study reported above demonstrated that associated conditions are reported very infrequently for deaths in which suicide is the underlying cause. To illustrate, suicide was considered the underlying cause in 16,627 deaths that occurred in the United States in 1955 and was the only condition reported on 80 percent of such deaths. For the other 20 percent of these deaths, 4,140 associated conditions were reported, and a mental disorder accounted for 1,734, or about one-half of such conditions. By relating the 1,734 deaths to the 16,627 deaths with suicide as the underlying cause it can be seen that only 10 percent of deaths with suicide as the underlying cause have a mental disorder recorded as an associated condition. The same study showed that suicide was reported only 112 times as an associated condition to deaths from all other underlying causes.

The Monroe County mortality study, mentioned above, demonstrates, however, that persons known to the psychiatric case register experience an excessive risk of death from suicide. When the ratios of deaths from specific causes among register patients to corresponding death rates in the general population were computed and ranked, suicide was that cause of death for which this relative risk ratio was the highest. The age-adjusted death rate from suicide among males known to the psychiatric case register was 8.0 times that for males in the general population; and 11.3 times for females (Babigian and Odoroff, 1969). Both this study and an earlier one (Gardner et al., 1964), emphasized that only one-third of the total suicides in the county were known to the case register. Although the national mortality statistics provide basic information on suicide, they do not serve a similar function for mental disorders. The data recorded on the death certificate with respect to mental disorders are not of direct value in studying either the distribution of mental disorders in the population or the relationship of mental disorder to suicide.

In summation, this chapter has expanded on some of the issues presented in the preface, namely: (1) the problems of developing morbidity rates for mental disorders; (2) the rates used to characterize patterns of use of psychiatric facilities and their relationships to true morbidity statistics; and (3) the cause of death statistics in relation to mental disorders and suicide. This material is essential background in understanding the detailed data presented in the several chapters comprising this monograph.

2 / Sources and Limitations of Data

Prior to 1946, the year in which Congress passed the National Mental Health Act (PL 79-487, 1946), national data on persons under psychiatric care consisted essentially of age, sex, and diagnostic descriptions of first admissions and resident patients in mental hospitals, particularly those under state and county control. These were the years when mental hospitals were the primary, and in many states the only, resource for the treatment of the mentally ill. During the 1950s increasing emphasis was placed on the development of alternatives to the mental hospital. Outpatient psychiatric clinics began to appear in substantial numbers in the 1950s (Bahn, 1961). In the 1960s other alternatives to the mental hospital began to appear in greater numbers. These included psychiatric services in general hospitals, residential treatment centers for emotionally disturbed children, halfway houses, day care centers, and nursing homes which were used increasingly for the aged mentally ill (Joint Commission, 1961). The passage of the Community Mental Health Centers Act in 1963 (PL 89-105) placed added emphasis on the treatment of persons in their own communities, maintaining them where possible in their own homes and providing continuity of care.

The following discussion describes the changes that have taken place in the number of psychiatric facilities in the United States during the period 1946-66. In 1946 the 586,333 beds in the 500 state, county, and private psychiatric hospitals accounted for 42 percent of all hospital beds in the United States. About 80 percent of the mental hospital beds were located in the state and county mental hospitals. In addition to these beds, there were only 500 outpatient psychiatric clinics and 109 general hospitals with psychiatric services. The situation changed quite dramatically during the next twenty years. In 1966, beds in state, county, and private psychiatric hospitals still accounted for 38 percent of all hospital beds, and 89 percent of the mental hospital beds were in state and county hospitals. But, in addition, 1,046 general hospitals routinely admitted psychiatric patients for diagnosis and treatment, another 2,137 general hospitals admitted such patients on an emergency basis only, and 2,148 outpatient psychiatric clinics were in operation.

Detailed statistics on the characteristics of patients under care in outpatient psychiatric facilities and psychiatric facilities in general hospitals are available for the United States in varying degrees of completeness for the period under consideration. However, by 1966 reports on the age, sex, and diagnostic characteristics of patients using the services of these other facilities had become sufficiently complete to provide a reasonably satisfactory basis for developing a quantitative description of the use of a universe of psychiatric facilities in the United States, defined by mental hospitals, outpatient facilities, and psychiatric services in general hospitals. The following sections describe the procedures that have been used for the collection of national data in mental hospitals and other psychiatric facilities.

THE NATIONAL REPORTING PROGRAM

The National Institute of Mental Health requests reports annually from all psychiatric facilities in the United States of the types indicated in Table 2.1. The data collected are basically of two types: (1) administrative data, such as type of facility, auspices under which it operates, staff, finances, and movement of patients; and (2) characteristics of patients by age, sex, and diagnosis. The numbers of

Table 2.1 Number of known psychiatric facilities 1959 and 1967 and average percent of facilities reporting detailed patient data over the period 1959-67: United States

Type of facility	Number of known facilities		Average percent of facilities reporting patient data, 1959-1967
	1959	1967	
State and county mental hospitals	279	307	90%
Private mental hospitals	270	180	70%
VA neuropsychiatric hospitals	39	41	99%
VA general hospitals	68	77	100%
General hospitals with psychiatric inpatient services	494	1,316	72%
Outpatient psychiatric clinics	1,429	2,213	79%

Source: Annual censuses of patients in mental institutions 1959-1967, National Institute of Mental Health.

facilities listed as reporting during the period 1959-67 in Table 2.1 represent those reporting data on characteristics of patients. The data are collected in the form of statistical tabulations prepared by the individual facility or by the statistical office in a state department of mental health responsible for collecting data on patients treated in the facilities over which it has jurisdiction.

The state and county mental hospitals are those which a state or county operates directly for the care and treatment of the mentally ill within their jurisdiction. The private mental hospitals are those designated as such by a reconciliation of the lists compiled by the American Hospital Association and the National Association of Private Psychiatric Hospitals. The list of general hospitals which admit psychiatric patients for diagnosis and/or treatment has been incomplete until recent years. In 1951 the NIMH conducted a survey to identify such hospitals, and the list was maintained thereafter by requesting additions and deletions from each state mental health authority. In 1964 when it became apparent that this procedure grossly underestimated the number of such facilities, the NIMH contracted with the American Hospital Association to survey all of the general hospitals in the United States to identify those which then admitted persons with a primary diagnosis of mental disorder. The number of hospitals so identified was more than double the number previously listed (Giesler et al., 1966). Since that time, such surveys are carried out on a regularly recurring basis.

At one time, schedules were sent directly to the individual Veterans Administration hospitals requesting data on their psychiatric patients. This practice was discontinued in the late 1950s. when the NIMH began to produce tabulations on neuropsychiatric patients resident in VA hospitals based upon individual patient data supplied by the Veterans Administration. A nation-wide statistical reporting program for outpatient psychiatric clinics was established by the NIMH in 1954 in cooperation with the state mental health authorities. The first nation-wide estimates of the number of patients according to specific characteristics are for the years 1955 and 1956 and were published in 1959 (Bahn and Norman, 1959). The first national survey of psychiatric day-night services was conducted in 1963 (Conwell et al., 1964) and of residential treatment centers for emotionally disturbed children in 1967 (National Association for Mental Health, 1967).

Until 1965 the inpatient and outpatient reporting activities of the NIMH were operated as separate programs. With the increasing emphasis on continuity of care, free-flow of patients between services, and the treatment of patients closer to their own homes, it became increasingly difficult to maintain a distinction between inpatient and outpatient facilities. Many state hospitals began to operate their own outpatient clinics, and some outpatient clinics developed day hospital programs. In 1965, therefore, all of the statistical reporting activities of the NIMH were combined and a first inventory of psychiatric facilities, for the year 1967, was conducted in 1968. Its purpose was to identify all of the various types of psychiatric facilities, to obtain a picture of their characteristics, to determine their staffing and the size of their caseloads and to provide a basis for both complete and sample surveys which would provide estimates of patients' characteristics. While this development is not reflected in the data presented in this volume, it indicates the direction in which national mental health statistics efforts are moving in an attempt to keep pace with developments in the field.

Limitations of the Data

The data collected nationally by the National Institute of Mental Health have a number of limitations. Since the reporting system is completely voluntary, the NIMH has no direct control over the extent to which schedules are submitted. It is apparent from Table 2.1 that reporting has been considerably more incomplete for the private facilities and the psychiatric services of general hospitals. For the state mental hospitals and the outpatient clinics, on the other hand, most states now have central statistical reporting systems in their state departments of mental health, and these agencies report the data requested directly to the NIMH for all of the facilities reporting to them. The reporting for state and county mental hospitals was sufficiently complete to permit in most cases an estimate of the age, sex, and diagnostic distributions for those instances in which the data were missing.

Because of the voluntary reporting system and of the method of record-keeping in many of the facilities, the NIMH has not been able to obtain data in the kind of detail desired from the non-state psychiatric facilities. Thus, data on the characteristics of first admissions by age, sex, and diagnosis were obtained only from the state and private mental hospitals. Since the general hospital record-keeping systems are primarily oriented toward discharges, it has been feasible to obtain data only on the characteristics of discharges. Furthermore, since psychiatric cases represent an average of only 3 to 5 percent of the total caseload of the general hospitals, it has not been possible to obtain such detail on discharges classified by both psychiatric diagnosis and age. Similarly, for outpatient psychiatric clinics it has proved to be more feasible to obtain characteristics of terminations rather than of admissions.

Perhaps one of the most difficult problems encountered in a national reporting system such as that maintained by the NIMH is to obtain data based on uniform definitions. Some degree of uniformity has been achieved only for the state mental hospitals and the outpatient psychiatric clinics. While the other facilities are provided with a detailed set of instructions and definitions, there is no evidence that these are followed by all of the facilities reporting. In 1951 the NIMH took steps to improve the quality of data supplied by the state mental hospital systems and to make possible the collection of additional tabulations basic to a fuller understanding of the population dynamics of the public mental hospitals. A Model Reporting Area for Mental Hospital Statistics was organized to: (1) develop a strong central statistical bureau in each state mental hospital system; (2) develop and use standardized definitions of the various categories of movement of mental hospital patients; (3) produce a standard set of basic tabulations that every state hospital system should have; and (4) use statistical methods appropriate to the analysis of data on patients followed for a long period of time. Eleven states participated in this program in the beginning, and the program grew to 35 states by 1963. At that time the Model Reporting Area was disbanded as a formal mechanism in order to permit more intensive work with the remaining 15 states in an attempt to achieve uniformity of definitions and tabulations across all 50 states.

A similar effort was launched in an attempt to obtain uniform outpatient psychiatric clinic statistics with a first Conference on Mental Health Clinic Statistics in April 1954 (U.S. Department of Health, Education, and Welfare, 1954). Agreement was obtained at that time on a uniform outpatient psychiatric clinic report form which would provide data on the number and location of outpatient psychiatric clinics; clinic auspices; professional staff and man-hours;

source of funds; number, age, and sex of patients served; amount and type of service received by patients; psychiatric disorders found; results of treatment; amount of professional time spent in community-oriented services; etc. Problems of definitions were indeed complex. Agreement was obtained on the definition of an outpatient psychiatric clinic and definition of a patient.

Although it has been possible to obtain age and diagnostic data from the Veterans Administration for resident patients over the years, the VA does not separate its admissions for mental disorders into first admissions and readmissions. Thus, it has not been possible to combine admission data for hospitalized VA psychiatric patients with those for other psychiatric hospitals. It is apparent that, because of these problems in national reporting of data on patients seen in psychiatric facilities, uniform data across all types of facilities do not exist. Therefore, it has not been possible to obtain a precise picture of the characteristics of all patients receiving psychiatric care during a defined period of time. Although attempts have been made to obtain crude estimates of these distributions, this problem is further complicated by the fact that certain individuals are seen in more than one type of facility during the year. Therefore, the addition of data from different types of facilities results in duplicated counts of individuals. Special studies have provided estimates of the amount of this duplication specific for patient characteristics, and, in more recent years, the development of psychiatric case registers has further refined the procedures for obtaining unduplicated counts of individuals receiving psychiatric care (Bahn et al., 1965).

Definition of First Admissions

The classification of admissions to mental hospitals as to whether they were first admissions or readmissions was first used on a national basis in the 1923 census of patients in mental institutions (U.S. Department of Commerce, 1926). The terms were defined essentially as follows: a first admission is a patient admitted for the first time to any hospital for the treatment of mental diseases except institutions for temporary care only. A readmission is a patient admitted who has been previously under treatment in a hospital for mental disease, excepting transfers and those who have received treatment only in institutions for temporary care. Thus, any patient with a prior course of hospitalization in a temporary care hospital, usually a general hospital with a psychiatric service, who was subsequently admitted to a prolonged care mental hospital would have been classified as a first admission to the latter.

These definitions remained essentially the same until 1952, when the Model Reporting Area attempted to make them more specific and to apply them more uniformly in the various state systems. The definition adopted at that time was as follows: A first admission is a patient who has not previously been admitted to a public or nonpublic hospital authorized or recognized for the treatment of mental disorders. A list of such hospitals was then compiled annually by the National Institute of Mental Health from lists submitted by each state mental hospital authority.

In 1962 the term "first admission" was discontinued for purposes of collecting data nationally on patients admitted to mental hospitals. In lieu of this, admissions to mental hospitals were classified according to the following categories:

A. No record of prior admission in an inpatient psychiatric facility
B. Prior admission to state system inpatient psychiatric facility in the state in question. This includes:
    1. State and county hospitals
    2. Institutions for mental defectives
    3. Psychopathic hospitals within the state system
C. Prior admission to other inpatient psychiatric facility. This includes:
    1. State psychiatric facility in other states
    2. VA hospitals
    3. Private hospitals
    4. All other inpatient psychiatric facilities, including psychiatric facilities in general hospitals
D. Combination of B and C

The category most comparable to the previous classification of "first admission" was that of admission with no record of prior admission in an inpatient psychiatric facility. Until 1962 a "first admission" to the New York State mental hospital system included categories (A) and (C,4), above. Included in (C,4) was a large number of patients who had spent a short time in one of the large general hospital psychiatric units in New York City prior to being admitted for the first time into the New York State mental hospital system. In 1962, those included in category (C,4) represented 58 percent of the so-called first admissions to the New York State system (New York State Department of Mental Hygiene, 1966). Since the New York State mental hospital system accounted for 13 percent of the state mental hospital first admissions in the nation immediately prior to the definition change (U.S. Department of Health, Education, and Welfare, 1963), this change in definition had a substantial effect on the comparability of mental hospital first admission data over time.

How well the definitions were adhered to over the years is difficult to determine. It is known that in some instances a first admission was considered as a person being hospitalized in a long-term hospital in that state for the first time regardless of how many previous hospitalizations he may have had in hospitals in other state systems or in private hospitals. In other instances where there were several mental hospitals in a state, each hospital reported a patient with respect to his admission status to that hospital. In others, a person admitted to a state hospital with a prior admission to a psychiatric service of a general hospital was considered a first admission to the state hospital, while in still others, he was considered a readmission. The degree to which each of these variations in definition was used is not known. Because of the incompleteness of reporting for private mental hospitals and because of the absence of data on first admission status of patients admitted to VA facilities, it is impossible to present data on first admission rates to all mental hospitals. Therefore, except where noted to the contrary, the data presented will pertain to first admissions to state and county mental hospitals only.

Definition of Resident Patients

Collection of national data on mental hospital resident patient rates by age, sex, and diagnosis has been much more difficult than collecting similar data for first admissions. This is due primarily to two factors: (1) the identification of resident patients as of a point in time and the tabulation of their characteristics requires the maintenance of a statistical system which permits the addition of information on persons entering the hospital and removal of information for those leaving the hospital; and (2) it has been difficult to obtain agreement on a uniform, nation-wide definition of "resident patient." In almost all the states, some form of statistical system on mental hospital patients is now maintained which permits the tabulation of data on resident patients. Through the Model Reporting Area an attempt was made to obtain a uniform national definition of resident patient. According to this definition, all of those patients present in the hospital on a given day, plus those on short-term leave with the expectation that they would return within seven days were considered resident patients. This is essentially the definition of resident patients used in the data to be presented in this volume. It should be kept in mind that while most of the states in the Model Reporting Area adhered to this definition, it was never adopted consistently by all states. Thus, the time patients spent on short-term leave, while they were considered residents of the hospital, ranged from three to thirty days. One element which all of these variations in definition of resident patient had in common, however, was the fact that patients out of the hospital on some form of short-term leave were considered resident patients, in addition to those physically present in the hospital.

COMPUTATIONS OF FIRST ADMISSION AND RESIDENT PATIENT RATES

The numbers and distributions of first admissions to various state mental hospital systems are subject to considerable annual variation. To obtain some stability in the first admission rates presented in this volume around the census years, average numbers of first admissions were prepared for each of the three-year periods 1939-41, 1949-51, and 1959-61. Estimates of the missing numbers were prepared for the state systems for which data were incomplete for one or more of these years. Similar estimating procedures were carried out for resident patient data from states for which incomplete data were reported for 1959-61. The population data obtained in each of the decennial censuses for the years 1940, 1950, and 1960 were used as the denominators of the various rates that were computed.

DIAGNOSTIC CLASSIFICATION OF MENTAL DISORDERS USED IN THIS MONOGRAPH

For purposes of national statistics, the reporting facilities are requested to use the primary diagnosis of mental disorder established for a patient by psychiatric staff as soon as possible after admission. Thus, the diagnosis on the records of patients admitted to a psychiatric facility – be it a mental hospital, psychiatric service in a general hospital, or outpatient clinic – is the basic item from which annual national statistics on the care of patients specific for type of mental disorder are produced.

Diagnostic nomenclatures based on two different classifications of mental disorders were used by psychiatrists during the period covered by this monograph. From 1934 to 1952 they used the nomenclature and definitions in the *Statistical Manual for Use of Hospitals for Mental Diseases* (American Psychiatric Association and National Committee for Mental Hygiene, 1942). From 1952 to 1970 they used the nomenclature and definitions in the *Diagnostic and Statistical Manual of the American Psychiatric Association,* to be referred to as DSM-1 (American Psychiatric Association, 1952). A historical description of the development of these classifications in the United States is given in Appendix C.

Section V of the fifth and sixth revisions of the International Classification of Diseases – to be referred to as ICD-5 and ICD-6, respectively – was not used to code the diagnostic data collected from the psychiatric facilities of the United States (W.H.O., 1948, 1957). This classification proved to be quite unsatisfactory for coding many of the diagnostic terms which were introduced in DSM-1 (see Appendix C). As a result of a very extensive international collaborative effort, the eighth revision of the ICD (ICD-8) now includes a section on mental disorders which eliminates many of the objections to the corresponding sections of ICD-6 and ICD-7 (W.H.O., 1967). The American Psychiatric Association has now developed a psychiatric diagnostic nomenclature which is compatible with ICD-8, and, starting in January 1, 1970, is being used in all psychiatric facilities throughout the United States (A.P.A., 1968). This now makes it possible to use ICD-8 in preparing statistical tabulations of mental disorders in the United States.

The categories of mental disorders used in this monograph are based on DSM-1. The conversion table given in Appendix D was used to convert diagnostic terms from the 1934 classification into the most appropriate term in DSM-1. The following categories are used:

*All Mental Disorders**

Brain Syndromes (01.0 - 19.43 except 02.1 & 13.00 - 13.03)

Diseases of the senium (15.0 & 17.1)

*The code numbers in parentheses are those that appear on pages 78-86 of DSM-1.

Cerebral arteriosclerosis (15.0)
Senile brain disease (17.1)
Syphilitic (11.0 - 11.2)
Other (except brain syndromes with alcoholism, 02.1 & 13.00 - 13.03)
Functional Psychoses (20-24)
Schizophrenic reaction (22)
Affective and Involutional (20-21)
Other (23-24)
Disorders associated with Alcoholism (02.1, 13.00-13.03, 52.3)
Brain syndromes (02.1 & 13.00 - 13.03)
Addiction (52.3)
Psychoneurosis (40)
Personality disorders (except alcoholism, 50-54 except 52.3)
Mental Deficiency (60-62)
All other

Accuracy and Consistency of Psychiatric Diagnoses

Although a single statistical classification has been used to summarize the diagnostic data reported by each type of facility over the years covered by this monograph, the use of such a classification *per se* does not assure that the diagnostic statistics are comparable. Various studies of the effect of observer variability on psychiatric diagnosis have demonstrated that differences among examining psychiatrists in their theoretical orientation, diagnostic procedures, and use of diagnostic terms can account for sizeable differences in the frequency with which a given diagnosis is reported as of a given moment in time or over time.* Thus, to insure comparability of diagnostic data within a given type of facility (e.g., a mental hospital), the clinical staff must take precautions to assure that they are consistent in the way they apply diagnostic criteria and utilize diagnostic terms with respect to all patients. Similar precautions

*See for example: Ash, 1949; Beck, 1962; Babigian et al., 1965; Cooper, 1967; Cooper et al., 1969; Foulds, 1955; Gurland et al., 1969, 1970; Norris, 1959; Pasamanick et al., 1959; Sandifer et al., 1964; Seeman, 1953; Hunt, 1953; Kreitman, 1961; Kreitman et al., 1961; Schmidt et al., 1956; Shepherd et al., 1968; Stengel, 1959; Ward et al., 1962; Zubin, 1967.

must be taken to assure comparability of diagnostic data between facilities of the same type, as well as between facilities of different types (e.g., the mental hospital vs. the outpatient clinic vs. the general hospital psychiatric service).

The distributions which were used to determine the age-specific rates for a given state by diagnosis were obtained by pooling the data for all hospitals within the state. The national totals were obtained by summing the appropriate diagnostic tables across all states, and the regional data by summing the totals for the states that comprise the region. However, it has not been possible to develop a practical procedure for making estimates of the extent to which differences within and among states in rates specific for diagnosis, either for a given year or over time, are due to variations resulting from observer biases and institutional procedures that affect the way in which patients are diagnosed. The basic reason why such estimates cannot be made is the absence of external standards and criteria for assessing the accuracy of most psychiatric diagnoses. The major exceptions are organic brain syndromes for which the etiology can be established (e.g., those associated with infections, trauma, and drugs).

Shepherd et al. (1968) have discussed the difficulties of assessing the reliability and validity of psychiatric diagnosis. They define the process of making a diagnosis as follows: "The psychiatrist interviews the patient, and chooses from a system of psychiatric terms a few words or phrases which he uses as a label for the patient, so as to convey to himself and others as much as possible about the etiology, the immediate manifestations and the prognosis of the patient's condition." These authors point out that although the same elements are found in diagnostic procedures in general medicine, "there the interview and clinical examination of the patient are usually followed by pathological or biochemical investigations which are expected to give specific and independent clues as to the diagnosis." They recognize that disagreements occur among experienced clinicians in interpretations of physical examinations of the chest, X-rays and electrocardiograms, need for tonsillectomy, etc. However, they state that: "whatever the situation in general practice, psychiatric procedures must be much more vulnerable to observer differences, for in dealing with most psychiatric patients there is a lack of external criteria by which psychiatrist's observations and decisions can be validated; it is usually necessary to rely upon what can be learned about the patient by means of interviews only. Until something is known about how to make the gathering and recording of interview information accurate and reliable, psychiatric diagnosis cannot rest upon a firm foundation."

Shepherd et al. (1968) specify four major elements of an interview conducted for the purpose of making a diagnosis: "These elements are: first, the interviewing technique of the psychiatrist; second, the perception of the patient's speech and behavior; third, the inferences and decisions made by the psychiatrist on the basis of what he has perceived; and fourth, the attachment of a particular diagnostic label to the patient. The second and third components together constitute a complex middle stage during which the psychiatrist perceives, classifies, summarizes, and to some degree interprets statements made by the patient. These processes go on in the psychiatrist's mind as the interview is proceeding, and are his guides in the choosing of further questions or lines of inquiry, which in turn result in more information."

Thus, the making of a psychiatric diagnosis is a process that is highly dependent on the characteristics of the psychiatrist and his techniques for carrying out an interview and for interpreting the information so obtained. This procedure is influenced by the clinician's training, the importance he attaches to diagnosis, his theoretical orientation to the etiology and treatment of specific mental disorders, and his clinical experience. Unless extraordinary precautions are taken, the whole process can be easily affected by the three types of biases that account for observer variability, as described by Reid (1960): "consistent bias which is a reflection of the type and intensity of training which the observer may have had; bias which is personal to himself; and the inconsistencies in his own judgment over a period of time which may be either erratic or regular." To these should be added a fourth type of bias that occurs in a reporting program that relies on diagnostic data from clinicians in hospitals and clinics operating under quite different administrative, fiscal, and clinical policies, as well as theoretical orientations: the bias resulting from formal processes and procedures which different institutions require their clinical staffs to follow in determining official diagnoses that are recorded in a patient's record.

Since no practical way exists at present for adjusting the reported diagnostic data for the various types of biases discussed above and since no external criteria exist for establishing a "correct" diagnosis in a uniform way for patients admitted to each type of facility, the diagnostic data in this monograph are presented as reported. Despite their inadequacies, they provide at least a quantitative description of the relative frequency of psychiatric disorders that a large proportion of the nation's psychiatrists state they are treating among the patients admitted to our major psychiatric facilities. Truly comparable data on the mental disorders will not be available until diagnostic standards and methods for their uniform application are developed. Some promising attempts have been made along these lines. These include:

(1) Activities under the auspices of the World Health Organization (W.H.O.):

a) Diagnostic seminars devoted to studies of observer variation and psychiatric diagnoses and the development of improved international statistical classification of mental disorders.*

b) A nine-country international pilot study of schizophrenia which is attempting to establish standards for a diagnosis of schizophrenia which can be applied uniformly across national boundaries (W.H.O.: *Report on International Pilot Study of Schizophrenia,* in preparation).

(2) Research being carried out by a bilateral team from the New York State Psychiatric Institute (New York City) and the Institute of Psychiatry (London):

a) Development and application of uniform diagnostic and patient assessment procedures for investigating diagnostic differences in admissions to mental hospitals in London and New York.†

b) Use of videotape.

c) Structured and unstructured interviews to investigate differences in diagnostic practice of British and American psychiatrists (Kendell et al., 1969; Gurland et al., 1969).

---

*The World Health Organization has convened 5 seminars on Psychiatric Diagnosis, Classification and Statistics. The overall program is described by Lin (1967) and Shepherd et al. (1968). The results of the first three seminars have been published (Shepherd et al., 1968, Ødegard and Astrup 1970, and Rutter et al., 1969). Mimeographed reports of the other seminars are available from the Mental Health Unit, W.H.O., Geneva (W.H.O., 1968, and W.H.O., 1969).

†Kramer, 1969; Zubin, 1969; Gurland et al., 1969, 1970; Cooper, 1969.

(3) Development of computer programs for producing psychiatric diagnoses by applying a logical decision-tree program, which simulates the way a clinician makes a diagnosis, to the analysis of patients' responses to questions in a standardized psychiatric interview (Spitzer, 1968; Wing, 1965).

The results of such research may provide in the future the instruments and procedures needed to resolve the difficult problems attendant to collecting uniform diagnostic data on the mental disorders.

3 / State and County Mental Hospitals, 1946-66

The care of the mentally ill in state and county mental hospitals has been documented extensively over the years, and the records of patients admitted to these hospitals have been a primary source of statistical data on the mental disorders. Statistics derived from these records have provided a first approximation to a descriptive epidemiology of the mental disorders. Studies of first admission rates to public hospitals by age, sex, migration factors, marital status, and other socioeconomic variables have demonstrated the high toll mental disorders take in every age group; in the lower socioeconomic groups; in nonwhites as compared to whites; in the highly urbanized areas as compared to the more rural; in migrant population groups as compared to the nonmigrant; and in the never married, separated, divorced, and widowed as compared to the married.*

Other studies have provided extensive documentation of the age, sex, marital, length of stay, and diagnostic characteristics of the populations resident in these institutions, and of the manner in which an increasing number of patients accumulated in these hospitals. Despite the fact that the proportion of first admissions being returned to their communities during the first twelve months following hospitalization increased from 50 percent in 1946 to about 63 percent in 1955, the chances of return to the community for those patients not released in the first year diminished rapidly with increasing length of hospitalization (H.E.W., 1962 and 1964). These patients became part of the hard core chronic population and grew old in the hospital. Table 3.1 illustrates the length of stay distribution of patients resident in the state and county mental hospitals of 23 states in the Model Reporting Area by selected diagnoses as of the end of 1962. The median length of hospitalization for all residents was 8.4 years, for schizophrenics 12.8 years; mental diseases of the senium (brain syndromes associated

*The following is a partial listing of such studies: American Psychopathological Association, 1945; Dayton, 1940; Faris and Dunham, 1939; Fowler et al., 1956; Group for the Advancement of Psychiatry, 1961; Jaco, 1960; Kramer et al., 1961; Locke et al., 1958, 1960a,b; McCaffery, 1955; Malzberg, 1955, 1958; Malzberg and Lee, 1956; Pollack et al., 1961; Pollock, 1941; Pugh and MacMahon, 1962.

Table 3.1 Number and percent distribution of patients resident in state and county mental hospitals at the end of year by length of stay for selected mental disorders: 23 selected states, 1962

Length of stay (in years)	All disorders	Schizo-phrenia	Mental diseases of senium	All other disorders
Number				
Total	359,654	184,449	46,890	128,315
Less than 1	66,302	24,923	13,499	27,880
1-4	79,012	31,162	20,337	27,513
5-9	52,514	24,711	8,251	19,552
10-19	73,451	41,431	3,855	28,165
20 & over	88,375	62,222	948	25,205
Median length of stay	8.4	12.8	3.0	8.3
Median age (years)	55.6	51.1	75+	75+
Percentage of diagnostic group				
Total	100.0	100.0	100.0	100.0
Less than 1	18.4	13.5	28.8	21.7
1-4	22.0	16.9	43.4	21.5
5-9	14.6	13.4	17.6	15.2
10-19	20.4	22.5	8.2	22.0
20 & over	24.6	33.7	2.0	19.6
Percentage of length of stay category				
Total	100.0	51.3	13.0	35.7
Less than 1	100.0	37.6	20.4	42.0
1-4	100.0	39.4	25.7	34.9
5-9	100.0	47.1	15.7	37.2
10-19	100.0	56.4	5.2	38.4
20 & over	100.0	70.4	1.1	28.5

Source: Kramer, Morton, Statistics of Mental Disorder in the United States. Journal of the Royal Statistical Society, Series A (general) Vol. 32, Part 3, Table 1, 1969.

with senile brain disease and cerebral arteriosclerosis) 3.0 years, and all other disorders 8.3 years. The accumulation of these patients, particularly the schizophrenics, was due not only to the severity of their illness but also to the depersonalizing effects of long-term institutionalization per se, due to such factors as inadequate treatment and rehabilitation programs, lack of psychosocial stimulation, insufficient staff, administrative problems related to organizational structure and size of hospital, insufficient community resources to bridge the gap between hospital and community, and decreased interest in patients on the part of relatives, friends, and the community at large.

The problems of providing medical and psychiatric care to the large number of aged with diseases of the senium also had their impact on the public mental hospitals. Studies underscored the high level of first admission rates of patients 65 years and over (Pollack et al., 1961). Between 1939-41 and 1956-58 the average annual number of first admissions of patients 65 years and over increased from 17,000 to 34,000 (a 100 percent increase), and the corresponding average annual age-specific first admission rates from 184 per 100,000 to 233 (a 27 percent increase). Although the duration of stay of the patients was relatively short, largely because of high mortality rates resulting from their poor physical condition at time of admission, the continuing admission of large numbers of aged patients contributed substantially to the growth of the public mental hospital population (Kramer et al., 1955; Pollack et al., 1959). Another factor that contributed to the increase in number of long-term patients was the reduction in patient mortality that occurred as the result of programs that provided better health care for patients and improved living conditions within the hospital setting. The general change in the mortality rates of the hospitalized mentally ill is illustrated by the experience of the New York State mental hospital system in Table 3.2, which presents the mortality rates for all patients, schizophrenics, and those with all other diagnoses specific for age along with the corresponding mortality rates in the general population for the years 1930 and 1962.

Although death rates in mental hospitals in 1962 were still higher than those in the general population, there was considerable improvement over the years in the mortality rates in every age group under 65 years. This reflects an overall improvement in the health situation in the hospitals. It was achieved by the application of advances in public health practice that resulted in better levels of environmental sanitation, control of tuberculosis and other infectious diseases, and improved diet, and of various advances in clinical medicine, such as the more effective treatment of pneumonia and acute infections by use of sulfonamides and antibiotics. While a reduction occurred in the mortality rates for schizophrenics in the age group 65 years and over, an increase occurred in the mortality in this age group for all other disorders combined. This is a reflection of

Table 3.2 Deaths per 1,000 population among the general population and deaths per 1,000 average annual resident patients among state mental hospital patients, with percent change, by selected diagnosis: New York State, 1930 and 1962

Age	New York State population		New York State Mental Hospitals: All disorders		Schizophrena		All other disorders	
	1930	1962	1930	1962	1930	1962	1930	1962
Total, 15 & over								
Adjusted[a]	20.0	13.4	78.4	51.4	35.4	22.3	132.6	76.9
Crude	13.5	13.7	87.0	99.0	32.4	29.9	165.6	191.1
15-24	2.8	0.9	51.2	4.7	32.2	5.1	84.2	4.2
25-34	4.1	1.4	41.3	8.0	24.8	6.5	80.7	12.3
35-44	6.6	3.0	45.7	13.9	19.5	9.7	103.3	26.1
45-54	13.7	7.6	58.6	26.2	21.1	15.7	122.3	51.9
55-64	28.5	17.4	92.8	58.9	39.5	31.9	156.5	96.9
65 & over	79.2	61.7	215.3	241.0	89.6	79.4	287.8	330.4
	Percent change (1930 to 1962)							
Total, 15 & over								
Adjusted[a]	-33.0		-34.4		-37.0		-42.0	
15-24	-67.9		-90.8		-84.2		-95.0	
25-34	-65.9		-80.6		-73.8		-84.8	
35-44	-54.5		-61.6		-50.3		-74.7	
45-54	-44.5		-55.3		-25.6		-57.6	
55-64	-38.9		-36.5		-19.2		-38.1	
65 & over	-22.1		+11.9		-11.4		+14.8	

[a]Adjusted to 1960 population of New York State.

the fact that the aged schizophrenics consist almost entirely of patients who have grown old in the hospital, while the other group is heavily weighted with newly admitted patients with mental disorders of the senium whose mortality rates are excessively high because of both their poor physical condition and their very high average age at admission. In effect, the mental hospital has had to deal with two types of aging problems. One was caused by the aging of the general population with a resultant increase of aged admissions with a high risk of mortality. The other resulted from the benefits of improved medical, psychiatric, and public health practices within the hospital, which resulted in a considerable saving of lives and led to an aging phenomenon for schizophrenics and other types of long-term patients similar to that occurring among persons in the general population.

The increasing size of the mental hospital population was a matter of much concern to public health officials, hospital administrators, other professionals, lawmakers, and the laity. This led to considerable action dedicated to changing the situation. During the ten-year period following the passage of the National Mental Health Act in 1946 (P.L. 79-487), many innovations were introduced to provide more effective psychiatric services to the nation, and additional facilities were developed to meet the rapidly increasing need and demand for services. Increasing numbers of outpatient clinics were opened (Bahn, 1961). Services were established in general hospitals at an accelerated rate. Additional nursing homes were opened and served to take some of the pressure off mental hospitals for beds for the aged. Many new approaches to the treatment and rehabilitation of the mentally ill appeared: intensive treatment for the acutely ill and increased staffing for more intensive treatment of the chronically hospitalized (Galioni et al., 1953), psychosurgery (Federal Security Agency, 1951, 1952, 1954), group psychotherapy, the open hospital and various programs for counteracting the dehumanizing effect of long-term institutionalization in the impersonal environment of the large state institutions (Milbank Memorial Fund, 1957). The introduction of the tranquilizers in the mid-1950s was an event of signal importance for developing further possibilities for improved treatment of the mentally ill (Cole and Gerard, 1959). The use of these drugs, which controlled agitated and excited behavior, provided increased opportunities for using additional treatment and rehabilitation procedures for returning many hospitalized patients to the community, for developing community programs to prevent hospitalization, as well as to treat and maintain the mentally ill in communities (Patton, 1958; Joint Commission, 1961). Such prospects engendered favorable changes in attitudes of staff, patients, their families, and the community toward each other.

During the years 1946-54, the numbers of patients in the state and county mental hospitals were increasing at an average annual rate of 2.1 percent (Figure 3.1). Although the changed attitudes toward the treatment of the mentally ill resulted in more and more patients being returned to the community, the rates of net release were still not sufficiently high to counterbalance the increasing number of admissions. So the mental hospital population continued to grow. A major turning point occurred at year-end 1955, when the patient population reached its peak of 558, 922. Between 1955 and 1956 the first drop occurred in this population. This was the year during which the use of tranquilizers became widespread in these hospitals. This decrease has continued consistently at an increasing rate, so that by year-end 1967 the resident population was 426,309 or 24 percent less than its peak number in 1955.

Changes in the number of patients in the year-end resident patient population are not occurring uniformly in every age group (Table

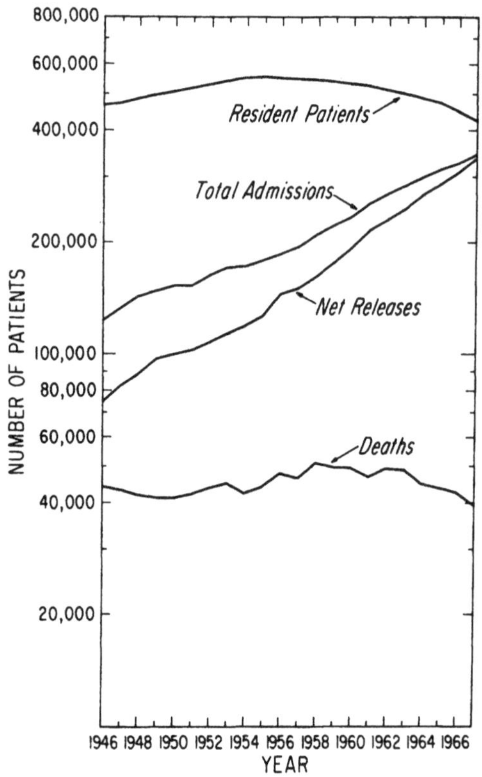

Fig. 3.1. Number of resident patients at end of year, total admissions, net releases, and deaths in state and county mental hospitals: United States, 1946-1967.

3.3). Decreases occurred in the number of patients 25 years and over, but the annual rate of decrease between 1955 and 1966 varied by age groups as follows: 25-34 years, 3.1 percent; 35-44 years, 4.1 percent; 45-54 years, 3.3 percent; 55-64 years, 1.0 percent; and 65 years and over, 1.8 percent. Marked increases have occurred in the number of patients under 25 years; the average annual rate of increase for patients under 15 years has been 10.3 percent, and for those 15-24 years, 5.9 percent. The extraordinary rate of increase in the number of patients in the age group under 15 years is due not only to the increase in the number of children in this age group in the general population but also to the increasing demand for services for seriously emotionally disturbed children and adolescents and

Table 3.3 Number and average annual rate of percent change in number of resident patients at end of year in state and county mental hospitals, by age: United States, 1955-66

Year	Total	Under 15	15-24	25-34	35-44	45-54	55-64	65+
1955	558,922	2,301	17,276	57,634	96,304	117,500	109,622	158,285
1956	551,390	2,617	16,785	53,642	91,714	115,857	110,929	159,846
1957	548,626	3,296	17,890	51,911	87,405	114,205	110,815	163,104
1958	545,182	3,577	18,657	49,562	83,848	113,527	110,630	165,381
1959	541,883	4,188	20,885	50,784	82,713	112,324	110,213	160,776
1960	535,540	4,417	21,350	48,133	79,468	110,341	111,125	160,706
1961	527,456	4,782	22,574	47,510	77,355	106,644	111,054	157,537
1962	515,640	4,860	23,485	45,876	74,582	103,429	110,099	153,309
1963	504,604	5,264	24,899	44,538	72,571	99,539	108,951	148,842
1964	490,449	5,118	26,369	43,521	70,098	95,360	106,150	143,833
1965	475,202	6,134	27,913	42,637	66,499	89,323	102,366	140,330
1966	452,089	6,289	27,280	41,434	62,114	82,925	97,337	134,710
Average annual rate of percent change 1955-1966	-2.0	10.3	5.9	-3.1	-4.1	-3.3	-1.0	-1.8

inadequate and insufficient services for them in other community resources.

On the other end of the age spectrum, the decrease in numbers of patients in the age group 65 years and over in the state and county mental hospitals has been accompanied by an increase in the numbers of aged mentally ill persons in nursing homes and related facilities for the aged. As of mid-1963, about 292,000 persons 65 years and over with specified mental disorders were resident in either long-stay psychiatric inpatient facilities or in nursing homes, geriatric hospitals, and homes for the aged and related facilities in the United States. This is a rate of 1,662 per 100,000 population 65 years and over. If one adds to these 292,000 persons those patients 65 and over resident in nursing homes and related facilities reported to be senile without mention of psychosis or to have ill-defined mental or nervous trouble, the total number of aged with some form of mental disorder is 364,000. Fifty-six percent of these were resident in nursing homes or related facilities, 39 percent in state and county mental hospitals, 4 percent in Veterans Administration hospitals and 1 percent in private mental hospitals (Figure 3.2). As a result of the increase in the number of nursing home beds throughout the nation since 1963 and the continued decrease in the number of aged mentally ill in state and county mental hospitals, the number of our elderly mentally ill citizens in nursing homes now exceeds that in the mental hospitals (Kramer et al., 1968).

Changes in age patterns of use of the state and county mental hospitals are affecting diagnostic composition of these hospitals. Decreases are occurring in the number of first admissions and resident patients with diseases of the senium, brain syndromes with central nervous system syphilis, the functional psychoses, and mental deficiency. Increases are occurring in disorders associated with alcohol, psychoneuroses, and personality disorders. The data reported in the following sections provide detailed information on average annual first admission and resident patient rates specific for age, sex, and diagnosis for the United States as a whole and its various geographic subdivisions for the years 1959-61. Trends are given for these rates both before and after these central years.

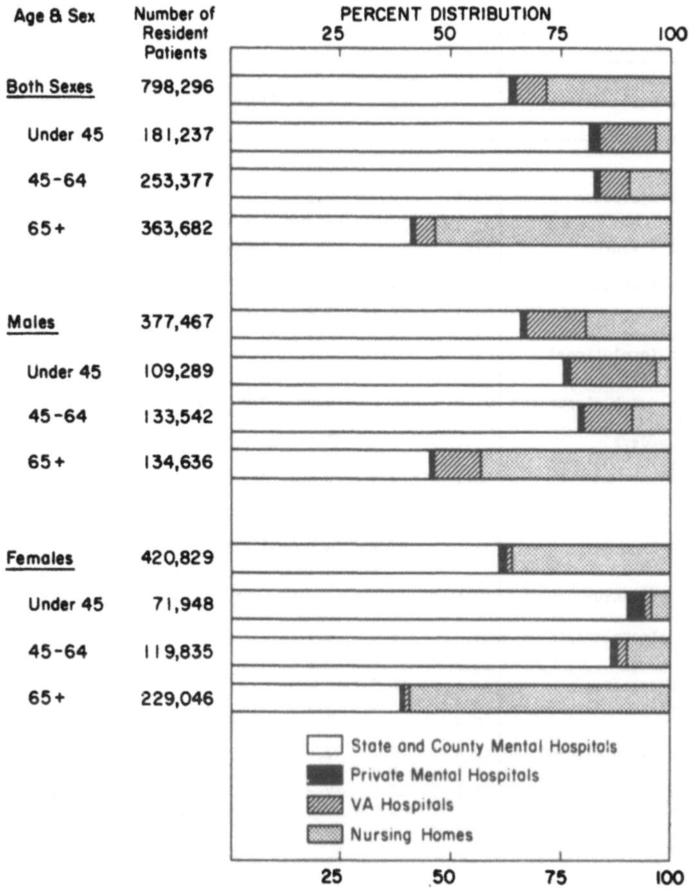

Fig. 3.2. Percentage distribution of patients with mental disorder resident in specified long-term institutions, by age and sex: United States, 1963.

FIRST ADMISSIONS 1959-61

Age, Sex, and Diagnoses

The average annual first admission rates to state and county mental hospitals by age, sex, and psychiatric diagnosis for the United States for 1959-61 are presented in Table 3.4 and Figure 3.3. For all mental disorders combined, the rates were low in the younger age group,

Table 3.4 Average annual first admission rates per 100,000 population to state and county mental hospitals by sex, age and diagnosis: United States, 1959-61

Diagnosis	All ages		< 15	15-24	25-34	35-44	45-54	55-64	65+
	Crude	Age adjusted							
Both sexes									
All mental disorders	77.6	80.3	6.3	75.4	104.6	102.8	100.4	96.3	200.4
Brain syndromes	22.0	20.5	0.8	4.5	4.6	5.7	10.7	31.1	172.8
Diseases of the senium	17.1	15.4	-	0.0*	0.1*	0.2	2.0	20.0	164.0
Syphilitic	0.4	0.4	0.0*	0.1*	0.2	0.5	1.1	1.4	0.8
Other (excl. alcoholics)	4.5	4.6	0.8	4.4	4.4	4.9	7.6	9.8	8.0
Functional psychoses	24.3	26.3	1.6	31.4	48.4	41.1	37.9	30.1	9.9
Schizophrenic reactions	17.8	19.7	1.5	29.2	43.5	33.1	20.5	10.1	2.5
Affective and involutional	5.7	5.9	0.0*	1.5	3.8	6.9	16.1	18.7	6.7
Other	0.7	0.8	0.0*	0.8	1.1	1.1	1.3	1.2	0.7
Disorders assoc. with alcoholism	11.3	12.0	0.0*	2.0	14.3	27.0	29.9	18.8	5.5
Psychoneurosis	5.8	6.3	0.3	6.2	12.6	10.5	8.4	6.9	3.1
Personality disorders	7.9	8.5	2.6	20.4	14.4	9.6	6.2	3.4	1.7
Mental deficiency	2.3	2.4	0.6	5.6	3.9	3.0	2.4	1.4	0.4
All other	4.1	4.3	0.5	5.3	6.5	5.9	4.9	4.7	7.1
Male									
All mental disorders	88.5	93.3	8.5	91.4	115.8	119.1	120.8	113.5	227.4
Brain syndromes	23.6	23.3	1.1	5.6	5.3	6.7	12.9	35.7	193.4
Diseases of the senium	17.6	17.1	-	0.0*	0.1*	0.3	2.4	22.3	181.8
Syphilitic	0.6	0.6	0.0*	0.1*	0.2	0.8	1.5	2.0	1.2
Other (excl. alcoholics)	5.4	5.6	1.1	5.5	5.0	5.6	9.0	11.4	10.4
Functional psychoses	21.9	24.0	2.0	35.5	44.7	33.6	29.6	25.4	8.9
Schizophrenic reactions	17.1	18.9	2.0	33.4	40.9	28.3	17.9	8.6	2.2
Affective and involutional	3.9	4.1	0.0*	1.0	2.3	4.0	10.2	15.4	5.9
Other	0.9	1.0	0.0*	1.1	1.5	1.4	1.6	1.4	0.7
Disorders assoc. with alcoholism	19.4	20.7	0.0*	3.4	24.1	45.6	52.3	34.4	11.0
Psychoneurosis	4.4	4.8	0.3	4.3	8.5	8.3	7.5	5.3	2.2
Personality disorders	11.1	12.0	3.7	27.5	20.6	14.2	9.6	5.0	2.4
Mental deficiency	2.8	3.0	0.8	7.7	4.6	3.3	2.7	1.5	0.4
All other	5.3	5.6	0.6	7.5	8.2	7.4	6.3	6.1	9.2
Female									
All mental disorders	67.0	67.9	4.1	59.7	93.9	87.2	80.6	80.2	177.9
Brain syndromes	20.5	17.9	0.5	3.4	3.9	4.8	8.5	26.8	155.6
Diseases of the senium	16.6	14.0	-	0.0*	0.1*	0.2	1.6	17.9	149.2
Syphilitic	0.2	0.2	-	0.0*	0.1*	0.3	0.7	0.7	0.4
Other (excl. alcoholics)	3.7	3.8	0.5	3.3	3.7	4.3	6.2	8.2	6.0
Functional psychoses	26.5	28.6	1.1	27.4	52.0	48.2	45.9	34.4	10.8
Schizophrenic reactions	18.6	20.4	1.0	25.0	46.0	37.7	23.0	11.6	2.7
Affective and involutional	7.4	7.6	0.0*	1.9	5.3	9.8	22.0	21.8	7.4
Other	0.5	0.5	0.0*	0.5	0.7	0.8	1.0	1.1	0.6
Disorders assoc. with alcoholism	3.4	3.6	0.0*	0.7	4.9	9.3	8.2	4.0	1.0
Psychoneurosis	7.1	7.7	0.3	8.1	16.5	12.5	9.3	8.4	3.8
Personality disorders	4.7	5.1	1.5	13.4	8.4	5.3	3.0	1.9	1.1
Mental deficiency	1.8	1.9	0.4	3.6	3.3	2.7	2.1	1.3	0.3
All other	3.0	3.1	0.3	3.1	4.9	4.4	3.6	3.3	5.4

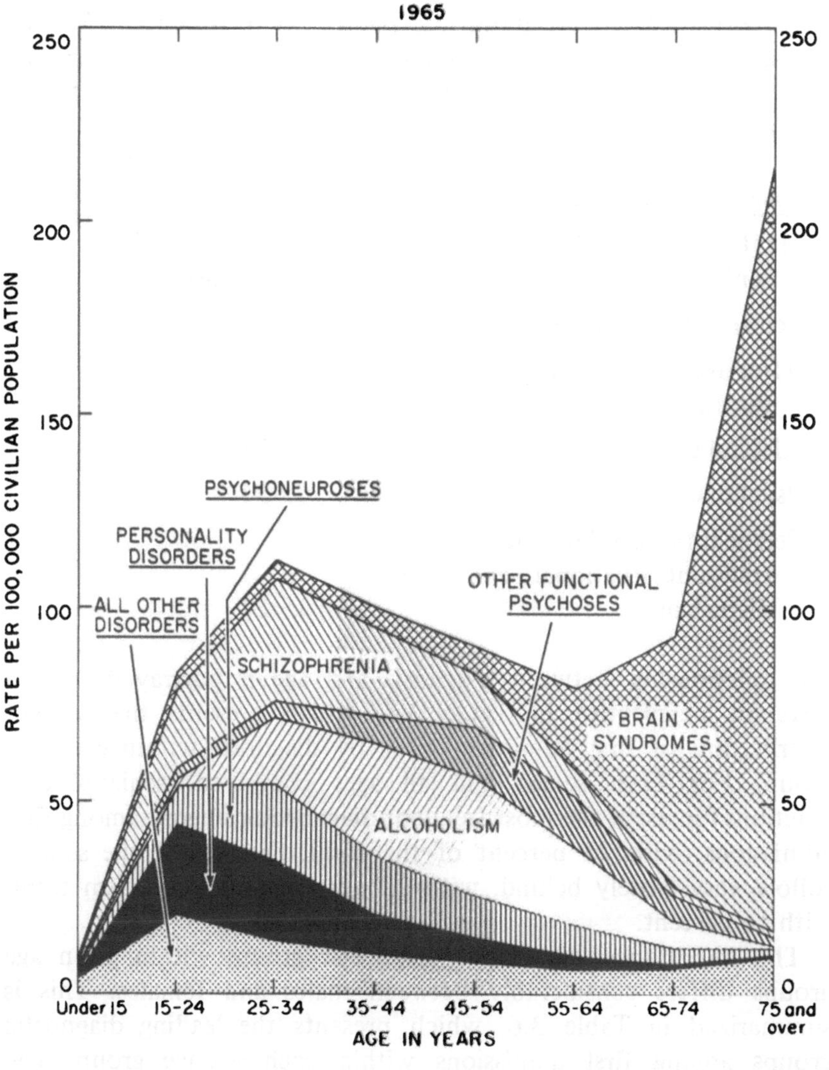

Fig. 3.3. First admissions per 100,000 population to state and county mental hospitals, by age and mental disorder: United States, 1965. (Note: First admission means no prior admission to any inpatient psychiatric facility.)

were fairly constant at about 100 per 100,000 from ages 25 to 64 years, and then double that amount for the age group 65 years and over. The age group in which the rate for each diagnostic category reached its maximum varied widely as follows:

Diagnostic category	Age group of maximum rate, yrs.
Mental disorders of the senium	65 and over
Schizophrenic reactions	25-34
Affective and involutional disorders	55-64
Alcoholism	45-54
Psychoneurosis	25-34
Personality disorders, including transient situational personality disturbances	15-24

The relationship between diagnosis and age is portrayed from a different perspective in Table 3.5, which presents the percent distribution of first admission rates by diagnosis within each age group. For both sexes, and all ages combined, schizophrenic reactions represent the most frequent diagnostic category among first admissions, with 23 percent of the total. Diseases of the senium follow very closely behind, with 22 percent and alcoholism third, with 16 percent.

The importance of various diagnostic groups within given age groups differs considerably between males and females. This is summarized in Table 3.6, which presents the leading diagnostic groups among first admissions within each sex-age group. The differences between the sexes appear most sharply in the age groups 35-64, where alcoholism appears consistently as the leading cause of first admission among males. Among females, on the other hand, schizophrenic reactions remain the leading cause of first admission through age 54, but affective and involutional disorders follow closely behind in the age group 45-54 and become the leading cause of first admission among females in the age group 55-64.

Table 3.5 Percent distribution by diagnosis of average annual first admissions to state and county mental hospitals by sex and age: United States, 1959-61

Diagnosis	All ages	<15	15-24	25-34	35-44	45-54	55-64	65+
Both sexes								
All mental disorders	100.0	100.0	100.0	100.0	100.0	100.0	100.0	100.0
Brain syndromes	28.4	12.9	5.9	4.4	5.6	10.6	32.3	86.2
Diseases of the senium	22.0	-	0.0	0.1	0.2	2.0	20.8	81.8
Syphilitic	0.5	0.1	0.1	0.1	0.6	1.1	1.4	0.4
Other (excl. alcoholics)	5.8	12.8	5.8	4.2	4.8	7.5	10.1	4.0
Functional psychoses	31.3	24.5	41.7	46.3	40.0	37.7	31.2	4.9
Schizophrenic reactions	23.0	23.7	38.7	41.6	32.2	20.4	10.5	1.2
Affective and involutional	7.4	0.4	2.0	3.7	6.7	16.0	19.4	3.4
Other	0.9	0.4	1.0	1.0	1.1	1.3	1.3	0.3
Disorders assoc. with alcoholism	14.6	0.1	2.7	13.7	26.3	29.8	19.5	2.8
Psychoneurosis	7.4	4.4	8.3	12.0	10.2	8.4	7.1	1.5
Personality disorders	10.1	41.7	27.0	13.7	9.4	6.2	3.6	0.8
Mental deficiency	2.9	8.9	7.4	3.6	2.8	2.4	1.5	0.2
All other	5.3	7.5	7.0	6.3	5.7	4.9	4.8	3.6
Male								
All mental disorders	100.0	100.0	100.0	100.0	100.0	100.0	100.0	100.0
Brain syndromes	26.7	13.0	6.1	4.5	5.6	10.7	31.5	85.0
Diseases of the senium	19.9	-	0.0	0.0	0.2	2.0	19.7	79.9
Syphilitic	0.7	0.2	0.1	0.2	0.7	1.3	1.8	0.5
Other (excl. alcoholics)	6.1	12.8	6.0	4.3	4.7	7.4	10.0	4.6
Functional psychoses	24.8	23.6	38.8	38.6	28.2	24.5	22.4	3.9
Schizophrenic reactions	19.4	23.0	36.5	35.3	23.8	14.8	7.6	1.0
Affective and involutional	4.4	0.2	1.1	2.0	3.3	8.4	13.6	2.6
Other	1.0	0.4	1.2	1.3	1.1	1.3	1.3	0.3
Disorders assoc. with alcoholism	22.0	0.1	3.7	20.8	38.3	43.3	30.3	4.8
Psychoneurosis	4.9	3.6	4.8	7.3	7.0	6.2	4.7	1.0
Personality disorders	12.6	43.8	30.0	17.7	11.9	7.9	4.4	1.0
Mental deficiency	3.0	8.8	8.4	4.0	2.7	2.2	1.3	0.2
All other	6.0	7.1	8.2	7.1	6.3	5.2	5.4	4.1
Female								
All mental disorders	100.0	100.0	100.0	100.0	100.0	100.0	100.0	100.0
Brain syndromes	30.6	12.8	5.7	4.2	5.5	10.5	35.5	87.4
Diseases of the senium	24.7	-	0.0	0.1	0.2	2.0	22.3	83.9
Syphilitic	0.4	0.1	0.2	0.1	0.5	0.9	0.9	0.2
Other (excl. alcoholics)	5.5	12.7	5.5	4.0	4.8	7.6	10.3	3.3
Functional psychoses	39.6	26.4	45.9	55.4	55.3	57.0	42.9	6.1
Schizophrenic reactions	27.8	25.2	41.9	49.0	43.2	28.5	14.5	1.5
Affective and involutional	11.0	0.8	3.2	5.6	11.2	27.3	27.1	4.2
Other	0.8	0.4	0.8	0.8	0.9	1.2	1.3	0.4
Disorders assoc. with alcoholism	5.0	0.2	1.2	5.2	10.6	10.2	5.0	0.6
Psychoneurosis	10.7	6.1	13.5	17.6	14.3	11.6	10.4	2.1
Personality disorders	7.0	37.1	22.5	9.0	6.1	3.7	2.4	0.6
Mental deficiency	2.6	9.0	6.0	3.5	3.1	2.6	1.7	0.2
All other	4.5	8.5	5.2	5.2	5.1	4.4	4.1	3.0

Table 3.6 Leading diagnostic groups among first admissions to state and county mental hospitals by age and sex: United States, 1959-61

Age	Male		Female	
All ages	Alcoholism	(22)	Schizophrenic reaction	(28)
	Diseases of the senium	(20)	Diseases of the senium	(25)
	Schizophrenic reaction	(19)	Affective & involutional	(11)
Under 15	Personality disorders	(44)	Personality disorders	(37)
	Schizophrenic reaction	(23)	Schizophrenic reaction	(25)
	Brain syndromes	(13)	Brain syndromes	(13)
15-24	Schizophrenic reaction	(37)	Schizophrenic reaction	(42)
	Personality disorders	(30)	Personality disorders	(23)
	Mental deficiency	(8)	Psychoneurosis	(14)
25-34	Schizophrenic reaction	(35)	Schizophrenic reaction	(49)
	Alcoholism	(21)	Psychoneurosis	(18)
	Personality disorders	(18)	Personality disorders	(9)
35-44	Alcoholism	(38)	Schizophrenic reaction	(43)
	Schizophrenic reaction	(24)	Psychoneurosis	(14)
	Personality disorders	(12)	Affective & involutional	(11)
45-54	Alcoholism	(43)	Schizophrenic reaction	(29)
	Schizophrenic reaction	(15)	Affective & involutional	(27)
	Personality disorders	(8)	Psychoneurosis	(12)
55-64	Alcoholism	(30)	Affective & involutional	(27)
	Diseases of the senium	(20)	Diseases of the senium	(22)
	Affective & involutional	(14)	Schizophrenic reaction	(15)
65 & over	Diseases of the senium	(80)	Diseases of the senium	(84)
	Alcoholism	(5)	Affective & involutional	(4)

Note: Percentages of total in each group are given in parentheses.

The ratios of male to female first admission rates for age-diagnostic groups are shown in Table 3.7. For all diagnoses combined, the male rates were consistently greater than the female rates in every age group, with the highest ratio in the under 15 age group (2.07) and the lowest in the 25-34 age group (1.23). This same pattern of higher male rates in every age group was observed in almost all diagnostic categories except schizophrenia, affective and involutional psychoses, and psychoneuroses. where female rates were generally greater. Male rates were noted to be particularly high for disorders associated with alcoholism, personality disorders, and brain syndromes associated with syphilis in comparison with the female rates for these disorders.

Table 3.7 Ratio of average annual male first admission rates to female first admission rates for state and county mental hospitals by age and diagnosis: United States, 1959-61

Diagnosis	All ages		< 15	15-24	25-34	35-44	45-54	55-64	65+
	Crude	Age adjusted							
All mental disorders	1.32	1.37	2.07	1.53	1.23	1.37	1.50	1.42	1.28
Brain syndromes	1.15	1.30	2.20	1.65	1.36	1.40	1.52	1.33	1.24
Diseases of the senium	1.06	1.22	-	*	*	1.50	1.50	1.25	1.22
Syphilitic	3.00	3.00	*	*	*	2.67	2.14	2.86	3.00
Other (excl. alcoholics)	1.46	1.47	2.20	1.67	1.35	1.30	1.45	1.39	1.73
Functional psychoses	.83	.84	1.82	1.30	.86	.70	.64	.74	.82
Schizophrenic reactions	.92	.93	2.00	1.34	.89	.75	.78	.74	.81
Affective and involutional	.53	.54	*	.53	.43	.41	.46	.71	.80
Other	1.80	2.00	*	2.20	2.14	1.75	1.60	1.27	1.17
Disorders assoc. with alcoholism	5.71	5.75	*	4.86	4.92	4.90	6.38	8.60	11.00
Psychoneurosis	.62	.62	1.00	.53	.52	.66	.81	.63	.58
Personality disorders	2.36	2.35	2.47	2.05	2.45	2.68	3.20	2.63	2.18
Mental deficiency	1.56	1.58	2.00	2.14	1.39	1.22	1.29	1.15	1.33
All other	1.77	1.81	2.00	2.42	1.67	1.68	1.75	1.85	1.70

*Ratios were not computed where rates were based on less than 20 admissions.

Geographic Distribution

The average annual first admission rates to state and county mental hospitals by diagnosis are presented for geographic regions in Table 3.8. There was considerable variation in the overall first admission rates among the four major regions. The rates ranged from a high of 91.5 per 100,000 in the Northeast region to a low of 74.4 in the North Central region. Among the subregions the highest rate occurred in the New England states (105.7) and the lowest in the West North Central states (67.7). Examination of the variation in rates for specific diagnostic categories for the major regions reveals that first admission rates for diseases of the senium, schizophrenia, and affective and involutional psychoses were substantially higher in the Northeast, whereas among the other three regions the rates showed little variation for these diagnoses. There was somewhat less regional variation among the other diagnostic categories, although the rate for alcoholism was lowest in the Northeast and the rate for personality disorders was highest in the Western region. A comparison of first admission rates for each of the diagnostic categories among the subregions reveals particularly high rates for diseases of the senium in the New England, Mid-Atlantic, and South Atlantic states, for schizophrenia in the Mid-Atlantic states, and for disorders associated with alcoholism in the New England states. Rates specific for diagnosis for each individual state are presented in Appendix Table 1.

Table 3.8 Average annual age-adjusted first admission rates per 100,000 population to state and county mental hospitals by diagnosis: United States and each region, 1959-61

Region	All mental disorders	Brain syndromes				Functional psychoses				Disorders assoc. with alcoholism	Psycho-nuerosis	Personality disorders
		Total	Diseases of senium	Syphilitic	Other	Total	Schizophrenic reactions	Affective and involutional	Other			
United States	80.3	20.5	15.4	0.4	4.6	26.3	19.7	5.9	0.8	12.0	6.3	8.5
Northeast Region	91.5	28.1	23.4	0.4	4.3	35.1	25.3	8.2	1.6	9.8	6.2	7.9
New England States	105.7	28.0	22.5	0.2	5.3	30.8	21.4	8.4	1.0	18.4	11.2	9.9
Mid-Atlantic States	89.4	28.1	23.6	0.4	4.1	35.8	25.9	8.2	1.7	8.5	5.5	7.6
North Central Region	74.4	16.6	12.0	0.4	4.2	21.5	16.7	4.3	0.6	12.4	6.6	9.6
East North Central States	77.5	18.5	13.7	0.4	4.4	22.7	18.0	4.1	0.6	11.6	6.7	9.8
West North Central States	67.7	12.9	8.8	0.3	3.8	18.8	13.5	4.8	0.4	14.2	6.5	8.9
Southern Region	80.2	20.9	14.9	0.6	5.4	26.2	19.9	5.8	0.5	12.7	5.7	6.2
South Atlantic States	84.6	24.6	18.0	0.7	6.0	27.5	20.5	6.4	0.5	12.1	6.8	6.1
East South Central States	79.9	18.6	12.9	0.5	5.4	26.6	19.5	6.4	0.6	12.5	5.0	6.7
West South Central States	72.8	16.2	11.4	0.5	4.4	23.5	19.0	4.2	0.2	14.2	4.5	6.0
Western Region	75.4	14.9	10.2	0.2	4.5	23.2	17.5	5.3	0.4	13.0	6.8	12.0
Mountain States	85.3	19.4	13.0	0.3	6.1	23.6	18.1	4.7	0.8	14.5	7.9	12.6
Pacific States	72.5	13.6	9.4	0.2	3.9	23.1	17.3	5.5	0.3	12.5	6.5	11.8

TRENDS IN FIRST ADMISSION RATES BY AGE, SEX, AND DIAGNOSIS

First admission rates to state and county mental hospitals for the three-year period around 1960 have been presented in some detail. To place these data in a time perspective, their trends are presented for the United States as a whole for the period 1950-65. In addition, average annual first admission rates are presented for three-year periods around the 1940 and 1950 censuses for purposes of comparison with the above rates. For all of the data presented, estimates have been made to adjust for underreporting.

It was pointed out in Chapter 2 that two changes were made in the definition of "first admission" over the period for which trends were analyzed, one in 1952 and the other 1962. Since the major aspect of the 1952 change was no longer to consider patients who had been hospitalized in another mental hospital as first admissions, the effect was to reduce somewhat the numbers of first admissions in the years since 1952 in comparison with the levels they would have reached under the old definition. The change in definition in 1962, on the other hand, represented a major break in the series, since the large number of first admissions who had been hospitalized for psychiatric disorders in a general hospital were no longer counted as first admissions. Therefore, the charts presenting trends over time will show breaks at 1962, where this change occurrred.

Age and Sex

The trends in age-specific first admission rates for the period 1950 to 1965 are presented in Figure 3.4. The rate for children under 15 years of age has been increasing, and that among persons 65 years of age and over has been decreasing. The rates for the age groups between age 25 and 64 years fall within a narrow range and have shown generally slight increases. These trends generally hold true for both males and females, as indicated in Figure 3.5. The rates for males were consistently higher than those for females in corresponding age groups. The average annual age-specific first admission rates around the 1940, 1950, and 1960 censuses, respectively, are presented in Table 3.9. Examination of the percent change over the entire 20-year period reveals that the greatest incease occurred in the rates for those under 15 years of age, although the

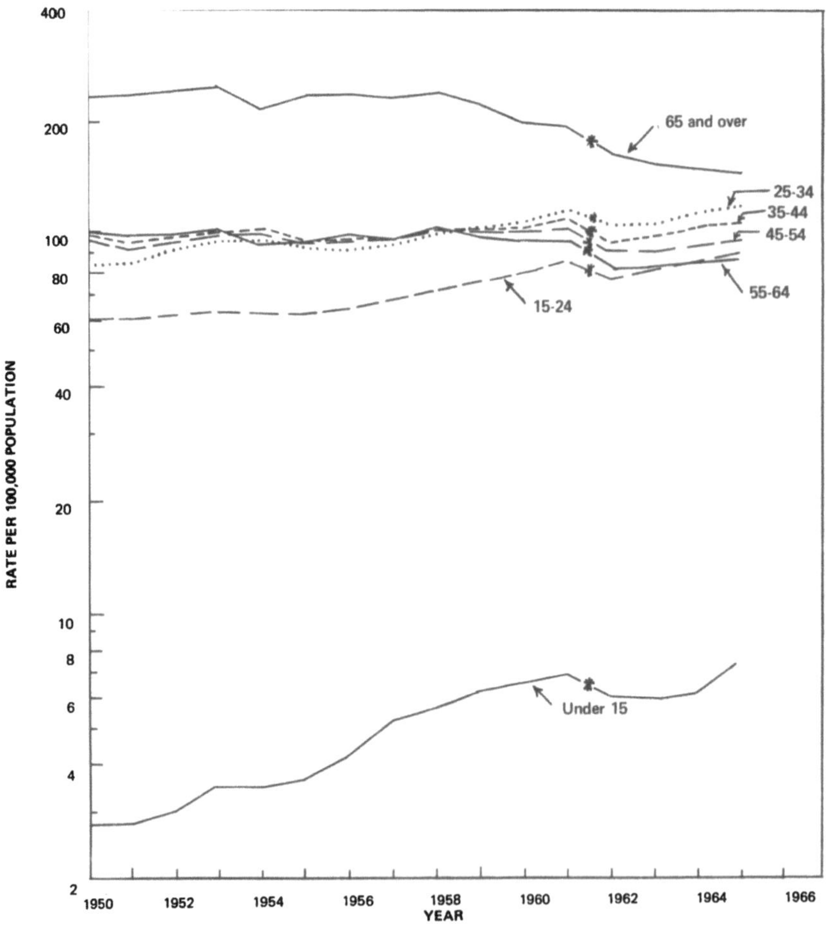

Fig. 3.4. First admissions per 100,000 population to state and county mental hospitals, by age: United States, 1950-1965. (Note: Break between 1961 and 1962 indicates change in definition to admission with no prior admission to any inpatient psychiatric facility.)

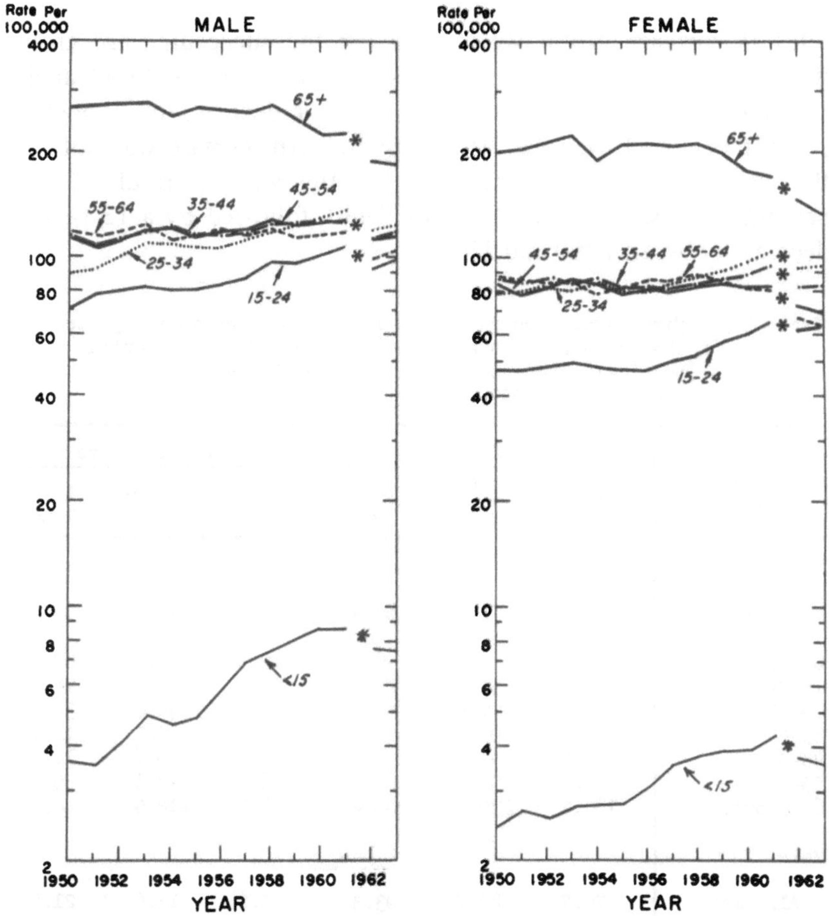

Fig. 3.5. First admissions per 100,000 population to state and county mental hospitals, by sex and age: United States, 1950-1963. (Note: Break indicates change in definition, as in Fig. 3.4.)

rates in this age group were small. In the succeeding age groups through age 54 years, the increases became smaller with advancing age, and in the age group 55-64 years, a decrease of almost 10 percent occurred over the 20-year period. An increase was noted in the age group 65 years and over, but this was the result of a 25 percent increase between 1940 and 1950, followed by a 13 percent decrease between 1950 and 1960.

Table 3.9 First admission rates per 100,000 population and percent change in rates over time in state and county mental hospitals, by age and sex: United States, 1939-41, 1949-51, and 1959-61

Sex and age	Rates			Percent change		
	1939-1941	1949-1951	1959-1961	1940-1950	1950-1960	1940-1960
Both sexes						
All ages	67.2	71.9	80.3	7.0	11.7	19.5
Under 15	2.4	2.7	6.3	12.5	133.3	162.5
15-24	42.9	51.9	75.4	21.0	45.3	75.8
25-34	77.9	77.6	104.6	-0.4	34.8	34.3
35-44	92.0	92.9	102.8	1.0	10.7	11.7
45-54	91.0	92.3	100.4	1.4	8.8	10.3
55-64	106.5	99.4	96.3	-6.7	-3.1	-9.6
65 & over	184.7	230.1	200.4	24.6	-12.9	8.5
Male						
All ages	76.7	80.7	93.3	5.2	15.6	21.6
Under 15	2.8	3.1	8.5	10.7	174.2	203.6
15-24	50.0	60.5	91.4	21.0	51.1	82.8
25-34	89.3	80.8	115.8	-9.5	43.3	29.7
35-44	105.6	104.5	119.1	-1.0	14.0	12.8
45-54	96.6	104.9	120.8	8.6	15.2	25.1
55-64	122.5	114.1	113.5	-6.9	-0.5	-7.3
65 & over	216.2	261.1	227.4	20.8	12.9	5.2
Female						
All ages	57.7	63.4	67.9	9.9	7.1	17.7
Under 15	2.0	2.2	4.1	10.0	86.4	105.0
15-24	35.9	43.5	59.7	21.2	37.2	66.3
25-34	66.7	74.7	93.9	12.0	25.7	40.8
35-44	78.4	81.6	87.2	4.1	6.9	11.2
45-54	85.0	79.7	80.6	-6.2	1.1	-5.2
55-64	89.7	84.6	80.2	-5.7	-5.2	-10.6
65 & over	154.3	202.0	177.9	30.9	-11.9	15.3

Diagnosis and Sex

Average annual age-adjusted rates for each of the three time periods are presented by diagnosis and sex in Table 3.10. The rates for diseases of the senium reflect the same pattern shown above for the age group 65 and over, namely, an increase between 1940 and 1950 followed by a decrease between 1950 and 1960. The dramatic decrease in the first admission rate with syphilitc psychosis is undoubtedly a reflection of measures taken in the general population for the control of syphilis. A consistent increase occurred in the rate for schizophrenic reactions, while a consistent decrease occurred in that for affective and involutional psychoses. The rates for alcoholism, psychoneurosis, and personality disorders all showed steady increases over the 20-year period. Table 3.10 also reveals that the changes in rates for specific diagnostic categories were strikingly similar between males and females.

Geographic Trends

The age-adjusted first admission rates around each of the three decennial censuses are presented in Table 3.11 for each of the four regions of the United States and their sub-regions. The Northeast and North Central regions showed essentially the same pattern of increase as that for the United States as a whole from 1940 to 1950 and 1950 to 1960. The Southern region showed practically no change between 1940 and 1950, but a 33 percent increase between 1950 and 1960, to arrive at a rate in 1960 which was approximately equal to that for the United States. The Western region, on the other hand, had an increase in first admission rates between 1940 and 1950 and a corresponding decrease between 1950 and 1960, to produce a net effect of no change over the 20-year period.

There was considerable heterogeneity in patterns of change in first admission rates for the subregions within each of the regions. In the Northeast region, the greatest amount of change occurred in the New England states. The smaller changes seen in the Mid-Atlantic states reflect the fact that very little change in rates occurred in New York and Pennsylvania over the entire 20-year period, as indicated in the Appendix Table 2. While the two subregions within the North Central region had substantially the same change over the 20-year period, the West North Central states had a 7 percent decrease between 1940 and 1950, followed by a 26 percent increase between

Table 3.10 Age-adjusted first admission rates per 100,000 population and percent change in rates over time to state and county mental hospitals, by diagnosis and sex: United States, 1939-41, 1949-51, and 1959-61

	Rate per 100,000 population			Percent change		
	1939-1941	1949-1951	1959-1961	1940-1950	1950-1960	1940-1960
Both sexes						
All mental disorders	67.2	71.9	80.3	7.0	11.7	19.5
Brain syndromes	30.2	28.3	20.5	-6.3	-27.6	-32.1
Diseases of the senium	16.9	19.4	15.4	14.8	-20.6	-8.9
Syphilitic	6.1	2.5	0.4	-59.0	-84.0	-93.4
Other (excl. alcoholics)	7.2	6.4	4.6	-11.1	-28.1	-36.1
Functional psychoses	22.5	24.6	26.3	9.3	6.9	16.9
Schizophrenic reactions	12.9	16.8	19.7	30.2	17.3	52.7
Affective and involutional	8.7	7.1	5.9	-18.4	-16.9	-32.2
Other	1.0	0.7	0.8	-30.0	14.3	-20.0
Disorders assoc. with alcoholism	6.4	8.8	12.0	37.5	36.4	87.5
Psychoneurosis	2.1	3.4	6.3	70.0	85.3	215.0
Personality disorders	1.3	2.0	8.5	66.7	325.0	608.3
Mental deficiency	3.2	2.6	2.4	-13.3	-7.7	-20.0
All other	1.9	2.2	4.3	15.8	95.5	87.5
Male						
All mental disorders	76.7	80.7	93.3	5.2	15.6	21.6
Brain syndromes	36.0	32.5	23.3	-9.7	-28.3	-35.3
Diseases of the senium	19.0	21.5	17.1	13.2	-20.5	-10.0
Syphilitic	8.8	3.6	0.6	-59.1	-83.3	-93.2
Other (excl. alcoholics)	8.2	7.5	5.6	-8.5	-25.3	-31.7
Functional psychoses	20.7	21.2	24.0	2.4	13.2	15.9
Schizophrenic reactions	13.5	15.6	18.9	15.6	21.2	40.0
Affective and involutional	6.3	4.8	4.1	-23.8	-14.6	-34.9
Other	1.0	0.8	1.0	-20.0	25.0	0.0
Disorders assoc. with alcoholism	11.0	15.1	20.7	37.3	37.1	88.2
Psychoneurosis	1.6	2.9	4.8	81.2	65.5	200.0
Personality disorders	1.6	2.9	12.0	81.2	313.8	650.0
Mental deficiency	3.3	3.0	3.0	-9.1	0.0	-9.1
All other	2.5	3.1	5.6	24.0	80.6	124.0
Female						
All mental disorders	57.7	63.4	67.9	9.9	7.1	17.7
Brain syndromes	24.4	24.2	17.9	0.8	-26.0	-26.6
Diseases of the senium	14.8	17.5	14.0	18.2	-20.0	-5.4
Syphilitic	3.4	1.4	0.2	-58.8	-85.7	-94.1
Other (excl. alcoholics)	6.2	5.4	3.8	-12.9	-29.6	-38.7
Functional psychoses	24.5	29.7	28.6	13.9	2.5	16.7
Schizophrenic reactions	12.3	17.9	20.4	45.5	14.0	65.9
Affective and involutional	11.1	9.3	7.6	-16.2	18.3	-31.5
Other	1.0	0.7	0.5	-30.0	-28.6	-50.0
Disorders assoc. with alcoholism	1.8	2.7	3.6	50.0	33.3	100.0
Psychoneurosis	2.4	3.9	7.7	62.5	97.4	220.8
Personality disorders	0.8	1.2	5.1	50.0	325.0	537.5
Mental deficiency	2.6	2.2	1.9	-15.4	-13.6	-26.9
All other	1.2	1.4	3.1	16.7	121.4	158.3

Table 3.11 Average annual age-adjusted first admission rates per 100,000 population and percent changes over time: United States and each region, 1939-41, 1949-51, and 1959-61

Region	Age-adjusted first admission rate per 100,000 population			Percent change		
	1939-1941	1949-1951	1959-1961	1940-1950	1950-1960	1940-1960
United States	67.2	71.9	80.3	7.0	11.7	19.5
Northeast Region	79.1	82.9	91.5	4.8	10.4	15.7
New England States	66.9	94.4	105.7	41.1	12.0	58.0
Mid-Atlantic States	81.0	81.2	89.4	0.2	10.1	10.4
North Central Region	61.7	67.5	74.4	9.4	10.2	20.6
E. No. Central States	63.8	74.1	77.5	16.1	4.6	21.5
W. No. Central States	57.5	53.7	67.7	-6.6	26.1	17.7
Southern Region	59.4	60.3	80.2	1.0	33.0	36.0
So. Atlantic States	60.3	61.2	84.6	1.5	38.2	40.3
E. So. Central States	66.5	62.4	79.9	-6.2	28.0	20.2
W. So. Central States	52.7	57.6	72.8	9.3	26.4	38.1
Western Region	75.1	87.0	75.4	15.8	-13.3	0.4
Mountain States	68.7	76.6	85.3	11.5	11.4	24.2
Pacific States	77.4	90.3	72.6	16.7	-19.6	-6.2

1950 and 1960. In the Western region the overall pattern of changes was influenced largely by the changes in rates in the Pacific states, which, in turn, reflect a 28 percent decrease in first admission rates in California between 1950 and 1960 (Appendix Table 2.). Appendix Table 2 reveals a wide variation in percent change in first admission rates among the states. Seven states showed decreases between 1940 and 1960. Sixteen states had decreases between 1940 and 1950, nine states had decreases between 1950 and 1960, but no state experienced a decrease in first admission rates in both of the 10-year periods.

RESIDENT PATIENTS

This section will present data on the resident patient population in the state and county mental hospitals as of 1959-61, and trends in this population, both before and after this period. To provide some background against which to view these data, a few comments will be made to illustrate some of the salient characteristics of this population and the factors that determine its composition.

Population Dynamics

As demonstrated in Chapter 1, the resident population of a mental hospital on any one day consists of survivors of groups of patients admitted over long periods of time. The number in each residual length of stay category specific for age, sex, and diagnosis depends on the initial size of the group of admissions and its subsequent rate of depletion. Figure 3.6 gives the distribution of all patients resident in state mental hospitals of 17 states in the Model Reporting Area by chronological age and time on the books for all mental disorders, schizophrenia, and mental disorders of the senium as of the end of 1955, the year when the mental hospital pupulation of the nation had reached its highest level. This distribution has been determined by the varying admission rates for specific disorders and the differential rates of release and mortality that have operated in the mental hospitals of these states over time.

Patients' experiences subsequent to admission vary markedly by age, sex, and diagnosis. For example, net release rates from mental hospitals, that is, the relative rate of change in the hospital population owing to the excess of patients released alive to the community over returns to the hospital, vary sharply with length of stay, being highest for the patients hospitalized for less than a year and lowest for those hospitalized 20 years or more. They also vary markedly by age, being highest for the youngest age groups (under 35 years) and lówest for the oldest (65 years and over). Mental hospital populations are heavily weighted with patients for whom release rates are quite low. In 1962, those hospitalized for less than one year accounted for only 20 percent of the resident population and those in the age group under 35 for only 15 percent. Deaths are an important factor in accounting for changes in the population in the age group 65 years and over. This age group, which accounted for 30 percent of the patient population in 1962, had a death rate of the order of 235 per 1,000 average resident population, or four times that of persons in the same age group in the general population. Patients in the 65 years and over age group consist essentially of two major categories: those who have grown old in the hospital setting (e.g., the schizophrenics) and those first admitted in the age group 65

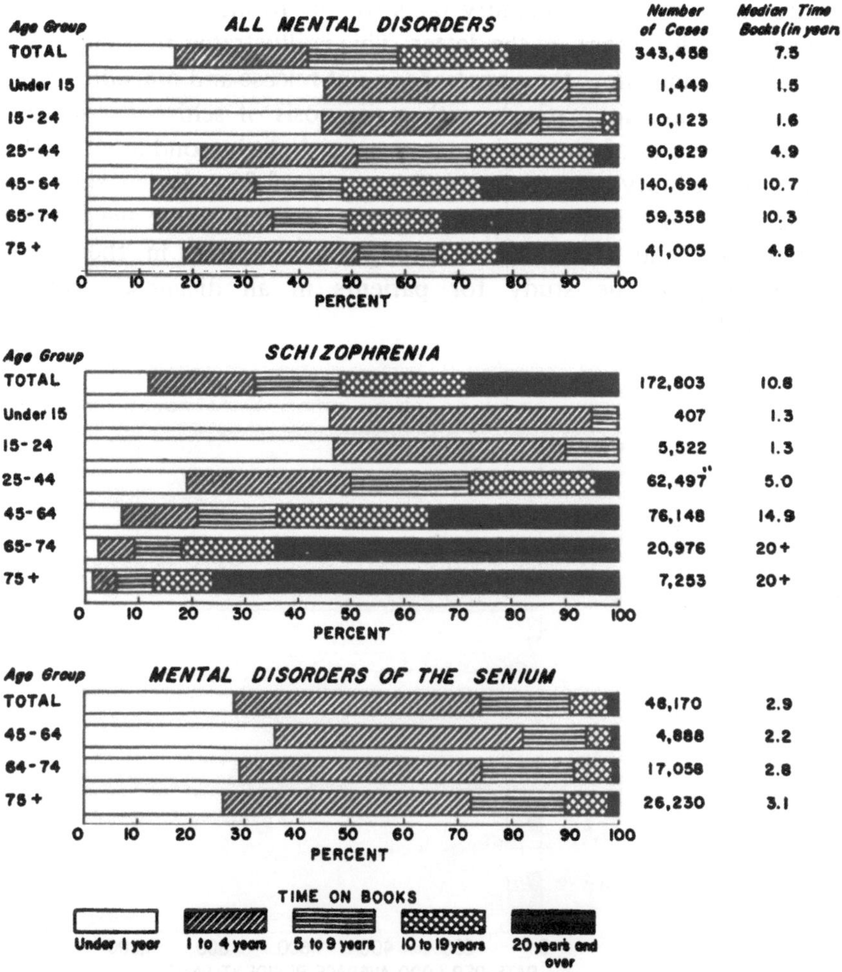

Fig. 3.6. Percentage distribution by time on books, with median time on books, of patients resident at end of year in public mental hospitals, by sex and age, for all mental disorders and selected diagnoses: 17 Model Reporting Area States, 1955.

Source: Unpublished data, National Institute of Mental Health, P.H.S., U.S. Department of Health, Education, and Welfare.

years and over. The mortality rates for the former group are much lower than for those in the latter. This is illustrated in Figures 3.7 and 3.8, which show the variations in net release and mortality rates specific for age for patients with a diagnosis of schizophrenia and mental disorder of the senium in a special study conducted in the state and county mental hospital systems of 23 selected states in 1962. Appendix Tables 3 and 4 show the variation in the age-specific net release and death rates among the hospitals in the states represented in the study for patients in all diagnostic groups combined.

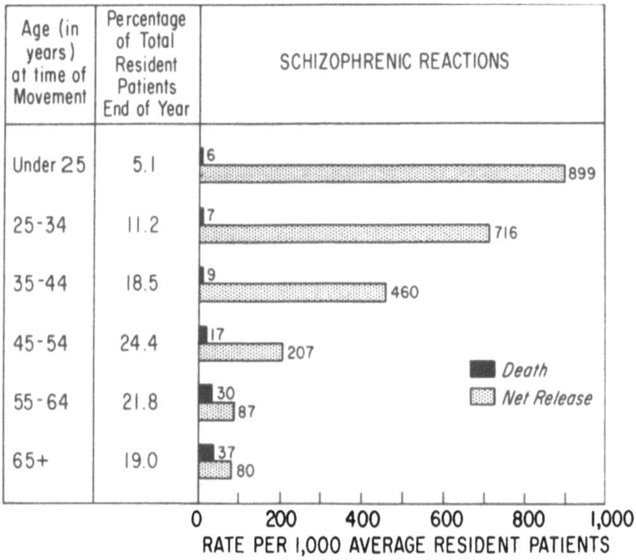

Fig. 3.7. Net releases and deaths per 1,000 average resident patients, and percentage distribution for schizophrenic patients resident at end of year, by age: 23 selected states, 1962.

Source: "Patient Movement Data, State and County Mental Hospitals, 1962," Washington, D.C., U.S. Department of Health, Education, and Welfare, Public Health Service Publication no. 1282, 1964.

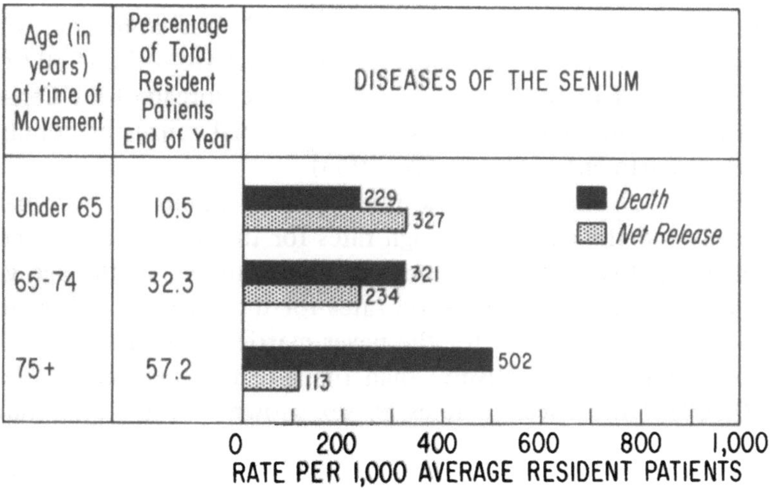

Fig. 3.8. Net releases and deaths per 1,000 average resident patients, and percentage distribution of patients suffering from mental disorders of the senium, resident at end of year, by age: 23 selected states, 1962.

Source: "Patient Movement Data, State and County Mental Hospitals, 1962," Washington, D.C., U.S. Department of Health, Education and Welfare, Public Health Service Publication no. 1282, 1964.

Patient movement rates are a function not only of age, sex, and diagnosis and of hospital programs that affect intake, release, and mortality of patients, but also of the demographic and socioeconomic characteristics of communities from which patients are drawn. The patients themselves also affect the rates by such characteristics as race, marital status, occupation, income, education, and the composition of household in which they live. Marital status exerts a considerable effect on the patterns of patient flow that determine the composition of the resident population of a mental hospital. To illustrate, consider the relationship of marital status to the first admission, release, readmission, and resident patient rates for functional psychotics. The data used are derived in part from a study carried out by the Biometry Branch of the National Institute of Mental Health in collaboration with 13 states in the Model Reporting

Area, yielding a combined total of 22,762 first admissions with a diagnosis of functional psychosis, and in part from the 1960 Census of Inmates of Institutions completed by the Bureau of the Census in April 1960, in conjunction with the decennial census of population (U.S. Department of Commerce, 1963).

Figure 3.9 shows the low rates of first admission for married persons and the excessively high rates for the never married and the separated, divorced, and widowed. For example, in the age group 25-44 years, the first admission rates for the divorced and separated (164 per 100,000), and for the never married (108) are about 6 and 4 times higher, respectively, than the rate for the married (28 per 100,000). Differences in rates by sex shown in Table 3.12 indicate

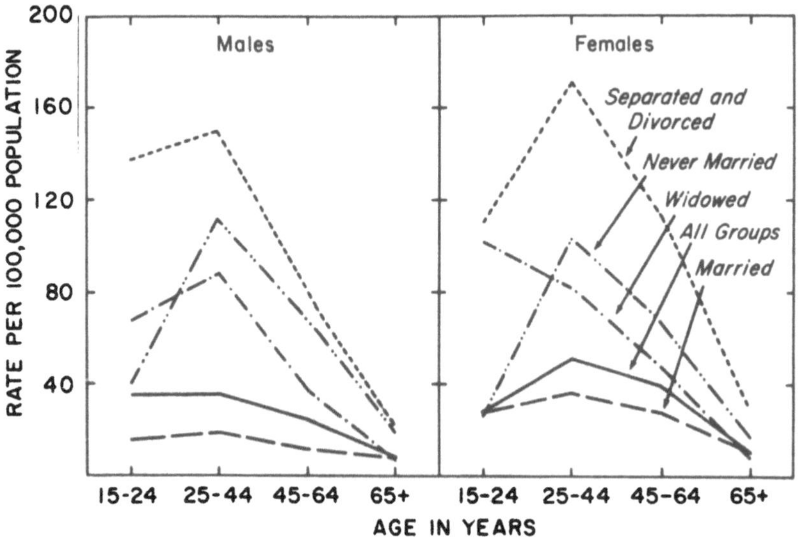

Fig. 3.9. First admission per 100,000 population for patients with functional psychoses, by sex, age, and marital status: 13 Model Reporting Area States, 1960.

Source: Kramer, M. "Epidemiology, biostatistics and mental health planning," *Psychiatric Research Report* no. 22, American Psychiatric Association, 1967.

Table 3.12 First admission rates per 100,000 population for patients with functional psychoses, specific for age, sex, and marital status: 13 Model Reporting Area states, 1960

Age	Marital status				
	Total	Never married	Married	Widowed	Separated & divorced
Both sexes					
Total[a]	33.7	70.5	22.8	64.7	117.8
15-24	31.8	33.3	23.2	95.2	118.7
25-44	43.8	108.4	27.8	83.3	163.6
45-64	32.3	68.5	22.0	46.3	99.1
65 & over	10.2	18.3	9.1	8.4	25.3
Males					
Total[a]	29.0	73.4	16.0	58.9	109.9
15-24	35.5	39.5	15.9	68.4	137.5
25-44	35.9	111.8	18.4	88.9	150.0
45-64	24.6	69.6	16.5	37.1	79.6
65 & over	9.3	19.3	7.9	7.6	22.2
Females					
Total[a]	38.2	66.7	29.0	66.2	124.1
15-24	28.3	25.6	27.1	102.5	110.8
25-44	51.3	103.3	36.7	82.1	171.9
45-64	39.6	67.4	28.2	48.3	113.5
65 & over	10.9	17.5	11.0	8.6	28.4

Source: Kramer, Morton, Epidemiology, Biostatistics and Mental Health Planning. Psychiatric Research Report No. 23, Table IV. Washington, D.C.: American Psychiatric Association, 1967.

[a] The age distribution of the population in the 13 states in the MRA Cohort Study was used as a standard population for the age adjustment of the total rates.

that in essentially all age categories for married, widowed, separated, and divorced, the female rates are considerably higher than the corresponding male rates. Only in the never married category are male rates higher than those for females.

The married not only have the lowest rates of admission but have also considerably higher probabilities of release than the other marital status groups, particularly the never married. Within six months following admission, about 80 percent of the married (all ages) have had a first significant release as compared to 56 percent of the single. The other two groups fall in between. Also, the never married and the separated and divorced who are released within the first three months following admission have slightly higher readmission rates within the six months following their release, with

18 percent of each group returning to the hospital as compared to 14 percent for the married. Figure 3.10 shows the relationship of marital status to probabilities of release following first admission, and Figure 3.11, probabilities of readmission for patients hospitalized less than three months specific for age.

The higher probability of retention for the never married, separated, divorced, and widowed results in the accumulation of disproportionately large numbers of these groups in the long-term or chronic population of the mental hospital. These phenomena are illustrated in two charts. Figure 3.12 demonstrates the way in which the number of persons with functional psychotic disorders in the first admission cohorts of married, never married, separated and divorced, and widowed changes within the first twelve months following admission. For example, of those aged 25-44 the married constitute 53 percent of the admission cohort, the never married 26 percent, and the other groups 21 percent. Among the one-year continuous-stay group the corresponding proportions are 27 percent, 47 percent, and 26 percent, respectively. Figure 3.13 shows the contribution that admissions for diseases of the senium make to the accumulation of widowed persons in the age groups 65-74 and 75 years and over. Thus, the proportion of widowed in each of these cohorts at time of admission is 37 percent and 58 percent, respectively. The corresponding proportion in the cohorts remaining at the end of one year are 43 percent and 60 percent, respectively.

The above data are only for first admissions for functional psychoses and diseases of the senium in the state mental hospitals of 13 states. Similar phenomena undoubtedly are occurring in other diagnostic groups in every other state in the nation, in both public and private mental hospitals. These differential rates of admission, release, and readmission by marital status, operating over the years, have produced an accumulative effect, portrayed in Figure 3.14, which shows the percent distribution of the population resident in all mental hospitals in the United States on April 1, 1960, by marital status and age. Forty-eight percent of the mental hospital population (all ages) consisted of never married patients. Another 13 percent are divorced or separated, 12 percent are widowed, and 27 percent are married. These are striking differences in the marital distribution by sex. Thus, the never married constitute 59 percent of the male patient population and 36 percent of the female, whereas the widowed account for 19 percent of the female population and only 6

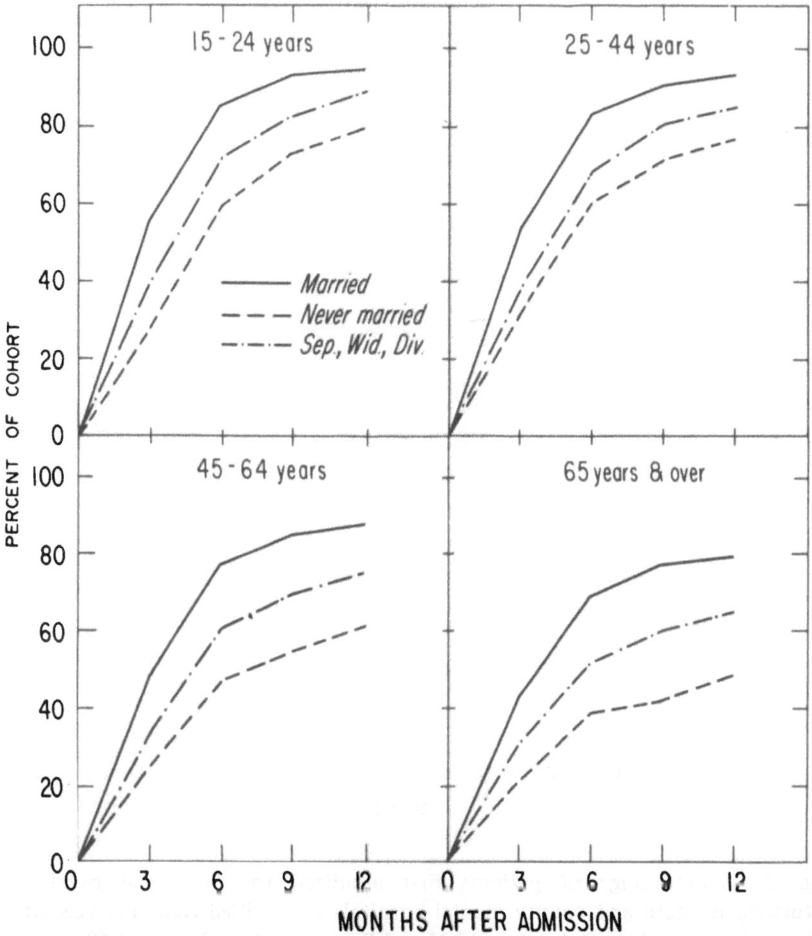

Fig. 3.10 Percentage of patients first admitted for functional psychoses released from state and county mental hospitals at specified time intervals, by age and marital status: 13 Model Reporting Area States, 1960.

Source: Kramer, M. "Some implications of trends in the usage of psychiatric facilities for community mental health programs and related research," Washington, D.C., U.S. Department of Health, Education, and Welfare, Public Health Service Publication no. 1434, 1967.

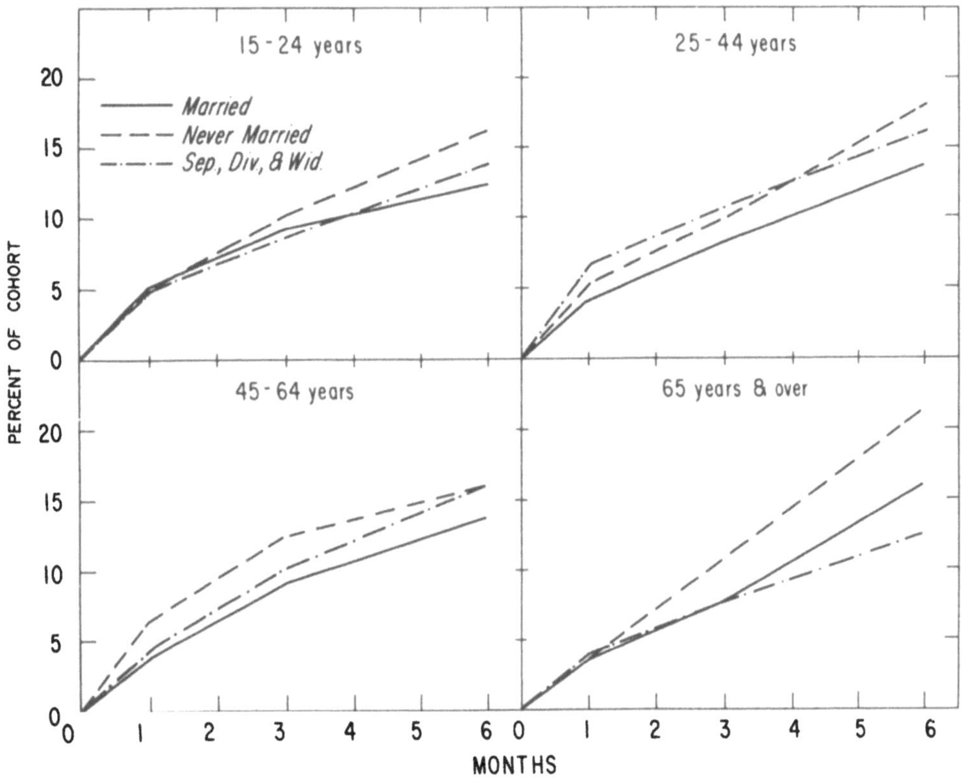

Fig. 3.11. Percentage of patients first admitted for functional psychoses returning to state and county mental hospitals at specified time intervals after release, by age and marital status: 13 Model Reporting Area States, 1960.

Source: Kramer, M. "Some implications of trends in the usage of psychiatric facilities for community mental health programs and related research," Washington, D.C., U.S. Department of Health, Education, and Welfare, Public Health Service Publication no. 1434, 1967.

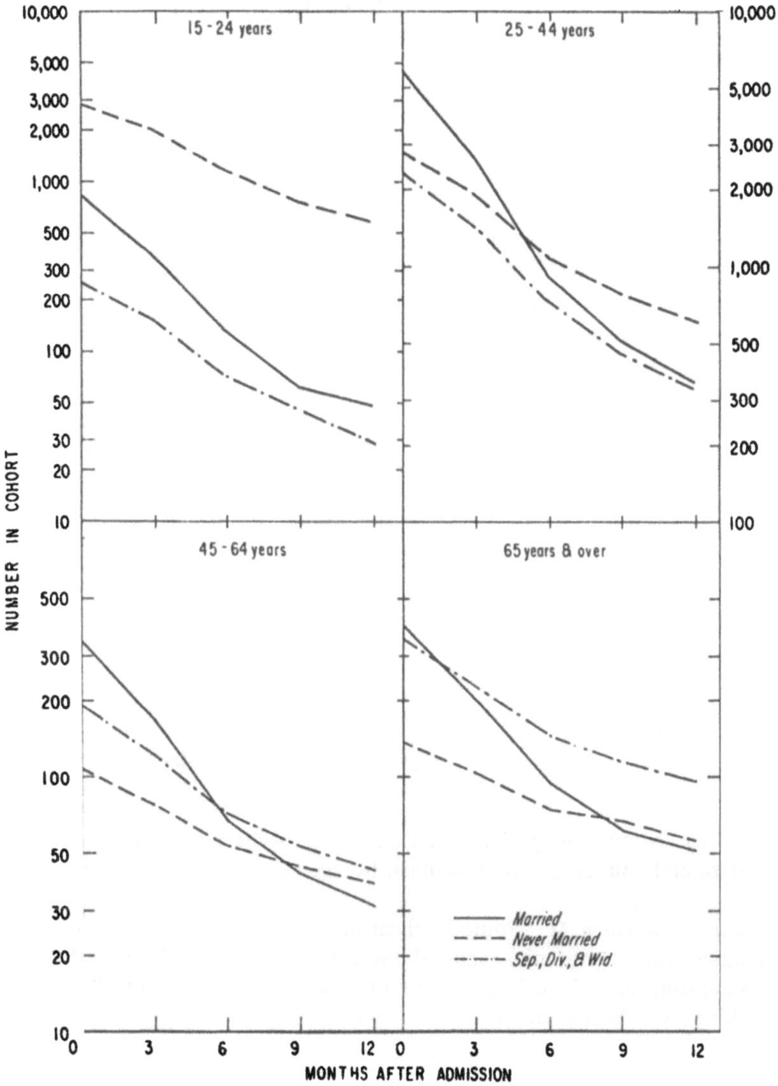

Fig. 3.12. Number of patients first admitted for functional psychoses retained in state and county mental hospitals at specified time intervals, by age and marital status: 13 Model Reporting Area States, 1960.

Source: Kramer, M. "Some implications of trends in the usage of psychiatric facilities for community mental health programs and related research," Washington, D.C., U.S. Department of Health, Education, and Welfare, Public Health Service Publication no. 1434, 1967.

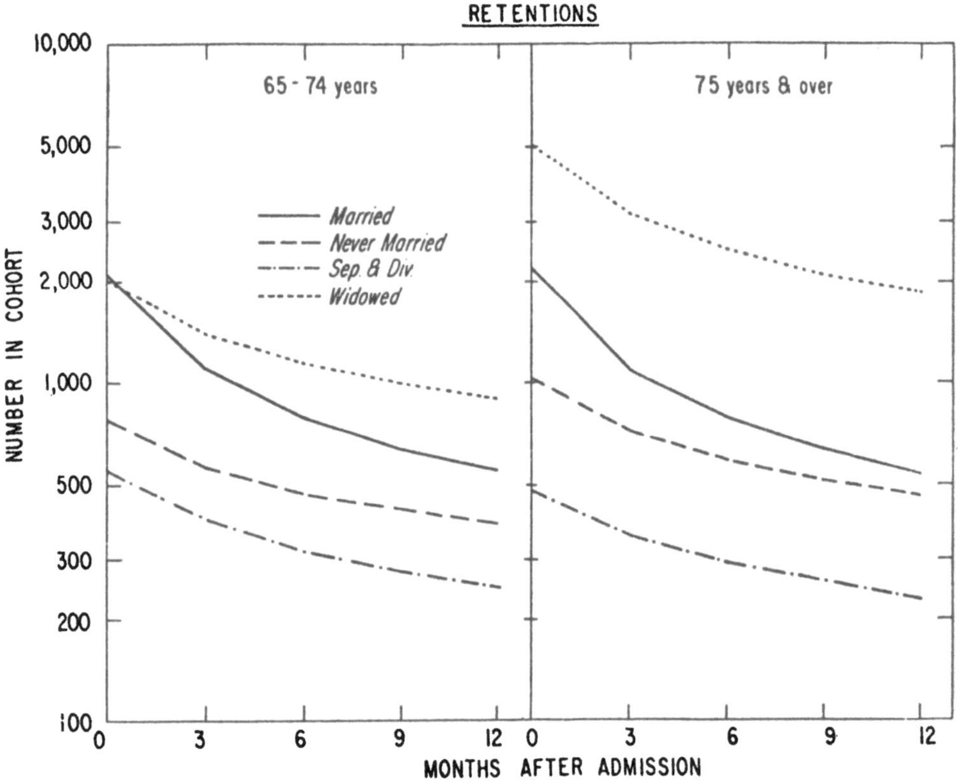

Fig. 3.13. Number of patients first admitted for diseases of the senium retained in state and county mental hospitals, by age: 13 Model Reporting Area States, 1960.

Source: Kramer, M. "Some implications of trends in the usage of psychiatric facilities for community mental health programs and related research," Washington, D.C., U.S. Department of Health, Education, and Welfare, Public Health Service Publication no. 1434, 1967.

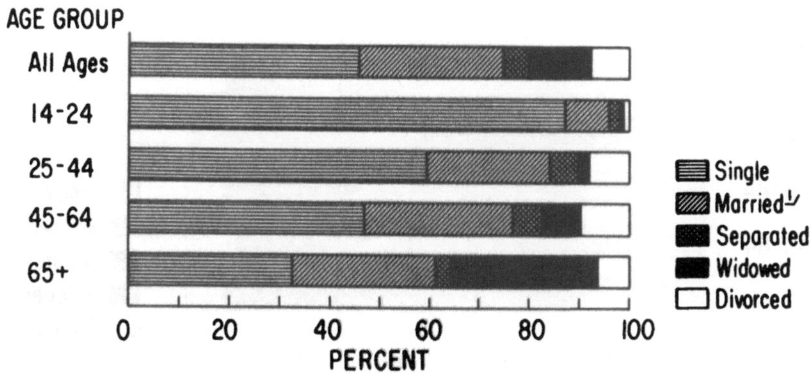

Fig. 3.14. Percentage distribution by marital status of patients in all mental hospital facilities, by age: United States, 1960.

Source: U.S. Census of Population, *Inmates of Institutions,* series PC (2) – 8A, Bureau of the Census, U.S. Department of Commerce.

[1] Excludes separated persons.

percent of the males. There is a somewhat higher proportion of the married among the females (32 percent) than among the males (23 percent). The proportion of separated and divorced is about the same among males and females (12 percent and 13 percent, respectively). Figures 3.15 and 3.16 show the variations in these proportions specific for age and sex.

Other important facts emerge when resident patient rates are computed specific for age, sex, and marital status. Figure 3.17 emphasizes the disproportionate representation of the never married, the divorced, and the separated in the mental hospital population compared to the general population. The rates for the never married among the males are particularly high. Their resident patient rate rises from 1,368 per 100,000 (1.4 percent) in the age group 25-34 years to 5,435 per 100,000 (5.4 percent) in the age group 45-54 years to 6,015 per 100,000 (6.1 percent) in the age group 75 and over.

Resident Patient Rates 1959-61 – Age, Sex, and Diagnosis

The age-specific and age-adjusted resident patient rates per 100,000 population for the United States for the three-year period 1959-61 are presented by mental disorder and sex in Table 3.13 and Figure 3.18. For all mental disorders combined, the age-specific resident

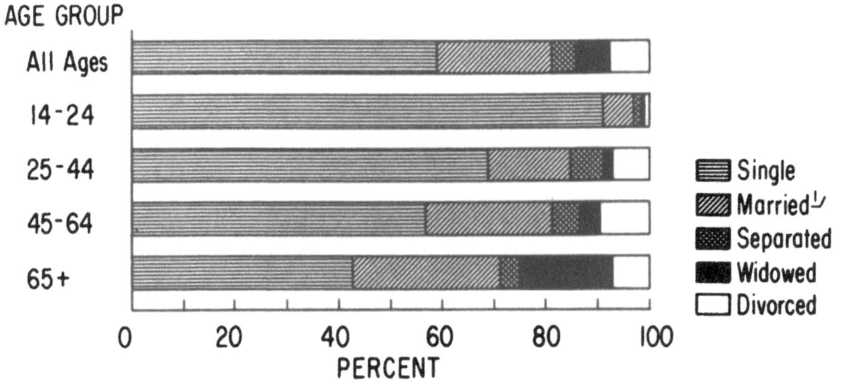

Fig. 3.15. Percentage distribution by marital status of male patients in all mental hospital facilities, by age: United States, 1960.

Source: U.S. Census of Population, *Inmates of Institutions,* series PC (2) – 8A, Bureau of the Census, U.S. Department of Commerce.

[1] Excludes separated persons.

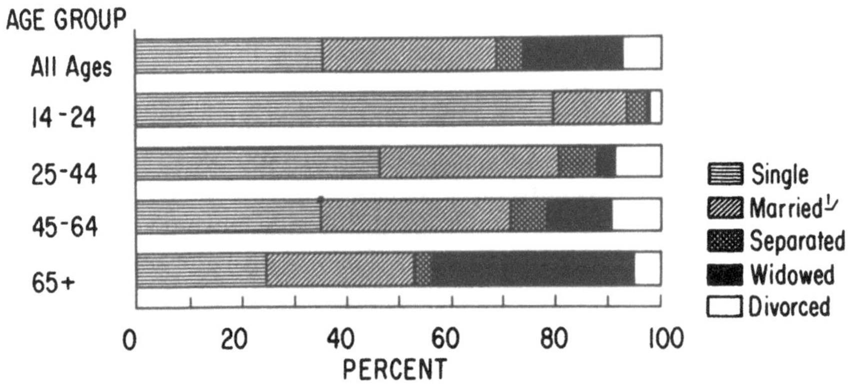

Fig. 3.16 Percentage distribution by marital status of female patients in all mental hospital facilities, by age: United States, 1960.

Source: U.S. Census of Population, *Inmates of Institutions,* series PC (2) – 8A, Bureau of the Census, U.S. Department of Commerce.

[1] Excludes separated persons.

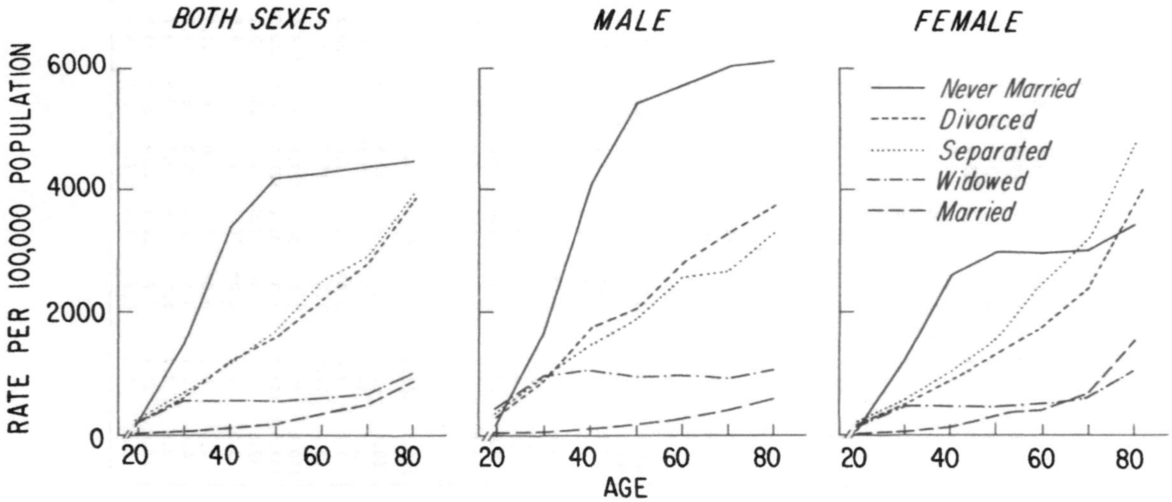

Fig. 3.17. Resident patients per 100,000 population in mental hospitals, by age, sex, and marital status: United States, 1960.

Source: U.S. Census of Population, *Inmates of Institutions,* series PC (2) – 8A, Bureau of the Census, U.S. Department of Commerce.

[1] Excludes separated persons.

Table 3.13 Average annual resident patient rates in state and county mental hospitals per 100,000 population by sex, age, and diagnosis: United States, 1959-61

Diagnosis	All ages		<15	15-24	25-34	35-44	45-54	55-64	65+
	Crude	Age adjusted							
Both sexes									
All mental disorders	295.8	296.7	7.9	90.0	212.8	329.6	530.3	706.0	952.7
Brain syndromes	70.8	67.3	1.6	11.1	20.6	33.7	72.4	140.5	447.8
Diseases of the senium	39.1	35.1	0.0*	0.0*	0.1	0.5	4.4	40.2	380.0
Syphilitic	11.6	11.5	0.0*	0.3	1.8	6.4	28.4	50.7	30.2
Other (excl. alcoholics)	20.2	20.8	1.6	10.8	18.6	26.8	39.6	49.6	37.6
Functional psychoses	175.9	178.8	2.3	46.5	141.2	226.8	365.2	456.0	424.3
Schizophrenic reactions	147.3	151.1	2.3	44.7	135.4	212.8	320.9	355.5	294.7
Affective and involutional	23.4	22.6	0.0*	0.8	3.5	10.4	37.6	85.9	104.7
Other	5.3	5.1	0.1	1.0	2.4	3.5	6.7	14.5	24.9
Disorders assoc. with alcoholism	11.2	11.3	0.0*	0.6	4.6	12.2	26.3	38.8	27.9
Psychoneurosis	3.7	3.8	0.2	2.1	4.3	5.3	6.6	8.3	6.8
Personality disorders	6.3	6.6	2.5	12.5	8.2	7.2	6.7	6.5	5.1
Mental deficiency	24.8	25.8	1.1	14.9	30.5	40.8	48.5	50.8	33.0
All other	3.1	3.1	0.3	2.3	3.3	3.7	4.6	5.2	7.9
Male									
All mental disorders	295.1	305.7	11.1	115.6	246.5	339.5	552.7	711.2	887.5
Brain syndromes	73.1	73.3	2.1	14.1	24.8	38.8	86.3	169.4	447.2
Diseases of the senium	34.9	33.8	0.0*	0.0*	0.1*	0.5	4.7	42.6	361.2
Syphilitic	15.4	15.7	0.0*	0.4	2.2	7.9	36.8	71.5	44.0
Other (excl. alcoholics)	22.8	23.9	2.0	13.7	22.4	30.4	44.8	55.2	42.0
Functional psychoses	160.6	168.1	3.2	58.6	155.2	215.3	351.6	402.8	337.5
Schizophrenic reactions	141.5	148.8	3.1	56.4	149.8	204.7	321.3	335.0	250.3
Affective and involutional	13.9	13.9	0.0*	0.7	2.1	6.0	22.8	53.3	65.2
Other	5.3	5.4	0.1*	1.5	3.4	4.6	7.6	14.6	22.0
Disorders assoc. with alcoholism	18.0	18.5	0.0*	0.9	7.3	18.6	41.0	65.3	50.0
Psychoneurosis	2.8	2.9	0.2	1.9	3.2	3.8	5.4	6.2	4.3
Personality disorders	9.0	9.5	3.7	17.3	12.9	10.8	9.7	8.8	6.3
Mental deficiency	28.0	29.8	1.4	19.6	39.0	47.9	53.6	52.6	33.5
All other	3.6	3.7	0.4	3.2	4.0	4.3	5.0	6.1	8.8
Female									
All mental disorders	296.5	287.1	4.7	64.8	180.4	320.3	508.5	701.0	1006.9
Brain syndromes	68.6	61.5	1.2	8.2	16.5	28.9	58.9	113.3	448.3
Diseases of the senium	43.1	36.1	0.0*	0.0*	0.1*	0.4	4.1	37.9	395.7
Syphilitic	7.8	7.6	0.0*	0.3	1.4	5.1	20.2	31.2	18.7
Other (excl. alcoholics)	17.7	17.8	1.2	7.9	15.0	23.4	34.6	44.2	34.0
Functional psychoses	190.8	188.1	1.4	34.6	127.8	237.7	378.4	506.0	496.5
Schizophrenic reactions	152.9	152.7	1.3	33.1	121.5	220.6	320.5	374.8	331.6
Affective and involutional	32.6	30.5	0.0*	1.0	4.8	14.6	52.1	116.7	137.7
Other	5.3	4.8	0.0*	0.6	1.4	2.5	5.8	14.5	27.3
Disorders assoc. with alcoholism	4.6	4.6	0.0*	0.2	2.0	6.0	11.9	13.8	9.4
Psychoneurosis	4.6	4.7	0.1	2.4	5.3	6.7	7.8	10.3	8.9
Personality disorders	3.6	3.7	1.1	7.6	3.7	3.9	3.7	4.2	4.0
Mental deficiency	21.6	22.1	0.7	10.3	22.4	34.0	43.6	49.0	32.6
All other	2.6	2.6	0.2	1.4	2.6	3.1	4.1	4.4	7.1

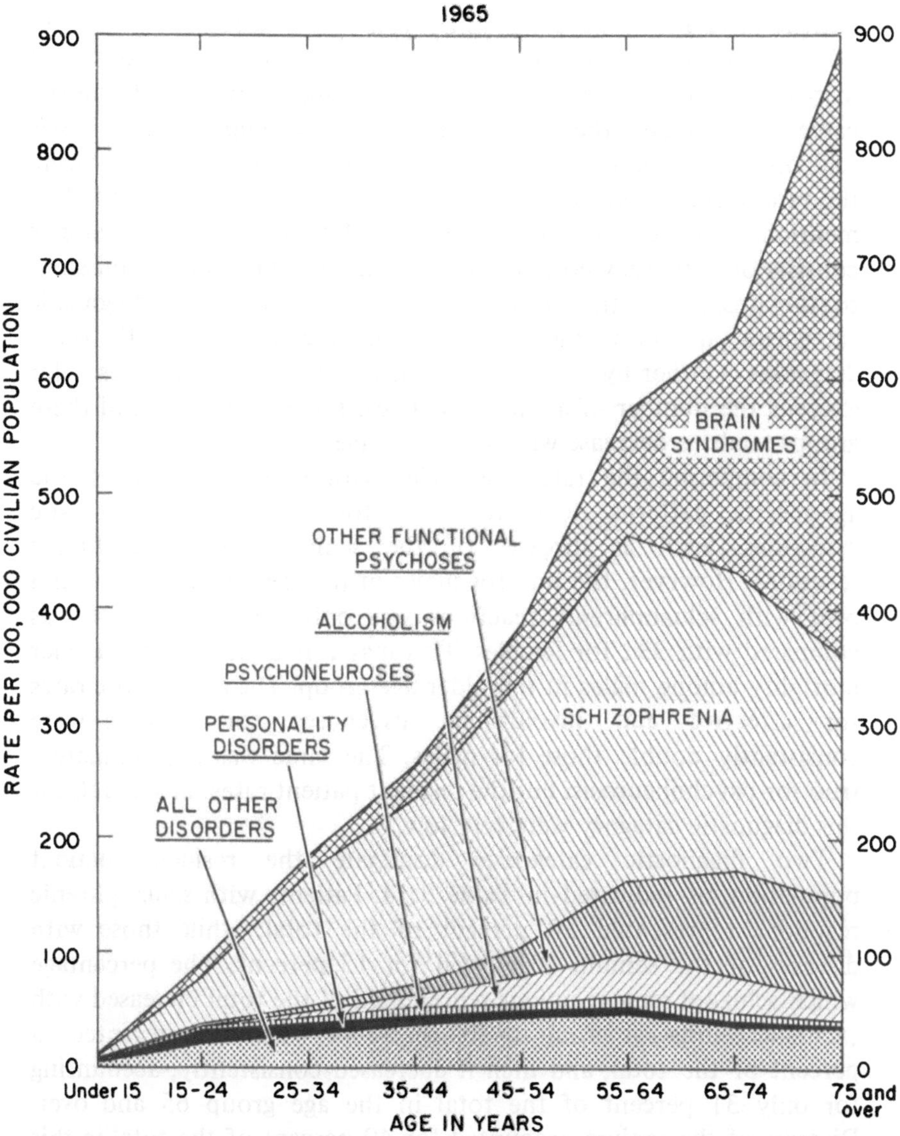

Fig. 3.18. Resident patients per 100,000 population in state and county mental hospitals for selected diagnoses, by age: United States, 1965.

patient rates increased consistently with age to a high of 952.7 per 100,000 population in the age group 65 and over. This consistent increase with age is characteristic of most of the diagnostic categories, except that for some, such as syphilitic psychoses, schizophrenic reactions, and disorders associated with alcoholism, the rate decreased in the age group 65 and over. This reflects the fact mentioned above that the resident population for these categories consists of patients who have aged in the hospital. Since admissions to the hospital in the age group 65 and over for these diagnostic categories are rare, the depletions in the patients with these diagnoses – either by death or by placement in other facilities – far exceeds the number of admissions. Thus, the numerical size of these groups tends to decrease with advancing age.

In comparing the rates for males with those for females, the age-specific patterns are quite similar for some of the diagnostic categories, such as diseases of the senium and schizophrenic reactions. However, the rate for males in the age group 65 years and over with schizophrenic reactions was only 250 per 100,000 as compared with 332 for females. This may reflect, in part, the higher mortality among males in the older age group. The age-specific rates for affective and involutional psychoses for females were consistently double those for males. The same was approximately true for psychoneurosis, but the resident patient rates, in general, for this diagnostic category were very low.

Two diagnostic categories dominate the resident patient population, as indicated in Table 3.14. Patients with schizophrenic reactions represented 50 percent of the total, while those with diseases of the senium accounted for 13 percent. The percentage which schizophrenic reactions represented of the total increased with each succeeding age group up to ages 35-44, where it represented 65 percent of the total, and then it decreased consistently, accounting for only 31 percent of the total in the age group 65 and over. Diseases of the senium accounted for 40 percent of the total in this latter age group.

Resident Patient Rates 1959-61 – Geographic Distribution

The average annual age-adjusted resident patient rates per 100,000 population are presented in Table 3.15 by geographic region and psychiatric diagnosis. As was true for first admission rates, the

Table 3.14 Percent distribution by diagnosis of patients resident in state and county mental hospitals by age: United States, 1959-61

Diagnosis	Total	< 15	15-24	25-34	35-44	45-54	55-64	65+
All mental disorders	100.0	100.0	100.0	100.0	100.0	100.0	100.0	100.0
Brain syndromes	24.9	20.6	12.4	9.7	10.2	13.7	19.9	47.0
Diseases of the senium	13.2	0.2	0.0	0.1	0.1	0.8	5.7	39.9
Syphilitic	3.9	0.2	0.4	0.9	2.0	5.4	7.2	3.2
Other (excl. alcoholics)	6.8	20.2	12.0	8.7	8.1	7.5	7.0	3.9
Functional psychoses	59.5	29.4	51.7	66.4	68.8	68.9	64.6	44.5
Schizophrenic reactions	49.8	28.4	49.6	63.6	64.6	60.5	50.4	30.9
Affective and involutional	7.9	0.2	0.9	1.6	3.2	7.1	12.2	11.0
Other	1.8	0.7	1.2	1.1	1.0	1.3	2.0	2.6
Disorders assoc. with alcoholism	3.8	0.1	0.6	2.2	3.7	5.0	5.5	2.9
Psychoneurosis	1.3	2.1	2.3	2.0	1.6	1.2	1.2	0.7
Personality disorders	2.1	30.9	13.8	3.9	2.2	1.3	0.9	0.6
Mental deficiency	8.4	13.3	16.6	14.3	12.4	9.1	7.2	3.5
All other	1.0	3.6	2.6	1.5	1.1	0.8	0.7	0.8

Table 3.15 Average annual age-adjusted resident patient rates per 100,000 population to state and county mental hospitals by diagnosis: United States and each region, 1959-61

Region	All mental disorders	Brain syndromes				Functional psychoses				Disorders assoc. with alcoholism	Psychoneurosis	Personality disorders
		Total	Diseases of senium	Syphilitic	Other	Total	Schizophrenic reactions	Affective and involutional	Other			
United States	296.7	67.3	35.1	11.5	20.8	178.8	151.1	22.6	5.1	11.3	3.8	6.6
Northeast Region	399.5	83.6	50.6	11.8	21.1	261.0	219.9	31.8	9.3	16.1	4.6	7.1
New England States	321.7	68.1	39.9	6.7	21.5	198.0	164.5	28.9	4.6	14.5	6.2	5.9
Mid-Atlantic States	411.4	86.0	52.3	12.6	21.1	270.7	228.4	32.3	10.0	16.4	4.4	7.3
North Central Region	281.8	61.7	29.3	12.4	19.9	166.8	143.3	17.9	5.6	11.7	4.1	8.4
East North Central States	306.7	69.2	34.0	14.4	20.8	181.1	154.9	19.0	7.2	13.5	4.1	8.5
West North Central States	226.8	46.2	20.1	8.0	18.1	134.3	116.3	15.8	2.2	7.7	4.2	8.0
Southern Region	262.8	65.6	30.4	11.9	23.4	146.3	120.5	22.9	3.0	5.9	3.2	4.3
South Atlantic States	296.1	79.2	39.4	13.3	26.5	162.0	131.0	27.2	3.7	7.8	3.9	4.8
East South Central States	242.4	55.5	26.2	9.9	19.5	140.1	115.5	22.2	2.4	3.1	2.2	2.7
West South Central States	226.9	52.6	20.2	11.2	21.2	126.7	107.6	16.8	2.2	4.9	2.8	4.8
Western Region	230.1	55.5	30.7	8.1	16.7	136.4	118.4	16.2	1.8	12.9	3.2	7.4
Mountain States	214.7	59.6	31.6	8.0	20.0	105.2	94.4	9.4	1.4	11.9	3.0	5.7
Pacific States	234.8	54.2	30.4	8.1	15.7	145.8	125.8	18.1	1.9	13.1	3.3	8.0

variation in resident patient rates among regions was considerable. The rates ranged from a high of 400 per 100,000 in the Northeast to a low of 230 in the Western region. Among the subregions, they ranged from a high of 411 in the Mid-Atlantic states to a low of 215 in the Mountain states – a differential of almost two to one. Examination of these rates for specific diagnostic categories reveals interesting variations among the four regions. Rates for diseases of the senium, schizophrenic reactions, and affective and involutional psychoses were all of considerably greater magnitude in the Northeast than those for the other three regions. The Northeast also had somewhat higher rates for other functional psychoses and disorders associated with alcoholism compared with the other regions, and the South exhibited the lowest rates for alcoholism and personality disorders. The regional differences were heavily influenced by differences in rates among individual states. Appendix Table 5 reveals that New York State had a resident patient rate of 499 for all disorders combined, compared with a low of 123 in New Mexico. Since New York State accounted for almost 20 percent of the resident patients in the United States, its high rate exerted a heavy influence on the rate both for the Mid-Atlantic states and for the Northeast. The low rate for the Mountain states, on the other hand, was due to the fact not only that New Mexico had the lowest rates but that most of the states in that region also had low rates. Examination of rates for specific diagnostic categories in Appendix Table 5 reveals that for diseases of the senium New York State had a rate of 67 compared with rates as low as 12 for Iowa and Utah, 11 for Kansas, and 4 for Oklahoma. For schizophrenic reactions New York State had a high of 291 compared with a low of 60 to 65 for Arizona, Utah, and Nevada.

Trends in Resident Patients

The trend of the number of resident patients at the end of the year and of the admissions, net releases, and deaths for the period 1946 to 1967 may be seen in Figure 3.1. As already indicated, the number of resident patients increased steadily between 1946 and 1955 at almost a constant 2 percent per year. Since that time, this number had decreased steadily from 558,922 at the end of 1955 to 426,309 at the end of 1967. The trend in the number of resident patients between 1946 and 1955 and the abrupt change between 1955 and

1956 has been analyzed in detail elsewhere (Kramer and Pollack, 1958). This sudden decrease has been attributed generally to the widespread introduction of the psychoactive drugs into the state mental hospitals in the mid-1950s. The acceleration of the decline in resident patients in the 1960s has resulted from the fact that the number of net releases has increased at a greater rate than the number of total admissions. This, in turn, may be due to the greater use of other facilities as alternatives to the mental hospital. This factor will be examined in more detail in Chapter 4.

The trend in the number of resident patients in state and county mental hospitals at the end of the year by age and sex for the period 1950 to 1965 is presented in Figure 3.19. The picture is generally one of increasing numbers for the age groups under 15 years and 15 to 24 years and decreasing numbers for the remaining age groups. An exception to this is the fact that the number of males aged 55 to 64 increased up to about 1962, after which it decreased slightly. Thus, with the exception of the younger age groups, which accounted for relatively small proportions of the resident patient population, the decrease in resident patient population appears to have occurred across all of the other age groups. This is also evident from the average annual rates of change in the number of resident patients for the period 1955-66 shown in Table 3.16. The magnitude of the average annual rates of change, however, is seen to vary by both age and sex. For example, males in the younger age groups (under 25 years) had higher average annual rates of increase than females. especially in the under 15-year age groups. In the older age groups where decreases in resident patients occurred, the average annual rates of decrease were greater for females in the 25-44 and 55-64 age groups, higher for males in the 65 and over age group, but of about equal magnitude for both of the sexes in the 45-54 age group.

Similar patterns were observed in the corresponding trend data for resident patient rates specific for age and sex as seen in Figure 3.20 and Table 3.17. These trends in the rates of change in number of resident patients in the various age-sex groups had impact on the trend in sex ratios in corresponding age groups. The ratio of males to females specific for age shown for the periods 1950-52, 1959-61, and 1964-66 in Table 3.18 indicate that overall the ratio changed very little over this time span, with females being slightly in excess of males. However, when examined by age, some dramatic changes have occurred in these ratios. The excess of males in the age groups under

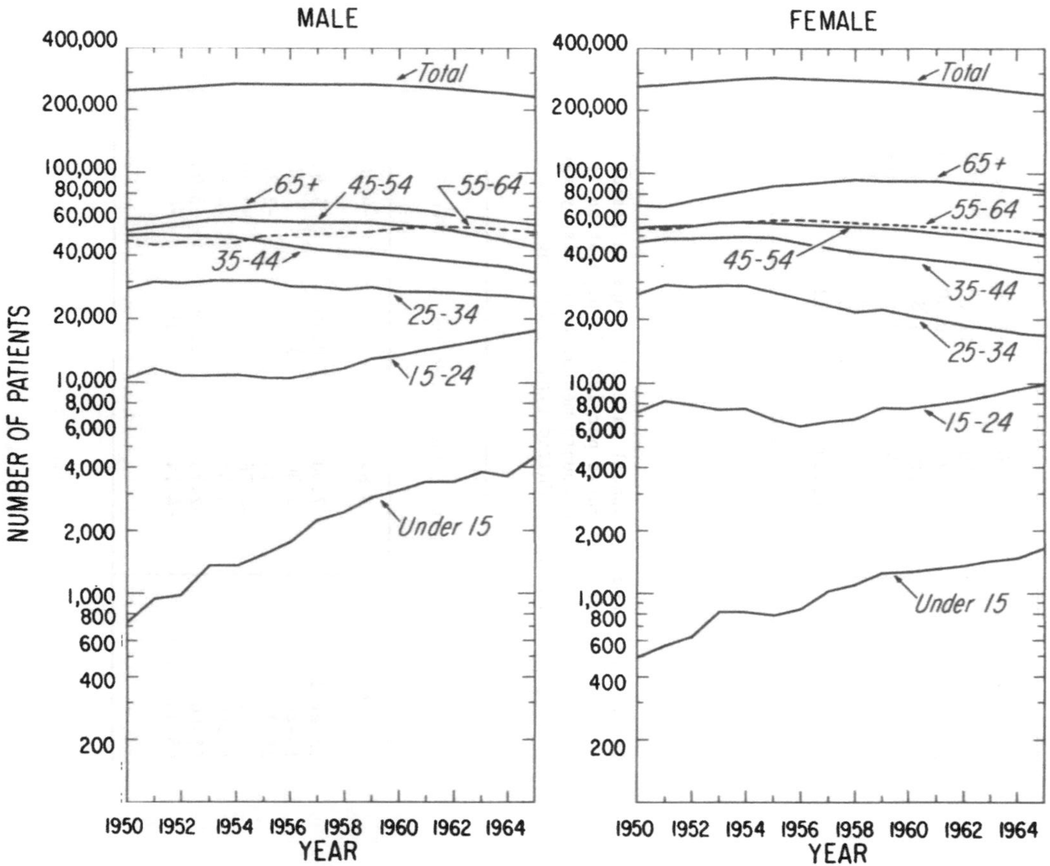

Fig. 3.19. Number of resident patients at the end of each year in state and county mental hospitals, by age sex: United States, 1950-1965.

Table 3.16 Average annual rate of change in number of resident patients in state and county mental hospitals: United States, 1955-66

Age	Both sexes	Male	Female
All ages	-2.00	-1.76	-2.21
Under 15	10.30	11.20	8.20
15-24	5.90	6.40	5.00
25-34	-3.10	-1.82	-4.72
35-44	-4.06	-3.66	-4.48
45-54	-3.31	-3.55	-3.08
55-64	-.96	0.0	-2.05
65 and over	-1.80	-2.93	-.99

Table 3.17 Average annual rate of change in resident patient rates per 100,000 population in state and county mental hospitals by age and sex: United States, 1955-66

Age	Both Sexes	Male	Female
All ages	-3.84	-3.55	-4.10
Under 15	7.90	8.80	5.90
15-24	1.30	1.40	.80
25-34	-2.19	-.89	-3.82
35-44	-4.76	-4.33	-5.20
45-54	-4.92	-4.98	-4.83
55-64	-2.73	-1.39	-3.95
65 and over	-4.74	-5.16	-4.50

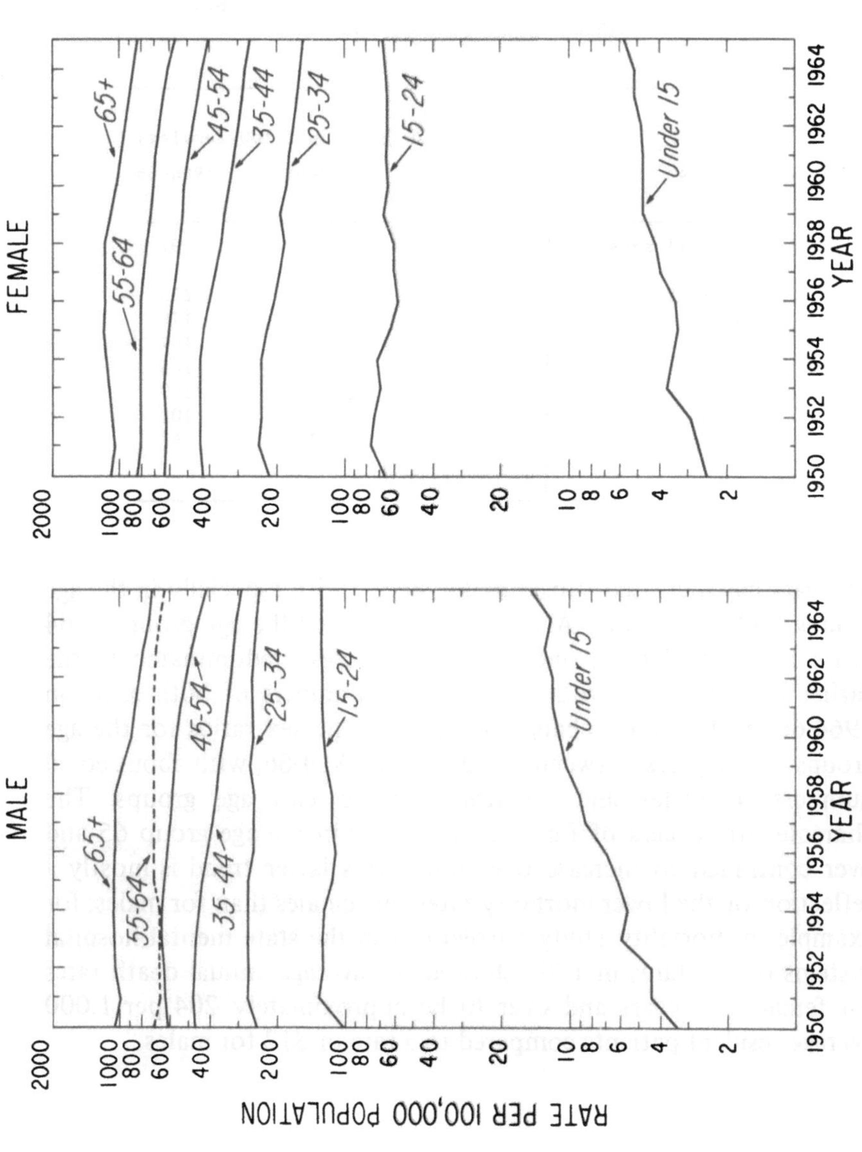

Fig. 3.20. Resident patients per 100,000 population in state and county mental hospitals, by age and sex: United States, 1950-1965.

Table 3.18 Ratio of number of male to female resident patients in state and county mental hospitals by age and sex: United States, 1950-52, 1959-61, and 1964-66

Age	Sex ratio (males per 100 females)		
	1950-52	1959-61	1964-66
All ages	95	97	97
Under 15	157	246	253
15-24	139	175	176
25-34	103	131	147
35-44	105	101	105
45-54	98	106	100
55-64	83	95	101
65 and over	85	73	67

35 years has increased substantially since 1950, especially in the age groups under 15 years. Also, the sex ratio for the age group 55-64 years has shifted from one in which females predominated in the earlier period to one with almost equal numbers of both sexes in 1964-66. Little or no change occurred in the sex ratios for the age groups 35-54 years between 1950-52 and 1964-66, with about equal numbers of males and females in these two age groups. The characteristic excess of females over males in the age group 65 and over continued to increase over time. This latter trend is mostly a reflection of the lower mortality rates for females than for males; for example, a mortality study carried out in the state mental hospital systems of 17 states in 1962 showed the average annual death rates for females 65 years and over to be approximately 204 per 1,000 average resident patients compared to a rate of 312 for males.

4 / Use of Psychiatric Facilities, 1966

Although the period 1955-66 was one of marked decline in the resident population of state mental hospitals, it was, as indicated in Chapter 3, one of marked increase in the establishment of outpatient clinics and of inpatient psychiatric services of general hospitals. Indeed, the downward trend in the mental hospital population is closely related to the upward trend in the use of other facilities. The availability and use of increased numbers of community-based services assisted in the reduction of the mental hospital population in several ways. In some instances the outpatient clinic or general hospital service served as an alternate facility for treatment which prevented, or at least delayed, the admission of certain types of patients to mental hospitals. In other instances, the outpatient or general hospital service served as a resource for follow-up care and thus facilitated the earlier discharge of some types of patients from the mental hospital.

Table 4.1 demonstrates the changes between 1955 and 1966 in the volume of services provided by each type of facility in the universe of psychiatric services consisting of the mental hospitals, outpatient clinics, and the general hospital inpatient services. The volume of services provided is summarized in terms of patient care episodes defined as follows: The sum of the number of patients under care in each facility as of the beginning of the year, plus the total admission actions to that facility during the following twelve months. These counts merely provide an index of the extent to which services are used by a given group.

PATIENT CARE EPISODES

In 1966 there were 2,764,000 patient care episodes. These episodes were generated by approximately 2,461,000 separate individuals, or about 1.2 percent of the total population of the United States. Of the total patient care episodes, 802,000 (29 percent) occurred in state and county hospitals, 123,000 (5 percent) in VA hospitals, and 104,000 (4 percent) in private mental hospitals. Thus, mental hospitals accounted for 1,029,000 patient care episodes, or about 37 percent of the total. The remaining 1,735,000 episodes (63 percent of the total) were accounted for by general hospitals with psychiatric

Table 4.1 Number and percent of patient care episodes[a] rate per 100,000 population and percent change in numbers and rates, by type of psychiatric facility: United States, 1955 and 1966

Type of psychiatric facility	Number		Percent		Rate per 100,000 pop.		Percent change 1955-1966	
	1955	1966	1955	1966	1955	1966	In number	In rate
All facilities	1,675,352	2,764,089	100.0	100.0	1,032.2	1,427.0	65.0	38.2
Mental hospitals	1,030,418	1,029,168	61.6	37.2	634.8	531.3	-0.1	-16.3
State and county	818,832	802,216	48.9	29.0	504.5	414.2	-2.0	-17.9
Veterans	88,355	122,979	5.3	4.4	54.4	63.5	39.2	16.7
Private	123,231	103,973	7.3	3.8	75.9	53.6	-15.6	-29.4
Psychiatric services of general hospitals	265,934	548,921	15.8	19.9	163.8	283.4	106.4	73.0
Outpatient psychiatric clinics	379,000	1,186,000	22.6	42.9	233.5	612.3	212.9	162.2

[a] Patient care episodes are equal to the number of persons resident in the specified facility as of the beginning of the year plus all admissions to that facility during the following twelve months.

services (549,000, or 20 percent of the total) and psychiatric outpatient clinics (1,186,000, or 43 percent of the total). This situation is in striking contrast to that in 1955, when mental hospitals accounted for 62 percent of the patient care episodes; outpatient clinics 22 percent; and general hospitals with psychiatric services 16 percent. In addition, the total number of episodes in all facilities in 1966 was 65 percent higher than the corresponding number in 1955, and the corresponding rates of patient care episodes 38 percent higher. The changes in the number of patient care episodes per 100,000 population specific for type of facility are also striking. The rate for mental hospitals decreased by 16 percent from 635 to 531, while that for psychiatric services in general hospitals increased by 73 percent (from 164 to 283), and for outpatient services by 162 percent (from 234 to 612).

As a result of more complete reporting from all psychiatric facilities in 1966, it is possible to present a composite picture of the pattern of use of the universe of psychiatric facilities, as defined above, and to illustrate the considerable differences in sex, age, and diagnostic composition of the patients admitted to each type of facility. These data are presented for patient care episodes during 1966 and the components of this index – admissions during the year and patients under care at the beginning of the year.

The rates of admission to the different types of facilities vary widely. Thus, in the public mental hospitals there were 74 annual admissions per 100 patients in the hospital at the beginning of the year. The corresponding ratios for private mental hospitals were 640, for general hospitals with psychiatric services 2,314, and for outpatient psychiatric clinics about 113 annual admissions per 100 patients under care at the beginning of the year.

Age and Sex

Of the total patient care episodes in 1966, 1,446,091 were accounted for by males (53 percent) and 1,317,998 by females (47 percent). The corresponding rates were 1,427 per 100,000 for both sexes combined: 1,542 per 100,000 males and 1,319 per 100,000 females. The distribution of patient care episodes by sex and type of facility is shown in Table 4.2. The rates of patient care episodes during 1966 are presented by age and type of facility in Figure 4.1 and in Appendix Table 6. For all services combined, the rates rise from 613

Table 4.2 Total patient care episodes by type of facility and sex: United States, 1966

Type of Facility	Patient care episodes (in thousands)		
	Both Sexes	Males	Females
All facilities	2,764	1,446	1,318
Mental hospitals	1,029	575	454
State and county	802	413	389
Veterans Administration	123	123	---
Private	104	39	65
Psychiatric inpatient services of general hospitals	549	220	329
Outpatient clinics	1,186	651	535

per 100,000 persons in the age group under 15 years to a maximum of 2,172 per 100,000 persons in the age group 35-44 years. From this peak, the rate decreases to 1,597 per 100,000 in the age group 55-64 years, and then increases slightly to 1,686 per 100,000 for persons 65 years and over.

Figure 4.1 also demonstrates the striking differences in the volume of services each type of facility provides to the different age groups. The outpatient clinics provide services predominantly to persons under 35 years of age and the mental hospitals to persons 35 years and over. The rate of patient care episodes for mental hospitals increases with advancing age, while that for outpatient clinics and general hospitals decreases. The high rate of patient care episodes in mental hospitals for the age group 65 years and over is accounted for by two factors mentioned earlier: The large number of patients in the resident population who grew old in the hospital setting (particularly patients with the functional psychoses) and the high admission rate for patients with mental disorders of the senium such as brain syndromes with cerebral arteriosclerosis and senile brain disease (Figure 4.2 and 4.3 and Appendix Tables 7 and 8).

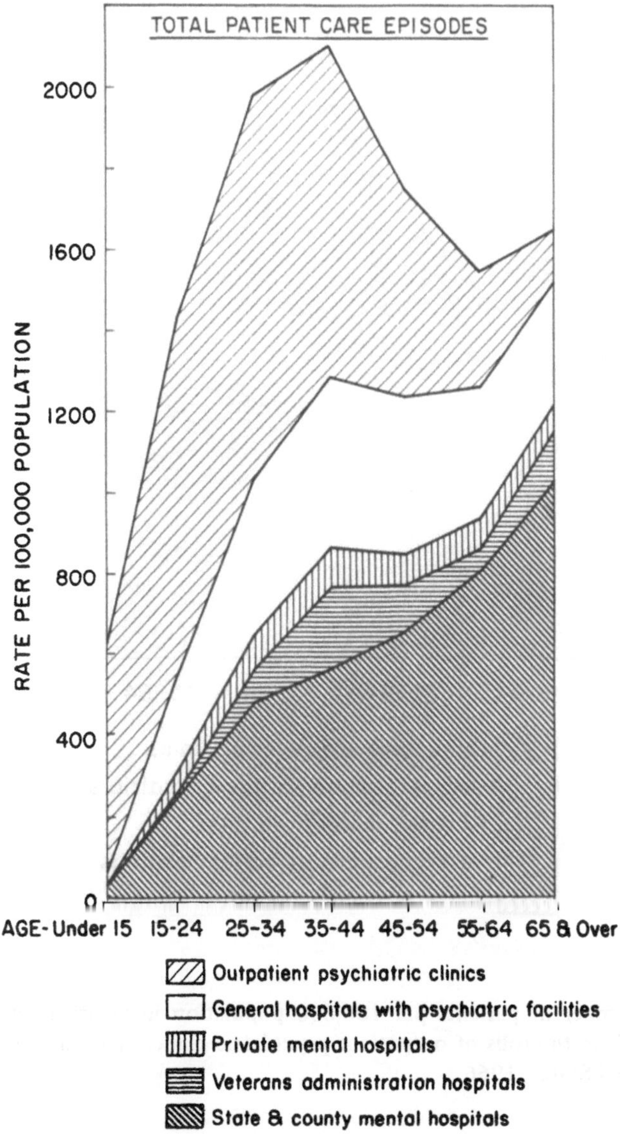

Fig. 4.1. Number of patient care episodes per 100,000 population in psychiatric facilities, by type of facility and age: United States, 1966.

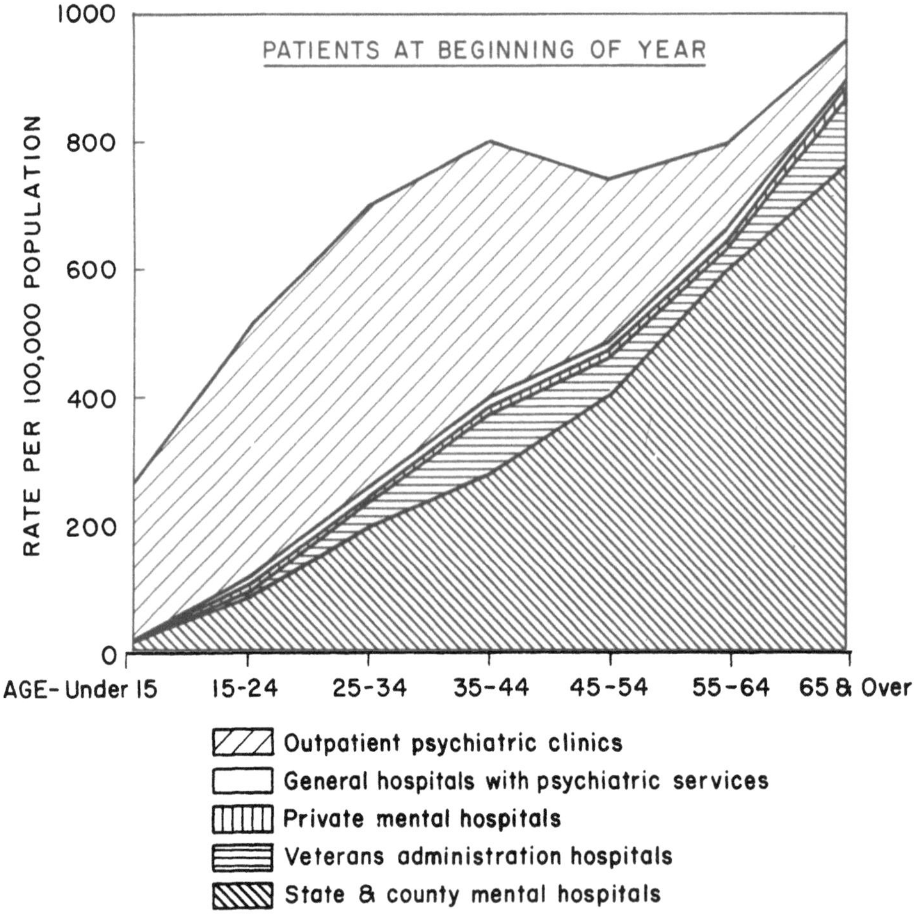

Fig. 4.2. Number of patients per 100,000 population in inpatient psychiatric facilities and on the rolls of outpatient psychiatric clinics at beginning of year, by age: United States, 1966.

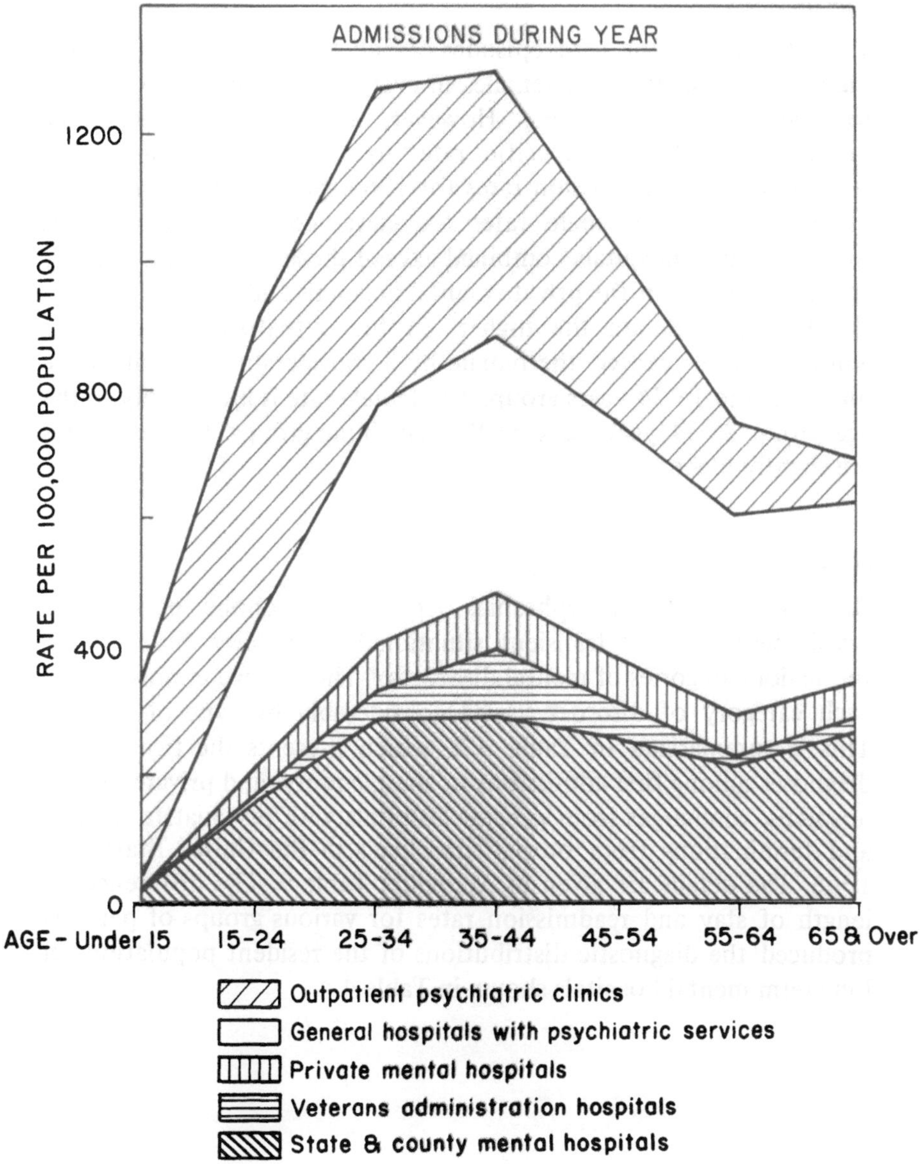

Fig. 4.3. Number of patients per 100,000 population admitted to psychiatric facilities, by type of facility and age: United States, 1966.

Age and Sex

The rate of patient care episodes for all facilities combined were higher for males than for females in every age group except the one for persons 25-34 years. However, there were considerable differences in the age-specific rates by sex and type of facility (Figure 4.4). The admission rates for 1966 specific for sex are given in Figure 4.5. The male rates for state, county, and Veterans Administration hospitals combined exceed those for females in every age group, while in the private mental hospitals and general hospitals the female rates are the higher. In the outpatient clinics, male admission rates exceed the female by a considerable amount in the under 15 and 15-24 years group. The female rate is higher only in the age group 25-34 years, and in the remaining groups, the male rates are slightly higher.

Diagnosis

Brain syndromes, schizophrenia, depressive, alcoholic, personality, psychoneurotic, and transient situational personality disorders are the major categories of mental disorders.* The relative importance of each category of disorder varied considerably by type of facility. This is summarized in Table 4.3, which presents the five leading diagnoses among first admissions to state, county, and private mental hospitals, discharges from general hospitals with psychiatric services and terminations from outpatient clinics in the United States for 1966. The details are given in Appendix Table 9. The differences in length of stay and readmission rates for various groups of patients produced the diagnostic distributions of the resident populations in long-term mental hospitals shown in Table 4.4.

---

*A more detailed description of each of these categories can be found in the definitions in the second edition of the *Diagnostic and Statistical Manual* of the American Psychiatric Association (1968) and in the Registrar General's *Glossary of Mental Disorders* (London, General Register Office, 1968).

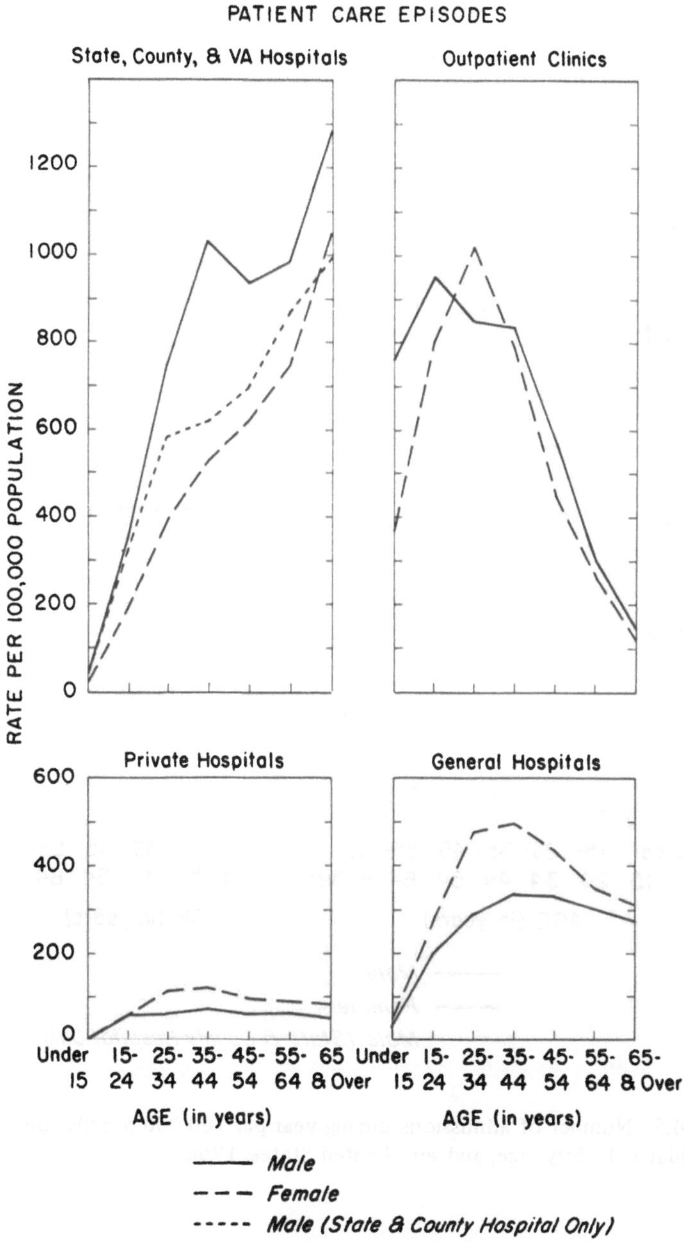

Fig. 4.4. Number of patient care episodes per 100,000 population, by type of psychiatric facility, age, and sex: United States, 1966.

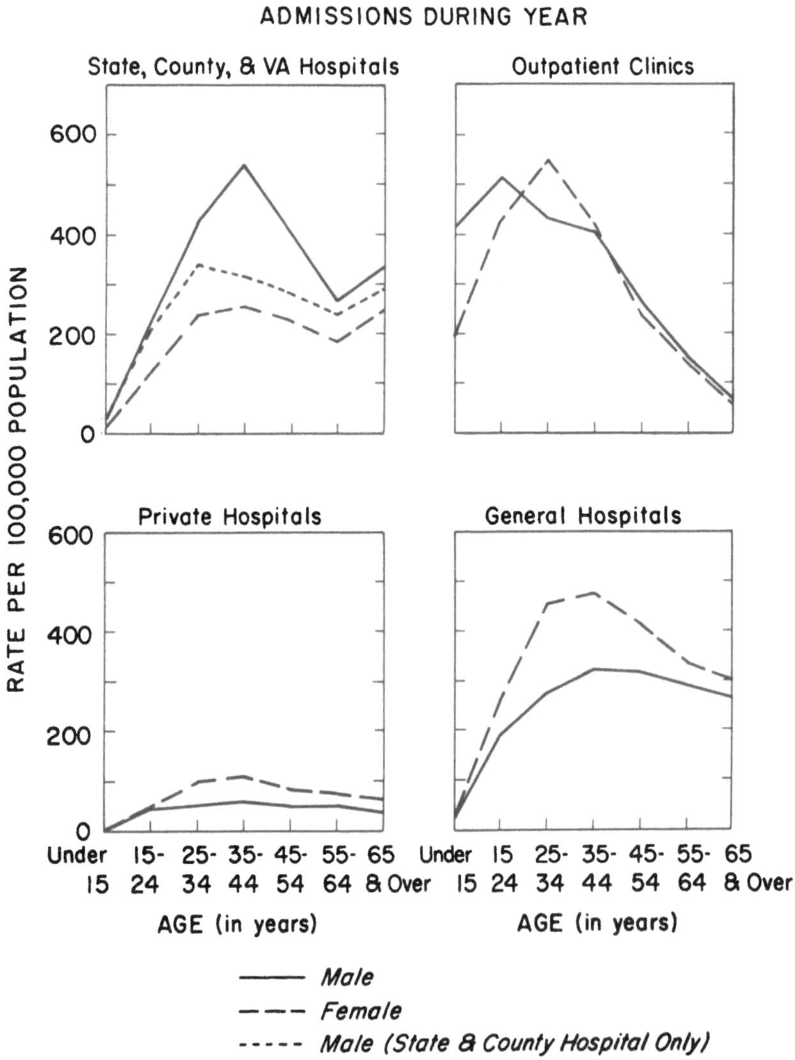

Fig. 4.5. Number of admissions during year per 100,000 population, by type of psychiatric facility, age, and sex: United States, 1966.

Table 4.3 Rank order and percent of total for five leading diagnoses among admissions to state, county, and private mental **hospitals,** discharges from general hospitals with psychiatric services, and terminations from outpatient clinics: United States, 1966

Diagnosis	State and county mental hospitals		Private mental hospitals		Psychiatric services in general hospitals		Out-patient clinics	
	Rank	% of total	Rank	% of total	Rank	% of total	Rank	% of total
Brain syndromes[a]	1	22	*		5	11	*	
Schizophrenia	2	19	2	19	3	15	3	16
Alcoholic disorders[b]	3	18	4	8	4	12	*	
Personality disorders[c]	4	11	5	8	*		1	23
Depressive disorders[d]	5	10	1	33	1	27	4	13
Psychoneurotic disorders[e]	*		3	10	2	15	5	12
Transient situational personality disorders	*		*		*		2	18

* Disorder not among first five for specified facility.

[a] Brain syndromes - excludes brain syndromes associated with alcoholism.

[b] Alcoholic disorders - includes brain syndromes associated with alcohol and the category of alcoholism from the personality disorders.

[c] Personality disorders - includes all personality disorders except alcoholism.

[d] Depressive disorders - includes all affective psychoses and psychoneurotic depressive reation.

[e] Psychoneurotic disorders - includes all psychoneurotic disorders except psychoneurotic depressive reaction.

Table 4.4 Rank order and percent of total for five leading diagnoses among resident patients of state, county, and private mental hospitals: United States, 1966

Diagnosis	State & county mental hospitals		Private mental hospitals	
	Rank	Percent of total	Rank	Percent of total
Schizophrenia	1	48	1	26
Brain syndromes	2	23	3	17
Mental deficiency	3	8	*	
Depressive disorders	4	5	2	20
Alcoholic disorders	5	5	*	
Personality disorders	*		4	9
Psychoneurotic disorders	*		5	5

* Disorder not among first five for specified facility.

VARIATIONS IN PATTERNS OF PSYCHIATRIC CARE BY SOCIOECONOMIC FACTORS

The differences in the age, sex, diagnostic and other characteristics of patients who are under care in the different types of psychiatric facilties described above result from the interaction of factors, described earlier in Chapter 1, that determine pathways by which an individual enters medical and psychiatric care and those that determine his length of stay in the facility. Briefly these factors include those that characterize: *(a)* the patient; *(b)* the physicians, psychiatrists, and social agencies that make specific referrals for admission; *(c)* the facility to which the patient was admitted; and *(d)* the community in which the patient lives.

It is not possible to develop rates of admission into psychiatric care facilities specific for every possible combination of factors that may determine which type of facility will be entered first by members of different subgroups of a population. However, admission rates to psychiatric facilities specific for such variables as race, sex, marital status, residence, place of birth, occupation, income, and living arrangements do illustrate the end result of the complex set of interactions that resulted in a specific pathway. Unfortunately, data are not available for the United States or its various states and regions on variations in patterns of care for persons with different disorders specific for the above-mentioned demographic factors. However, they are available from intensive studies carried out in three states – Ohio, Maryland, and Louisiana. Data will be presented for Ohio in Chapter 5 and for Maryland and Louisiana in Chapter 6 to illustrate how admission rates are influenced by these factors. These data will demonstrate important differences in the way existing services are being utilized. Although it is not possible to generalize satisfactorily from them to the nation as a whole or to states other than those represented in these studies, the facts to be reported are not atypical.

In 1963 the Congress enacted the Community Mental Health Centers Act (PL 88-164), which, inter alia, is attempting to change the patterns of delivery of mental health services so as to make such services readily available to all regardless of race, creed, color, residence, and socioeconomic status. Thus, rates specific for various social and economic factors will provide some indication of types of major problems which the states face in improving the delivery of mental health services. The data to be presented in Chapters 5 and 6 are for the year 1960. Thus, they document certain conditions that existed prior to the introduction of the new programs and provide benchmarks against which to measure subsequent change.

5 / Patterns of Use of Psychiatric Facilities in Ohio, 1950-60

This chapter describes changes that occurred between 1950 and 1960 in first admission rates to state mental hospitals in Ohio. The basic data consisted of first admissions to the state hospitals during two periods – January 1, 1948, through June 30, 1952, and July 1, 1958, through December 31, 1961.* For the second period, data were also obtained for admissions to private mental hospitals, VA neuropsychiatric hospitals, general hospitals with psychiatric services, and outpatient psychiatric clinics in Ohio, making it possible to describe patterns of first admissions to this universe of psychiatric facilities. Average annual first admission rates, centered on each of the census years 1950 and 1960, were computed for two broad geographic areas of the state (metropolitan and nonmetropolitan counties)† specific for diagnosis, age, sex, race, marital status, occupation, and, for state mental hospital patients, education and place of birth. Data on the demographic variables listed were obtained from the patients' record of admission to the specific facility. In the collection of demographic data on first admissions the state hospitals used the same definitions as those used by the Bureau of the Census. Thus, the specified distributions of first admissions and corresponding distributions of the population were used to compute the rates. For the most part, this chapter will be concerned with descriptive profiles of characteristics of patients diagnosed as having schizophrenia, mental diseases of the senium, alcoholism, and psychoneurosis. The question pursued is: What are the characteristics

---

*See the following bibliographic references (29), (74), (79), (80), (81), (82), (83), (84), (85), (86), (87), (88), (89), (90), (141), for studies based on these data.

†A metropolitan area is a county or group of contiguous counties containing at least one city of 50,000 inhabitants or more or "twin cities" with a combined population of at least 50,000. In addition to the county or counties containing such a city or cities, contiguous counties are included in a metropolitan area if, according to certain criteria, they are essentially metropolitan and are socially and economically integrated with the central city. U.S. Bureau of the Census: U.S. Census of the Population; 1960, vol. II, *Characteristics of the Population,* part 37, Ohio, (Washington, D.C.: U.S. Government Printing Office, 1962).

Because these studies were concerned with Ohio only, certain counties in the SMSA's which crossed state lines were classified as nonmetropolitan if the Ohio portion did not contain the central city of 50,000 or more inhabitants.

of the patients within each such diagnostic group who used the specific types of psychiatric services in Ohio in each time period, and what are the differences in patterns between time periods? Time period comparisons are limited to state mental hospitals, since, in 1950, data were available only for these hospitals.

OVERALL FINDINGS

In both time periods under review, the majority of facilities were located in the metropolitan counties (Table 5.1). During the decade the nonmetropolitan counties increased their psychiatric services through the provision of outpatient clinic services, whereas the metropolitan counties had increases in both inpatient and outpatient psychiatric facilities. Table 5.2 summarizes the 1950 and 1960 data by type of facility, residence, and diagnosis. The impact on admissions to the state mental hospitals from metropolitan and nonmetropolitan counties due to the increase in other psychiatric facilities can be noted. For example, on the basis of admission data to state mental hospitals alone, it would seem that between 1950 and

Table 5.1 Number of psychiatric facilities available, by type and geographic location: Ohio, 1950 and 1960[a]

Type of facilities	State total		Geographic location			
			Metrop. counties		Nonmetrop. counties	
	1950	1960	1950	1960	1950	1960
Total facilities	62	104	54	85	8	19
Inpatient facilities						
Total	38	52	31	45	7	7
State mental hosp.	16	20	11	14	5	6
General with psychiatric	11	21	10	21	1	0
Private and V.A.	11	11	10	10	1	1
Outpatient clinics	24	52	23	41	1	11

[a] Data are derived from such sources as Veteran's Administration Statistical Summaries, Hospitals Guide Issues, Report Schedules sent to Biometrics Branch, NIMH, and Directories of Outpatient Psychiatric Clinics compiled by the National Association for Mental Health and the National Institute of Mental Health for appropriate study years.

Table 5.2 Average annual first admission rates per 100,000 population by residence, diagnosis, and specified psychiatric facilities during two study periods: Ohio, January 1, 1948, through June 30, 1952 (1950) and July 1, 1958, through December 31, 1961 (1960)

Residence and diagnosis	Relevant age group	1950 State mental hospitals average annual first admissions		1960 State mental hospitals average annual first admissions		1960 All reporting psychiatric facilities[a] average annual first admissions		Ratio of 1960 rates to 1950 rates - State mental hospitals
		Number	Rate	Number	Rate	Number	Rate	
All counties[b]								
Schizophrenic reaction	15-64	1308	25.2	1942	33.8	3278	57.2	1.34
Mental diseases of the Senium	45+	1260	52.3	1303	46.7	1611	57.6	.89
Alcoholism	25-64	388	9.5	879	19.6	1270	28.3	2.06
Psychoneurosis	10+	-	-	865	11.4	5477	72.6	-
Metropolitan counties								
Schizophrenic reaction	15-64	979	27.3	1453	37.3	2501	64.2	1.37
Mental diseases of the Senium	45+	913	57.7 (64.1)[c]	789	40.3 (43.1)[c]	1021	55.0 (58.0)[c]	.70
Alcoholism	25-64	285	9.9	538	17.5	873	28.3	1.77
Psychoneurosis	10+	-	-	567	11.2	3989	79.0	-
Nonmetropolitan counties								
Schizophrenic reaction	15-64	329	20.5	489	26.7	777	42.4	1.30
Mental diseases of the Senium	45+	347	43.2 (37.3)[c]	514	55.0 (49.1)[c]	590	62.9 (56.4)[c]	1.27
Alcoholism	25-64	103	8.4	341	24.4	397	28.3	2.90
Psychoneurosis	10+	-	-	297	11.9	1488	60.1	-

[a] All reporting psychiatric facilities includes 1960 first admissions to State mental hospitals.

[b] Some counties shifted metropolitan or nonmetropolitan status between the 1950 and 1960 censuses.

[c] Figure in parenthesis represents age-adjusted rates based on Ohio population 45 years of age and older in 1950 or 1960 U.S. Census.

1960 some shift had occurred in admission rates from metropolitan and nonmetropolitan counties. In 1950, admission rates from the metropolitan counties were higher than those for nonmetropolitan counties, whereas in 1960 this was true only for schizophrenia. The 1960 data for all psychiatric facilities, however, showed similar rates of admission for alcoholism and mental diseases of the senium, for both areas of residence, but for schizophrenia and psychoneurosis, rates of admission were higher for the metropolitan counties. The following tabulation illustrates these findings by presenting the ratio of metropolitan to nonmetropolitan rates for specified diagnoses, time periods, and facilities.

Diagnosis	*State mental hospitals*		*All psychiatric facilities*
	1950	*1960*	*1960*
Schizophrenia	1.33	1.40	1.51
Mental diseases of the senium	1.34(1.72)	0.73(.88)	0.87(1.03)
Alcoholism	1.18	0.72	1.00

( ) Ajusted rates based on Ohio population aged 45 years or older.

It has been hypothesized that the increased availability of psychiatric facilities other than the state mental hospitals would result in an alteration of diagnostic profiles between the two study periods. This did not occur, and the reason can be readily seen from data presented in Table 5.3. Except for psychoneurosis, the state mental hospitals, even in 1960, cared for the largest proportions of patients admitted in the study categories. Thus, it was not surprising that the diagnostic profiles found in the 1950 study of first admissions to the state mental hospitals were, in general, supported by the 1960 study of first admissions to all psychiatric facilities. Distinctive characteristics of these patient profiles will be discussed later.

Although they are not the main focus of this chapter, the data presented in Table 5.3 can be viewed from another perspective, which shows that of the nearly 70,000 total first admissions in 1960, schizophrenia represented 16.3 percent, mental diseases of the senium, 8.0 percent; alcoholism, 7.1 percent; and psychoneurosis, 23.4 percent.

Table 5.3 First admissions to psychiatric facilities by type of facility and diagnosis: Ohio, July 1, 1958 - December 31, 1961[a]

Type of facilities	Diagnoses				
	All diagnoses[b]	Schizophrenia	Mental disorders, senium	Alcoholism	Psychoneuroses
	Numbers				
All facilities	69,990	11,425	5,634	4,939	16,361
State mental	29,905	6,998	4,443	3,339	3,042
Gen'l hospitals with psychiatric facilities	12,366	1,579	570	703	6,629
Private and V.A.	4,868	796	411	304	1,993
Outpatient clinics	22,851	2,052	210	588	4,697
	Percent distribution				
All facilities	100.0	100.0	100.0	100.0	100.0
State mental	42.7	61.2	78.9	67.6	18.6
Gen'l hospitals with psychiatric facilities	17.7	13.8	10.1	14.3	40.5
Private and V.A.	7.0	7.0	7.3	6.2	12.2
Outpatient clinics	32.6	18.0	3.7	11.9	28.7

[a] Among all first admissions during this 3 1/2 year data collection period, only 376 or 0.5% first admissions were to VA neuropsychiatric facilities. In this and all tables that follow VA data will be combined with private mental hospital data.

[b] Data for this category includes first admissions with diagnoses not shown in this table.

As a final part of the overview, prior to considering the diagnostic groups separately, it should be noted that certain population groups experienced a greater risk of first admission to mental hospitals in both 1950 and 1960. When marital status was considered, the divorced and separated exhibited the highest rates; when occupation was analyzed, laborers had excessive rates. By race, nonwhites* had

*In Ohio the overwhelming majority of nonwhites are Negroes. Census underenumeration of the nonwhite (and of persons living alone) may contribute to some extent here. An estimate of this is to be found in the results of the studies evaluating the 1960 census (Taeuber and Hansen, 1963).

higher rates than whites in all diagnostic categories except for psychoneurosis; by sex, women had higher admission rates than men for schizophrenia and psychoneurosis, and men the highest rates for alcoholism and mental diseases of the senium. On the basis of state mental hospital data, it seems that U.S.-born migrants to Ohio incur higher rates of illness than Ohio-born persons, except in the case of psychoneurosis for nonwhites (both sexes) and alcoholism for nonwhite females.

SCHIZOPHRENIA

Residence, Facility, Sex, Color, and Age

Table 5.2 shows that there has been a substantial increase in the first admission rates for schizophrenia in Ohio between 1950 and 1960 and that this increase is somewhat more pronounced in the metropolitan area. The 1960 study based on data from all psychiatric facilities reinforces the findings of both the 1950 and the 1960 studies confined only to admission data from state mental hospitals, namely, that proportionately more first admissions for schizophrenic reactions* come from metropolitan areas. This is consistent with findings in other studies of admissions to mental hospitals (Malzberg 1940, Dunham 1964).

Table 5.3 indicates that state mental hospitals were the primary resource for treating schizophrenics. Of all reported first admissions for schizophrenia, 61 percent were to the state hospitals, 14 percent to the general hospitals with psychiatric facilities, 7 percent to the private and Veterans Administration neuropsychiatric hospitals, and 18 percent were seen in the outpatient psychiatric clinics. Within each facility, first admissions for schizophrenia comprised 23 percent of all first admissions to the state mental hospitals, 13 percent of all general hospital psychiatric admissions, 16 percent of all admissions to private mental hospitals and VA neuropsychiatric hospitals, and 9 percent of all clinic admissions. The total rate for females was higher than that for males in both study periods. In 1960 the rate for women (66.6) exceeded that for men (50.3) by one-third (Table

*Throughout this monograph "first admission" and "first admitted" for schizophrenia or any other diagnosis indicates the first admission to any psychiatric facility, not just the first admission for that diagnosis.

5.4). Exceptions are found in higher rates among single men and men 15-24, to be discussed below. The first admission rates by sex, color, residence, and type of facility presented in Table 5.4 indicate that female schizophrenics had higher first admission rates to each of the various types of facilities shown. When examined by color, first admission rates for schizophrenia among nonwhites to Ohio state hospitals were about three times the rates for whites. This disparity was reduced slightly when data from other psychiatric facilities were studied. The rate for nonwhites to all facilities then exceeded the whites by two and one-half times.

Table 5.4 Average annual first admission rates per 100,000 population aged 15-64 years to psychiatric facilities for schizophrenia, by sex, color, residence, and type of facility: Ohio, 1958-61

Sex, color, & residence	Total	State mental hospitals	General with psychiatric facilities	Private and V.A. hospitals	Outpatient clinics
Males	50.3	31.3	7.5	2.7	8.8
White					
Metrop.	45.7	28.2	6.4	3.5	7.7
Nonmetrop.	38.2	25.6	2.0	1.5	9.0
Nonwhite					
Metrop.	109.2	80.9	10.5	(1.4)	16.4
Females	66.6	36.4	13.6	5.0	11.6
White					
Metrop.	62.4	33.7	11.2	7.1	10.4
Nonmetrop.	43.2	26.9	4.0	2.2	10.1
Nonwhite					
Metrop.	141.2	94.3	19.5	(.1)	27.3
Ratio: M/F					
White					
Metrop.	.7	.8	.6	.5	.7
Nonmetrop.	.9	1.0	.5	.7	.9
Nonwhite					
Metrop.	.8	.9	.5	(N.A.)	.6

( ) Indicates less than 10 admissions a year; for this reason the nonwhite male to female ratio for admissions to private and V.A. hospitals was omitted as not appropriate.

The 1950 data for state mental hospitals and the 1960 data for all psychiatric facilities emphasize that the highest first admission rates for schizophrenia were concentrated in the 20-44 age group and that the rates peak higher at an earlier age among men than among women. This is shown in Table 5.5, which indicates that in 1960 the highest first admission rates for males in metropolitan areas, regardless of color, occurred in the 20-24 year age group, and for males in nonmetropolitan areas in the 25-29 year group. For women, regardless of residence and color, the highest rates prevailed between 25 and 34 years of age. It is only for the youngest age groups 15-19 and 20-24 that male rates exceeded or approximated female rates.

Table 5.5 Average annual first admission rates per 100,000 population to psychiatric facilities for schizophrenia, by age, sex, color, and residence: Ohio, 1958-61

Sex, color, & residence	Total	Adj.[a]	15-19	20-24	25-29	30-34	35-44	45-54	55-64
Males									
White									
Metrop.	45.7	46.1	50.6	77.0	67.1	66.9	47.4	27.2	11.2
Nonmetrop.	38.2	38.5	38.2	53.2	62.2	58.6	38.3	25.1	12.6
Nonwhite									
Metrop.	109.2	106.5	93.3	234.7	183.0	138.7	98.5	54.9	(27.0)
Females									
White									
Metrop.	62.4	62.4	36.3	79.0	99.8	100.8	75.7	42.6	18.2
Nonmetrop.	43.2	43.7	25.0	53.1	63.3	72.0	54.7	29.2	16.3
Nonwhite									
Metrop.	141.2	133.0	93.3	158.7	226.1	227.7	146.0	83.5	46.9
Ratio:M/F									
White									
Metrop.	.7	.7	1.4	1.0	.7	.7	.6	.6	.6
Nonmetrop.	.9	.9	1.5	1.0	1.0	.8	.7	.9	.8
Nonwhite									
Metrop.	.8	.8	1.0	1.5	.8	.6	.7	.7	.6

a Adjusted rate on total Ohio population 15-64 years of age.
( ) Indicates less than 10 admissions per year.

Marital Status

In 1950 and 1960 the highest admission rates for schizophrenia occurred among the divorced and separated, irrespective of residence or sex. The lowest rates were among the married, as indicated in Table 5.6 for 1960. It can be noted that among women, the differential between the admission rates of single and married is not so marked as among men – perhaps due to the earlier age at which women marry. Sixty percent of the females admitted were married, compared to 42 percent of the males, and their corresponding rates of admission were almost 50 percent higher than those for married men. This was the greatest disparity between the sexes by marital status. Table 5.7 illustrates the distribution of admissions by sex and marital status to the various psychiatric facilities in Ohio in 1960. These data reemphasize the greater use of facilities other than state mental hospitals by women and the high admission rates to the state mental hospitals of divorced and separated persons.

Occupation and Employment

Excessively high rates of admission to Ohio psychiatric facilities were found among unskilled workers – laborers and domestics among women, and laborers, farmers, and service workers among men (Table 5.8). Admission rates for women classed as laborers were 60 percent higher than for male laborers. The rates for women were much higher than for men in 1950 in all occupational categories for which comparisons were made, whereas the 1960 data showed a number of exceptions. Over one-fourth of the females first admitted for schizophrenia were employed. Among these women, the major occupation was clerical work. However, the admission rates for these women were less than the overall female admission rate (66.6). Admission rates were consistently higher in the metropolitan area than in the nonmetropolitan area.

Table 5.9 depicts the distribution of male admissions from metropolitan areas by major occupation groups among the various types of facilities in Ohio in 1960. From data not tabulated here, it can be stated that by taking facilities other than the state mental hospitals into account, rates for professionals (including men and women in both types of residences areas) were double the rates obtained from state hospital data alone, and in metropolitan areas female clerical workers and male managers and proprietors also

Table 5.6 Average annual first admission rates per 100,000 population to psychiatric facilities for schizophrenia, by age, sex, marital status, and residence: Ohio, July 1, 1958 - December 31, 1961

Sex, residence, and age	Single	Married	Widowed	Divorced and separated
Males				
Metropolitan[a]				
Total[b]	104.1	31.5	(33.9)	168.1
Adjusted[b]	133.1	33.4	(79.2)	198.1
15-24	76.8	41.9	-	288.5
25-34	230.9	47.8	(277.4)	253.5
35-44	179.0	37.1	(44.6)	207.9
45-54	92.5	20.5	(43.8)	128.7
55-64	(56.9)	7.7	(11.4)	(34.8)
Nonmetropolitan[a]				
Total[b]	63.0	21.5	(44.0)	121.5
Adjusted[b]	98.1	21.7	(54.3)	123.4
15-24	44.5	22.3	-	(74.5)
25-34	173.9	32.7	(68.7)	253.5
35-44	131.5	24.7	(119.2)	138.1
45-54	80.7	15.2	(47.1)	(87.3)
55-64	(41.3)	7.6	(28.7	(29.7)
Females				
Metropolitan[a]				
Total[b]	82.4	60.9	49.5	199.8
Adjusted[b]	126.7	60.7	87.4	199.3
15-24	54.5	74.6	(46.9)	187.8
25-34	238.2	95.7	(186.8)	283.2
35-44	170.7	65.4	95.0	263.1
45-54	105.9	32.2	59.8	144.0
55-64	(33.7)	13.1	27.3	58.8
Nonmetropolitan[a]				
Total[b]	44.0	38.3	38.6	119.0
Adjusted[b]	88.0	37.1	75.1	118.1
15-24	28.9	37.8	(72.7)	94.6
25-34	149.1	61.2	(128.8)	161.2
35-44	141.9	44.3	82.7	152.9
45-54	(66.9)	20.0	46.9	94.2
55-64	(34.7)	9.7	20.9	(66.6)

[a] In order to use available Census data metropolitan counties Allen, Butler, Clark and Lorain were shifted to the metropolitan area. This was true for all subsequent tables showing a metropolitan -nonmetropolitan breakdown.

[b] Total and adjusted rates based on Ohio population 15-64 years old.

( ) Indicates less than 10 admissions per year.

Table 5.7 Average annual age-adjusted[a] first admission rates per 100,000 population aged 15-64 to psychiatric facilities for schizophrenia, by sex, residence, marital status, and type of facility: Ohio, 1958-61

Sex, residence, and marital status	Total	State mental hospitals	General with psychiatric facilities	Private and V.A. hospitals	Outpatient clinics
Males					
Metropolitan					
Single	133.1	87.5	15.3	10.2	20.1
Married	33.4	20.3	4.4	1.9	6.8
Divorced & separated	198.1	151.2	(15.2)	(5.8)	26.0
Nonmetropolitan					
Single	98.1	66.3	4.8	(6.2)	20.8
Married	21.7	14.3	(1.2)	(0.9)	5.3
Females					
Metropolitan					
Single	126.7	69.7	23.7	16.0	17.3
Married	60.7	32.6	11.3	5.6	11.3
Divorced & separated	199.3	129.6	19.2	(5.3)	45.2
Nonmetropolitan					
Single	88.0	54.8	10.3	(3.5)	19.5
Married	37.1	23.5	3.6	2.1	7.9

[a] Age adjusted rates based on total Ohio population 15-64 years of age.

( ) Indicates less than 10 admissions per year.

showed a tendency to use other facilities. Although the data showed the state mental hospitals were not the only psychiatric resource for the unskilled worker and laborer, this resource was used more by these groups than by the other occupational groups. Nevertheless, the more complete facility reporting for 1960 did not invalidate the 1950 findings derived from state mental hospital information as to relative size of admission rates by occupation.

Table 5.8 Average annual first admission rates per 100,000 population aged 15-64 years to psychiatric facilities for schizophrenia, by sex, residence, and occupation of employed patients: Ohio, 1958-61

Occupation	Males		Females	
	Metrop.	Nonmetrop.	Metrop.	Nonmetrop.
Professional, technical, and kindred workers	41.1	26.9	51.9	26.1
Managers, officials, and proprietors except farm	30.8	13.6	--	--
Clerical and kindred workers	43.3	26.7	46.4	24.9
Sales workers	36.0	22.2	--	--
Service workers except domestics	73.4	45.7	68.2	40.3
Domestics (private household workers)	--	--	117.4	75.0
Farmers and farm laborers	97.8	41.8	--	--
Craftsmen, foremen, and kindred workers	32.9	20.7	--	--
Operatives and kindred workers	27.5	19.7	19.9	6.3
Laborers	147.8	128.8	382.0	335.6

Education

Data on years of school completed were available only for admissions to the state mental hospitals. The median number of school years completed by the general population of Ohio (10.9 years) was about the same as that for persons admitted to the state mental hospitals for schizophrenia (11.1 years). A detailed analysis by residence (of the 1950 and 1960 data) showed no consistent pattern for different educational levels. However, when counties were consolidated to use available census data by age, an inverse relationship emerged between educational level and first admission rates. Table 5.10 indicates that males in metropolitan areas with at least 8 years of school had admission rates one and one-half times in excess of those with some high school and twice that for those with some college. Among women and nonmetropolitan men the differences were not as striking. Since educational level is so highly correlated with occupation, data in Tables 5.3 and 5.9 would seem to indicate that the inverse correlation might be strengthened had information been available for admissions to all facilities in the 1960 study.

Table 5.9 Average annual first admission rates per 100,000 population aged 15-64 years to psychiatric facilities for schizophrenia, by type of facility and major occupational group of employed metropolitan male residents: Ohio, 1958-61

Occupation	State mental hospitals	General with psychiatric facilities	Private and V.A. mental hospitals	Outpatient clinics
Professional, technical, and kindred	20.1	6.4	(5.0)	9.5
Other white collar [a]	22.2	5.0	2.9	6.1
Service and operatives	25.8	3.0	(1.8)	5.0
Craftsmen, foremen, and kindred	22.0	3.5	3.5	3.9
Laborers	113.1	14.1	(6.3)	14.4

[a] Managers, officials, proprietors, clerical, and sales.

( ) Indicates less than 10 admissions per year.

Table 5.10 Average annual age-adjusted[a] first admission rates per 100,000 population to state mental hospitals for shizophrenia, by years of school completed, residence, and sex: Ohio, 1958-61

Years of school completed	Metropolitan		Nonmetropolitan	
	Male	Female	Male	Female
Elementary	48.0	52.8	29.9	32.2
0-4 years	66.2	55.6	28.7	29.9
5-7 years	44.2	50.7	26.7	27.4
8 years	46.6	53.6	32.3	35.1
High school	32.3	38.5	21.2	25.4
1-3 years	34.9	40.6	22.3	27.4
4 years	30.7	37.9	21.0	24.9
College (1 or more years)	23.3	28.5	19.4	19.3

[a] Age-adjusted rates based on total Ohio population 15-64 years of age.

Migration

Data on migration were available only for admissions to state mental hospitals. Table 5.3 indicates the degree to which the data may apply to all schizophrenia admissions. Among the foreign-born whites, only 14 percent of the first admissions were for schizophrenia, compared to the 23 percent of all first admissions to the state mental hospitals among native-born whites. Table 5.11 indicates that admission rates, when adjusted for age, were slightly higher among the immigrants. This finding is in agreement with that reported in other studies of schizophrenia among the foreign born and suggests that the extremely high rates found in past studies are a decreasing area of concern (Locke, Kramer, and Pasamanick 1960; Lazarus, Locke, and Thomas 1963; Locke and Duvall 1964).

When U.S.-born patients are examined by state of birth, migrants to Ohio showed higher rates of first admissions than did native Ohioans (Table 5.12). Among women, the native-born migrant to Ohio had higher rates than the foreign-born immigrant, whereas the reverse was true for the men. Higher rates among the migrants were consistent with the 1950 findings. As a further check, metropolitan and nonmetropolitan counties were subdivided by migration rates and compared. Among the nonmetropolitan counties the areas with the highest migration rates had the lowest admission rates for schizophrenia; higher admission rates among the highest migration rate metropolitan counties were barely discernible. It would appear that areas characterized by high migration (as an index of extreme population mobility) are not necessarily high risk areas for schizophrenia.

Discussion

A descriptive study of schizophrenia as reflected in the Ohio data raises more questions than it answers and suggests areas where other epidemiological tools and techniques must be created and used in investigating schizophrenia with the objective of public health intervention. It is clear that first admissions rates for schizophrenia in Ohio increased. To what extent this was due to an increased ability to make differential diagnoses and a willingness to classify patients as schizophrenics, to an increase in the number of facilities to treat mental illness, or to an increase in the true incidence of this disease is not known. These are important questions to be answered in

Table 5.11 Average annual first admission rates per 100,000 to state mental hospitals for schizophrenia, by sex, age, residence, and nativity of white persons: Ohio, 1958-61

Sex and age	Metropolitan		Nonmetropolitan	
	Native-born	Foreign-born	Native-born	Foreign-born
Males (15-64)	28.1	21.8	25.0	22.7
Adjusted total[a]	27.7	34.8	25.1	30.9
15-24	35.5	58.6	28.7	50.7
25-34	38.9	47.5	39.6	45.1
35-44	30.1	29.8	24.6	14.4
45-54	18.8	19.8	16.2	23.9
55-64	6.5	6.7	9.5	14.5
Females (15-64)	33.4	26.8	26.4	29.2
Adjusted total[a]	33.1	35.4	26.6	35.1
15-24	27.8	29.5	22.1	55.5
25-34	50.1	61.1	40.6	11.3
35-44	42.0	42.6	34.7	47.0
45-54	25.2	22.9	17.9	42.8
55-64	10.9	9.6	10.4	10.9

[a] Adjusted rate based on total Ohio population 15-64 years of age.

Table 5.12 Average annual age-adjusted[a] first admission rates per 100,000 population to state mental hospitals for schizophrenia, by sex, color, and state of birth for native-born patients 15-64 years of age: Ohio, 1958-61

Color and place of birth	Male	Female
White		
Born in Ohio	26.0	29.4
Born in other States	29.9	36.5
Nonwhite		
Born in Ohio	72.8	80.2
Born in other States	81.9	93.0

[a] Age adjusted rates based on total Ohio population 15-64 years of age.

planning for preventive actions or the provision of psychiatric services. In addition to conducting community surveys and utilizing psychiatric registers to develop the data to answer these questions, the findings with regard to those groups most consistently vulnerable to admission merits investigation.

It has been shown that rates of admission were higher for persons living in metropolitan area counties, higher for persons aged 20 to 44, generally higher for females than for males, and excessively higher for nonwhites. These are the groups which have been shown to be most vulnerable to admission to state mental hospitals. It appears that when the spectrum of services is broadened, these groups are still judged to be most in need of care. Higher rates of schizophrenia continue to be found among those groups considered to have higher proportions of individuals in the lower social and economic strata of society – the unskilled workers and laborers, as well as in those groups considered highly mobile – those who change their residence and those who because of an absence of marital ties (the separated, divorced, and single) can be considered on the move. However, the positive association of poverty and family stress with a chronic disorder like schizophrenia, which has a prolonged onset, may relate to a biological, genetic, or physiological predisposition with a socioeconomic effect rather than to a socioeconomic, or (even) cultural cause. For example, Warren Dunham's hypothesis of the effect of the disease process on occupational achievement was suggested by his study of social class of schizophrenics controlled by their father's social class, which showed that the social class of the fathers of this patient group was more evenly distributed than was that of the patients (Dunham 1964).

More detailed comparisons of population groups with high admission rates versus those with low admission rates may provide other clues to etiology in addition to the measurable demographic and socioeconomic variables, as, for example, the kinds of marital discord that might result in divorce among some population groups but not among others. Studies are needed with regard to pathways of admission to the various psychiatric facilities and also on the extent to which the availability of a custodial relative may be a determinant of hospital admission (whether short or long term) or outpatient treatment. Information on whether admission to a facility (particularly the outpatient clinics) results in diagnostic evaluation or treatment is necessary in planning community services. For example, as more and more community mental health centers come into existence, evaluation is needed as to which groups consistently are evaluated and referred elsewhere and which receive outpatient treatment.

MENTAL DISEASES OF THE SENIUM

Residence, Facility, Sex, Color, and Age

The first admission rates to state mental hospitals for mental diseases of the senium showed a decrease between 1950 and 1960 from 52.3 to 46.7 per 100,000 population (Table 5.2). This decrease was accounted for essentially by the decrease in rates for metropolitan counties (from 64.1 to 43.1), since the rate for the nonmetropolitan counties had increased between 1950 and 1960 (from 37.3 to 49.1). These changes in rates also resulted in changes in the relative level of rates for the metropolitan and nonmetropolitan counties. In 1950 the metropolitan rate was 1.7 times higher than the nonmetropolitan, whereas in 1960 the corresponding ratio was 0.9. Data for all facilities in 1960 indicated little overall difference in admission rates for diseases of senium between the two residential areas, suggesting that higher rates of use of facilities other than the state mental hospitals by residents of metropolitan areas tend to equalize the rates (Table 5.13).

Over 96 percent of the 5,634 Ohio patients first admitted for diseases of the senium were hospitalized during the 1960 study period, and 82 percent of these, or 4,443 patients, were admitted to the state mental hospitals. Only 210 individuals were seen at psychiatric outpatient clinics (Table 5.3). For state mental hospitals, patients with mental diseases of the senium constituted 15 percent of the total first admissions, as opposed to outpatient care, where these patients made up less than 1 percent of all new admissions: In 1950, mental diseases of the senium comprised 21 percent of all first admissions to state mental hospitals.

In contrast to the changes in admissions by geographic area and by facility during the two study periods, data on admissions by sex and race remained relatively unchanged between 1950 and 1960. The 1960 rates for men were seen to have been consistently higher than for women, whether observed by residence or by color for most age groups (Table 5.14). This was also true in 1950. These higher rates

Table 5.13 Average annual age adjusted[a] first admission rates per 100,000 population aged 45 and over to specified psychiatric facilities for mental diseases of the senium, by residence: Ohio, 1958-61

Type of facilities	Geographic location	
	Metrop. counties	Nonmetrop. counties
Total facilities	58.0	56.4
Inpatient facilities		
State	43.1	49.1
General with psychiatric	7.6	2.4
Private and V.A.	5.8	1.7
Outpatient clinics	1.6	3.2

[a] Age adjusted rates based on total Ohio population 45 years of age and over.

Table 5.14 Average annual age-adjusted[a] first admission rates per 100,000 population aged 45 and over to psychiatric facilities for mental diseases of the senium, by sex, color, residence, and type of facility: Ohio, 1958-61

Sex, color, residence	Total	Adj.	45-54	55-59	60-64	65-69	70-74	75-79	80-84	85 & over
Males										
White										
Metrop.	51.9	60.0	3.1	(7.0)	34.0	71.2	133.6	244.1	290.1	447.8
Nonmetrop.	74.9	70.1	(2.9)	(12.2)	51.6	94.0	175.1	233.7	349.8	402.4
Nonwhite										
Metrop.	93.0	126.6	(7.8)	(32.0)	103.6	173.7	279.8	477.6	(598.1)	(545.1)
Females										
White										
Metrop.	50.3	49.1	1.8	8.9	29.7	73.5	123.3	172.7	244.8	250.7
Nonmetrop.	50.7	43.8	(1.9)	(11.2)	38.4	77.3	100.6	136.3	186.1	186.3
Nonwhite										
Metrop.	83.4	104.7	(5.4)	(49.3)	(72.3)	166.9	264.2	376.5	(348.7)	(386.1)
Ratio: M/F										
White										
Metrop.	1.0	1.2	1.7	0.8	1.1	1.0	1.1	1.4	1.2	1.8
Nonmetrop.	1.5	1.6	1.5	1.1	1.3	1.2	1.7	1.7	1.9	2.2
Nonwhite										
Metrop.	1.1	1.2	1.4	0.6	1.4	1.0	1.1	1.3	1.7	1.4

[a] Age adjustment based on Ohio population 45 years of age and older.

( ) Rates based on less than 10 admissions per year.

are in keeping with the generally higher male morbidity and mortality rates at advanced ages. The overall age-adjusted 1960 admission rate for men in Ohio, 68.7, was 30 percent higher than the female rate, 53.0 (Table 5.15). However, admission rates to psychiatric facilities other than the state mental hospitals were of almost equal magnitude for the two sexes. The data at both time periods indicate that the nonwhite first admission rates were more than double the rates for whites. This is evident in Tables 5.14 and 5.15, which are based on the 1960 data. Admission rates for white males and females appear to differ by residence: for white males, the rate was higher in the nonmetropolitan counties, while the reverse was true for white females (Table 5.15).

Table 5.15 depicts the differential use of the various psychiatric facilities available in 1960 by sex, race, and residence. Admissions to general hospitals and outpatient clinics were few, especially for nonwhites, for whom admissions numbered less than 10 per study year in 1960 (Table 5.3). No nonwhite admissions were noted to the

Table 5.15 Average annual age-adjusted[a] first admission rates per 100,000 population aged 45 and over to psychiatric facilities for mental diseases of the senium, by sex, color, residence, and type of facility: Ohio, 1958-61

Sex, color, & residence	Total	State mental hospitals	General with psychiatric facilities	Private and V.A. hospitals	Outpatient clinics
Males	68.7	54.1	8.7	3.8	2.0
White					
Metrop.	60.0	45.6	7.2	5.9	(1.2)
Nonmetrop.	70.1	63.0	2.3	(1.8)	3.0
Nonwhite					
Metrop.	126.6	110.3	(12.8)	-	(3.1)
Females	53.0	37.8	8.3	4.5	2.3
White					
Metrop.	49.1	34.3	7.1	6.4	1.2
Nonmetrop.	43.8	36.2	2.6	(1.6)	3.4
Nonwhite					
Metrop.	104.7	82.5	(13.9)	-	(8.4)

[a] Age adjustment based on Ohio population 45 years of age and older.

( ) Rates based on less than 10 admissions per years.

private and VA neuropsychiatric hospitals. It is known that other facilities, such as proprietary homes for the aged, admitted few Negroes, e.g., in 1958 only 4 of some 600 such homes licensed by the states accepted Negroes. To what extent excess rates of first admissions to state mental hospitals among nonwhites can be attributed to inability (due to financial or discriminatory causes) to use other treatment facilities in the community remains a question which cannot be answered with the data at hand.

Marital Status

For the divorced and separated, both men and women experienced the highest rates of admission (Table 5.16). Among admissions to outpatient psychiatric clinics and state mental hospitals the percentage of divorced or separated was especially high (9.5 and 8.0 percent), respectively, whereas, in the general Ohio population 45 years and older, only 5.0 percent are divorced and or separated. The corresponding percentages for general hospitals and private hospitals were 5.4 percent and 2.7 percent respectively. Admission rates for the widowed and the single were next highest and were of about equal magnitude, and rates for married were lowest. This was true for both males and females. Admission rates in each marital status category for women were consistently lower in the nonmetropolitan areas, whereas for men the admission rates for the single and the divorced and separated were higher in the nonmetropolitan areas.

Occupation

Over 41 percent of the employed men admitted to psychiatric facilities were farmers and laborers, yet these two occupational groups comprise only 14 percent of employed male labor force aged 55 years and over. Laborers had the highest admission rates and farmers the next highest, as seen in Table 5.17. Men with white collar occupations had the lowest rates of admission, although operatives had a lower rate than two of the three major white collar occupational categories in the metropolitan area. These findings cannot be interpreted conclusively, since the rates are not adjusted for age other than by the gross grouping of the age groups 55 years and older. The relative position of the rates by occupational grouping were about the same at both time periods, 1950 and 1960.

Table 5.16 Average annual first admission rates per 100,000 population to psychiatric facilities for mental diseases of the senium, by age, sex, marital status, and residence: Ohio, 1958-61

Sex, residence and age	Single	Married	Widowed	Divorced and separated
Males				
Metropolitan				
Total[a]	95.0	54.5	94.5	143.1
45-54	1.3	3.3	19.5	6.5
55-64	61.9	17.6	38.7	69.6
65-74	184.8	82.4	173.3	230.5
75 & over	337.2	276.6	352.8	644.8
Nonmetropolitan				
Total[a]	102.9	53.3	88.3	180.8
45-54	10.9	1.9	-	6.7
55-64	62.0	20.0	49.2	76.3
65-74	215.7	95.3	180.7	335.5
75 & over	316.3	239.5	322.9	766.9
Females				
Metropolitan				
Total[a]	60.6	43.6	65.3	108.2
45-54	5.7	1.3	7.6	1.1
55-64	21.1	17.0	34.6	42.5
65-74	106.9	79.7	128.9	171.8
75 & over	267.1	192.1	226.0	532.2
Nonmetropolitan				
Total[a]	47.4	39.4	47.3	51.0
45-54	2.4	1.5	3.7	2.7
55-64	21.4	19.9	30.8	35.3
65-74	101.3	74.8	91.3	109.5
75 & over	170.4	155.7	158.5	149.7

[a] Age adjusted rates based on 1960 Ohio population 45 years of age and over.

Table 5.17 Average annual first admission rates per 100,000 male population aged 55 and over to psychiatric facilities for mental diseases of the senium, by residence and occupation: Ohio, 1958-61

Occupation	Metropolitan	Nonmetropolitan
Professional, technical, and kindred workers	44.5	40.7
Farmers, farm managers, and farm workers	187.4	129.7
Managers, officials, and proprietors	19.4	46.2
Clerical, sales, and kindred workers	39.4	49.7
Craftsmen and kindred workers	61.9	92.7
Operatives and kindred workers	31.5	73.0
Service workers except private household	99.2	72.6
Laborers except farm and mine	245.1	272.5

Education

Data on years of school completed were obtained only from state mental hospital records and are presented in Tables 5.18 and 5.19 for 1960. Age adjustment indicated that highest rates of admission to the state mental hospitals occurred for those with elementary education and generally declined as educational level increased. As in the 1950 study, higher rates for men and for nonwhites were found at every educational level.

Migration

Data on migration are available only for admissions to the state mental hospitals. Inasmuch as these admissions represent 79 percent of all admissions to psychiatric facilities in 1960 it is unlikely that the findings would be greatly altered were data on admissions to other psychiatric facilities available (Table 5.3). In the 1960 study, among the foreign-born patients first admitted, 43 percent had

Table 5.18 Average annual age-adjusted[a] first admission rates per 100,000 population 45 years and over to state mental hospitals for mental diseases of the senium, by years of school completed, residence, and sex: Ohio, 1958-61

Years of school completed	Metropolitan		Nonmetropolitan	
	Male	Female	Male	Female
Elementary	51.8	39.4	60.6	36.6
0-4 years	45.4	35.9	60.3	38.9
5-7 years	41.1	29.4	34.2	21.9
8 years	68.5	49.2	80.2	44.4
High school	30.7	25.7	31.0	24.7
1-3 years	19.4	12.1	23.9	14.0
4 years	45.6	39.9	41.5	36.5
College (1 or more years)	25.6	14.1	32.4	20.2

[a] Age-adjusted rates based on total Ohio population 45 years of age and older.

Table 5.19 Average annual first admission rates per 100,000 population 45 years and over from 11 metropolitan counties[a] to state mental hospitals for mental diseases of the senium, by years of school completed, sex, and color: Ohio, 1958-61

Years of school completed	Male		Female	
	White	Nonwhite	White	Nonwhite
Elementary (0-8)	56.9	82.2	49.6	65.8
High school (9-12)	15.1	(26.9)	16.1	(24.4)
College (1 or more)	13.1	(20.8)	(8.0)	(32.1)

[a] Cuyahoga, Franklin, Greene, Hamilton, Lake, Lucas, Mahoning, Miami, Montgomery, Summit, and Trumbull.

( ) Indicates less than 10 admissions per year.

mental diseases of the senium, and this was the most prevalent diagnosis among this group. Although age adjustment for the most part reduces the differences noted in crude rates of admission between native and foreign born, a considerable differential remained among males in the nonmetropolitan area, with the foreign born showing an admission rate 50 percent higher than the native born (Table 5.20). When data on state mental hospital admissions were analyzed by state of birth in the United States, age-adjusted rates by sex and race were higher for those born in states other than Ohio (Table 5.21 and Figure 5.1). These findings are consistent with other analyses of admissions to state mental hospitals (Locke, Kramer, and Pasamanick 1960; Lazarus, Locke, and Thomas 1963; Locke and Duvall 1964). They also parallel findings reported in Chapter 7 in the section on mobility and suicide.

Table 5.20 Average annual first admission rates per 100,000 population to state mental hospitals for white persons for mental diseases of the senium, by age, residence, nativity, and sex: Ohio, 1958-61

Sex and age	Metropolitan		Nonmetropolitan	
	Native-born	Foreign-born	Native-born	Foreign-born
Males (45+)	33.2	64.7	62.6	145.0
Adjusted total [a]	43.8	48.5	62.1	95.3
45-54	(1.5)	(3.5)	(2.1)	(0)
55-64	14.9	(17.0)	21.8	(82.3)
65-74	69.1	72.1	115.9	144.1
75-84	204.3	189.2	252.2	346.9
85 and over	289.4	505.7	386.0	(469.9)
Females (45+)	30.2	53.3	40.9	(45.7)
Adjusted total [a]	32.1	37.6	36.8	28.0
45-54	(1.1)	(1.1)	(1.4)	(0)
55-64	12.3	(14.8)	18.9	(10.9)
65-74	59.5	65.2	65.9	(58.0)
75-84	133.8	153.2	145.5	(118.2)
85 and over	169.6	262.2	180.1	(89.0)

[a] Adjusted rate based on total Ohio population 45 years of age and and older.

( ) Indicates less than 10 admissions per year.

Table 5.21 Crude and age-adjusted[a] average annual first admission rates per 100,000 population 45 years of age and over to state mental hospitals for mental diseases of the senium, by age, color, and state of birth of native born: Ohio, 1958-61

Color and place of birth	Crude[a]		Adjusted[a]	
	Male	Female	Male	Female
White				
Born in Ohio	46.6	34.7	51.1	32.7
Born in other states	43.5	35.9	61.6	41.6
Nonwhite				
Born in Ohio	74.8	(34.2)	93.3	(37.0)
Born in other states	83.7	72.0	113.0	93.1

[a] Crude and age-adjusted rates based on total Ohio population 45 years of age and over.

( ) Indicates less than 10 admissions per years.

Discussion

Despite the substantial increase of psychiatric facilities other than state mental hospitals during the decade under review, almost 80 percent of the first admissions for mental diseases of the senium were to the state mental hospitals. Outpatient psychiatric clinics apparently are rarely used as a resource for the care of these mentally ill. It may be that the increase in first admission rates to the state mental hospitals between 1950 and 1960 for the nonmetropolitan areas resulted from the fact that few other facilities were available. In metropolitan areas, general hospitals with psychiatric facilities were increasingly available to partially reduce admissions to state mental hospitals. Although sufficient information was not available concerning the role of nursing homes and related facilities, such facilities are more likely to be found in metropolitan than in nonmetropolitan areas. Some studies of nursing home and chronic disease hospital populations have indicated a high proportion of mental confusion among their aged patients, but these studies did not focus specifically on types of care provided nor did they distinguish between patients diagnosed as having mental diseases of the senium and those classified as senile.

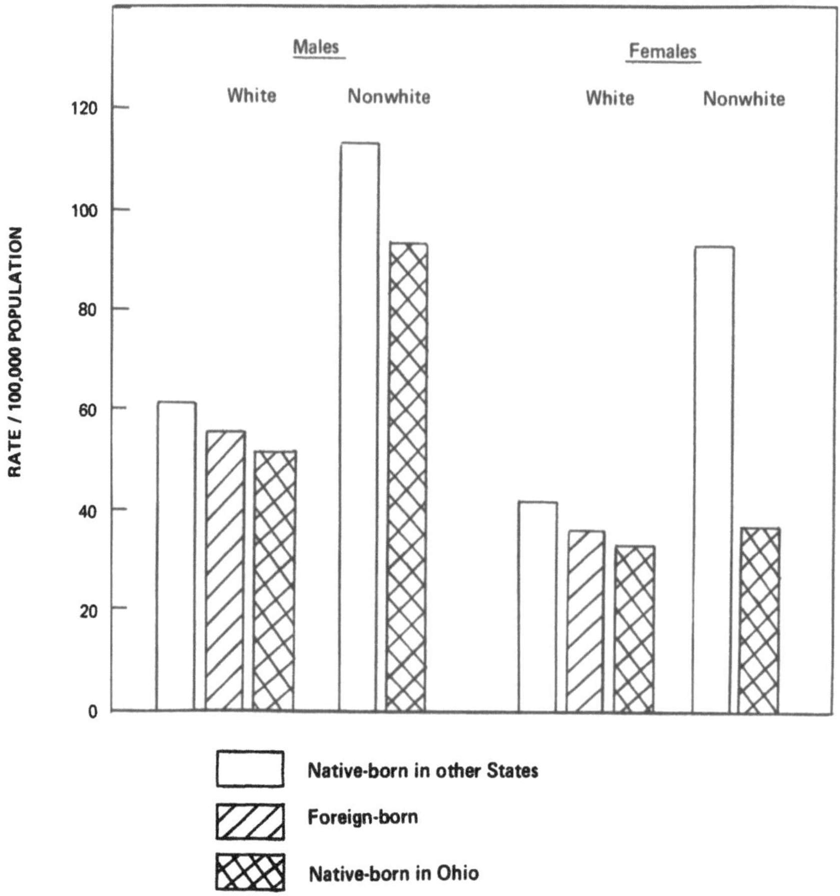

Fig. 5.1. Average annual age-adjusted first admissions per 100,000 population 45 years of age and older to state mental hospitals for diseases of the senium, by nativity, sex, and color: Ohio, July 1, 1958 - December 31, 1961.

During both study periods it was consistently found that admission rates for white and nonwhite males were higher than those for women throughout all categories studied, with greater relative differences in the nonmetropolitan area. This phenomenon of higher admission rates for men is in keeping with higher mortality rates from all causes for males. Retirement and lessening of activity may have a greater impact on men than on women, who are accustomed to being at home. Some evidence related to this was noted in the 1950 study, when women who were housewives were seen to have had substantially lower age-adjusted admission rates than employed women.

Nonwhite rates were excessively high in both study periods. It is known that few Negroes were admitted to nursing homes in the state, and the data showed little or no use of private facilities for inpatient care of this group. If studies were to demonstrate that nursing homes cared for large numbers of white patients whose behavior and diagnosis was equivalent to that of the first admissions to psychiatric facilities, one could conclude that the high rates noted in Ohio for nonwhites were due primarily to differential use of facilities rather than to greater susceptibility to these illnesses because of a variety of social, economic, and even nutritional reasons.

ALCOHOLISM

Residence, Facility, Sex, Color, Age

Even when based solely on state mental hospital data, the first admission rate for alcoholism doubled between 1950 and 1960. The increase of about 80 percent in the metropolitan area and nearly threefold in the nonmetropolitan was partially a reflection of the differences in availability of other psychiatric facilities in the two areas. Alcoholism admission data in 1960 for all psychiatric facilities show equal rates for the two areas (Table 5.2). Despite the increase in other psychiatric facilities 2 out of every 3 first admissions for alcoholism were to a state mental hospital (Table 5.3). The differences in alcoholism admission rates by facility, residence, race, and sex are shown in Table 5.22 and suggest, as do data from the other diagnostic groups studied, that the state mental hospitals are used more by nonmetropolitan white males and metropolitan nonwhites.

Table 5.22 Average annual first admission rates per 100,000 population aged 25-64 to psychiatric facilities for alcoholism, by sex, color, residence, and facility: Ohio, 1958-61

Sex, color, & residence	Total facilities	State mental hospitals	Private, general with psychiatric and V.A. hosps.	Outpatient clinics
Males				
White				
Metrop.	40.6	24.2	12.1	4.3
Nonmetrop.	49.7	43.2	3.1	3.4
Nonwhite				
Metrop.	82.9	61.6	12.3	9.0
Females				
White				
Metrop.	9.6	5.2	3.6	0.8
Nonmetrop.	6.6	5.1	(0.6)	(0.9)
Nonwhite				
Metrop.	34.5	23.0	7.4	(4.1)

( ) Indicates less than 10 admissions per year.

Table 5.23 presents the first admission rates of alcoholics to all psychiatric facilities by age, sex, color, and residence in 1960. These profiles differ little from the 1950 findings, even though there has been a substantial increase in psychiatric facilities and the admission rate to all such facilities in 1960 was three times the rate in 1950 (9.5 and 28.3 per 100,000 population aged 25-64, respectively). Overall, the data indicated that the male rates were uniformly and substantially greater than the female, that nonwhite rates for each sex greatly exceeded the corresponding white rates, and that nonwhite women in the metropolitan area had an overall rate of admission approaching that of white metropolitan men. In addition, it is clear that the peak ages of admission differ by race. Men comprised 81 percent of the 4,444 alcoholic admissions between the ages of 25 and 64 to all Ohio psychiatric facilities in 1960. The highest admission rates for alcoholism among nonwhites occurred at an earlier age than those for whites. This was particularly true for nonwhite women, who show very high rates between ages 25 and 39. Forty percent of the first admissions for nonwhite women were for patients under 30 years of age – more than double the corresponding percentage for white women. For nonwhite men, over 50 percent were admitted under 40 years of age as compared to 35 percent of white men.

Table 5.23 Average annual first admission rates per 100,000 population to psychiatric facilities for alcoholism, by age, sex, color, and residence: Ohio, 1958-61

Sex, color & residence	Total	Adj.[a]	25-29	30-34	35-39	40-44	45-49	50-54	55-59	60-64
Males										
White										
Metrop.	40.6	40.3	18.1	31.4	45.6	50.0	54.8	49.3	43.4	28.3
Nonmetrop.	49.7	49.4	21.0	32.5	49.5	65.5	77.6	58.7	58.7	31.3
Nonwhite										
Metrop.	82.9	81.9	78.7	94.9	90.0	103.8	88.1	78.6	(54.6)	(40.5)
Females										
White										
Metrop.	9.6	9.6	(4.8)	7.0	13.2	11.2	14.8	11.2	(6.4)	(6.1)
Nonmetrop.	6.6	6.6	(2.2)	(5.9)	(8.8)	11.6	(9.7)	(7.0)	(2.9)	(1.8)
Nonwhite										
Metrop.	34.5	33.0	44.1	40.3	41.0	(37.4)	(30.2)	(26.0)	(19.7)	(10.3)

[a] Adjusted rates based on total Ohio population 25-64 years of age.
( ) Indicates less than 10 admissions per year.

Marital Status

The highest rates of first admissions for alcoholism in Ohio occurred among the separated and divorced, who comprised more than one-fourth of the alcoholic admissions (Table 5.24). Particularly high rates for the divorced and separated occurred among men in the nonmetropolitan area. The widowed had higher rates than the single, and the lowest rates occurred among the married. These findings are from the 1960 study based on admissions to all psychiatric facilities and are similar to the findings of the 1950 study of admissions to the state mental hospitals.

Occupation and Education

Laborers, comprising 24 percent of the first admissions of employed male alcoholics, had the highest rates, and those in the professional occupations the lowest rates in both metropolitan and nonmetropolitan areas. The only information available on years of

Table 5.24 Average annual first admission rates per 100,000 population aged 25-64 to psychiatric facilities for alcoholism, by age, sex, marital status, and residence: Ohio, 1958-61

Sex, residence, and age	Single	Married	Widowed	Divorced and separated
Males				
Metropolitan				
Total	76.0	30.7	112.7	240.9
Adjusted[a]	81.7	30.6	113.6	239.6
25-34	57.3	22.2	(69.4)	203.2
35-44	84.3	37.9	(156.0)	297.6
45-54	101.8	37.8	(121.6)	270.3
55-64	88.6	27.8	102.6	161.0
Nonmetropolitan				
Total	74.8	29.9	125.5	331.8
Adjusted[a]	81.3	29.8	99.6	321.2
25-34	46.9	18.3	(-)	167.5
35-44	102.4	35.3	(71.5)	407.4
45-54	102.4	39.9	(111.4)	426.2
55-64	(72.3)	29.0	(82.0)	219.7
Females				
Metropolitan				
Total	14.2	8.5	22.2	53.8
Adjusted[a]	14.4	8.4	37.0	54.1
25-34	(17.5)	5.7	(53.4)	74.5
35-44	(18.1)	11.5	(22.8)	58.7
45-54	(17.1)	10.1	(29.4)	50.9
55-64	(-)	(4.8)	(12.7)	(19.6)
Nonmetropolitan				
Total	(7.2)	4.3	(13.7)	40.6
Adjusted[a]	7.8	4.2	14.4	41.6
25-34	(6.3)	(3.2)	(-)	(48.4)
35-44	(12.7)	6.5	(24.4)	(61.2)
45-54	(7.2)	4.8	(24.4)	(32.3)
55-64	(2.7)	(1.3)	(7.2)	(11.8)

[a] Adjusted rate based on total Ohio population 25-64 years of age.

( ) Indicates less than 10 admissions per year.

Table 5.25 Average annual first admission rates per 100,000 male population aged 25-64 to psychiatric facilities for alcoholism, by residence and occupation: Ohio, 1958-61

Occupation	Metropolitan	Nonmetropolitan
Professional, technical, and kindred workers	17.5	20.1
Farmers, farm managers, and farm laborers	25.8	34.3
Managers, officials, and proprietors	31.7	31.3
Clerical and sales workers	28.2	28.2
Skilled craftsmen and foremen	34.7	38.7
Operative and kindred workers	29.1	33.3
Service workers except private household	72.5	53.2
Laborers, except farm and mine	137.7	197.0

school completed is derived from first admission to state mental hospitals. Among these patients, there appeared to be an inverse relationship, particularly for whites and especially for the men, between the level of education and alcoholism. This finding is consistent with the 1950 data (Table 5.26 and 5.27). When color was controlled, however, nonwhite men with at least one year of high school had higher rates than those with an elementary school education or at least one year of college, and among nonwhite women there seemed to be no appreciable difference in rates relative to education. These findings are not in accord with the 1950 data, which showed greater similarity between white and nonwhite with regard to admission profiles by education. The median years of school completed among the alcoholics admitted (9.5 years) was less than that for the Ohio population in general (10.9 years). However, correlating the 88 counties of Ohio by the median years of school completed the alcoholic first admission rates indicated that the educational level of a community cannot be used as a successful predictor of its rate of hospitalization for alcoholism in state mental hospitals.

Table 5.26 Average annual first admission rates per 100,000 population aged 25-64 to state mental hospitals for alcoholism, by residence, sex, and years of school completed: Ohio, 1958-61

Years of school completed	Metropolitan		Nonmetropolitan	
	Male	Female	Male	Female
Elementary	40.0	9.1	53.9	7.8
0-4 years	41.9	13.2	52.7	10.2
5-7 years	34.0	7.0	44.0	6.2
8 years	43.7	9.4	60.1	8.4
High school	26.8	6.5	33.8	4.1
1-3 years	32.6	9.1	40.7	5.2
4 years	21.2	4.7	28.6	3.5
College (1 or more years)	10.1	4.7	14.7	1.7

Table 5.27 Average annual first admission rates per 100,000 population aged 25-64, from 11 metropolitan counties[a] to state mental hospitals for alcoholism, by years of school completed, sex, and color: Ohio, 1958-61

Years of school completed	Male		Female	
	White	Nonwhite	White	Nonwhite
Elementary (0-8)	37.5	60.2	7.0	18.8
High school (9-12)	23.5	66.2	4.9	21.9
College (1 or more)	10.0	16.8	3.5	21.1

[a] Cuyahoga, Franklin, Greene, Hamilton, Lake, Lucas, Mahoning, Miami, Montgomery, Summit, Trumbull.

Migration

Data on nativity were available only for state mental hospital admissions, which constituted two-thirds of the admission to all psychiatric facilities in 1960. Only 7 percent of the foreign-born white males first admitted were diagnosed as alcoholics. In the metropolitan counties the native-born white male admission rate of 24.2 was more than triple the 7.9 of the foreign-born; corresponding rates in the nonmetropolitan counties were 42.3 to 19.0. These findings are consistent with those of a selected population in New York City (Malzberg, 1940). Cultural attitudes and traditional uses of alcohol doubtless play an important role in the observed lower admission rates among the foreign-born. In Ohio, over half of the foreign-born came from Italy and the Balkans and another quarter were from northern and western Europe.

Analysis of the native-born males admitted for alcoholism in regard to birth in Ohio or elsewhere in the United States yielded interesting observations on the role of migration. There was a distinct difference by color in the native-Ohio versus native-other-state admissions. Among whites, migrants to Ohio had higher first admission rates (40.0) than nonmigrants (27.0), a finding consistent with results in the 1950 study. However, among nonwhites, the rates, when residence was controlled, were not significantly different (nonmigrants 65.6 and migrants 61.7). The age-specific rates of male alcoholics by nativity and race are shown in Figure 5.2.

Discussion

Although many more psychiatric facilities became available in the period between 1950 and 1960 and the first admission rate for alcoholism trebled during this period, the profile of patients so diagnosed remained fairly constant. Undoubtedly there are other community facilities, medical and social, which contributed to meeting special needs of alcoholics in the community. Family doctors, health clinics in industry, general hospitals without psychiatric facilities per se, to say nothing of family service agencies, Alcoholics Anonymous, etc., see patients similar in many ways to those enumerated in the studies reported here.

The difference by sex in admission rates may be related to cultural prohibitions on excessive drinking among women. In our society much more opprobrium is attached to women than to men who drink to excess. Thus, the use of alcohol as a coping device is more acceptable for men than for women. Among the nonwhites, however, admission rates for women were closer to rates for white men than to rates for white women. In both study periods the sex ratio for nonwhites was smaller than for whites. Among nonwhites the excessive rates suggest that marginal economic status and other social conditions are factors that affect admissions for alcoholism. Perhaps also a lower nutritional level produces an earlier onset of the

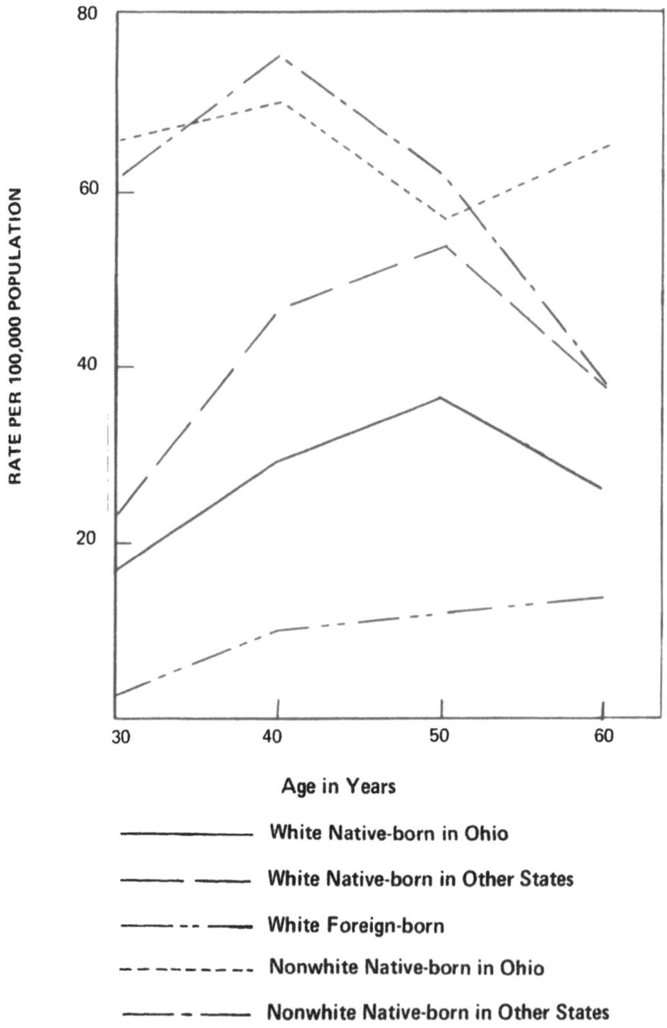

Fig. 5.2. Average annual first admissions of males per 100,000 population to state mental hospitals for alcoholism, by nativity, age, and color: Ohio, July 1, 1958 – December 31, 1961.

physiological effects of alcohol. Other factors contributing to the high nonwhite rates may be (1) the unavailability of a custodial relative in the home to provide care for a nonwhite alcoholic owing to the earlier entrance of nonwhites into the working world, (2) the high proportion of out-of-state immigrants among the nonwhites (75 percent among the age group considered here are from other states), and (3) the greater percentage of women in the labor force. The fact that nonwhite males with some high school education have higher admission rates than those with only elementary education may reflect the greater frustration felt by this group due to lack of appropriate work opportunities.

PSYCHONEUROSIS

Residence, Facility, Sex, Color, Age

Psychoneurosis was investigated in Ohio in 1960, when it was possible to ascertain first admissions in this diagnostic category throughout the psychiatric services of the state. As seen in Tables 5.2 and 5.3, less than one out of every five first admissions for psychoneurosis were to a state mental hospital. The 1960 data show the first admission rates were higher in the metropolitan than in the nonmetropolitan counties. Table 5.28 shows quite clearly that the facilities contributing most to the high rate in the metropolitan areas were those generally found in such areas, that is, the short-term inpatient care facilities of the general hospitals and the private mental hospitals. Rates of admissions to the general hospitals for metropolitan area residents were 60 percent higher than the rates for the nonmetropolitan area residents – this percentage would have been higher if only whites had been examined.

In view of the importance of the short-term community-oriented inpatient facilities in the treatment of the neurotic disorders, it is of interest to note that almost 10 percent of the admissions to state mental hospitals from nonmetropolitan areas (constituting 72 counties) were from the one nonmetropolitan county which contains a hospital designed to accomodate patients on a short-term basis. Among all the diagnostic categories studied, psychoneurosis lends itself most easily to the assumption of a close relationship between availability of facilities and high admission rates.

Table 5.28 Average annual first admission rates per 100,000 population aged 10 years and older to psychiatric facilities for psychoneurosis, by sex, color, residence, and type of facility: Ohio, 1958-61

Sex, color, & residence	Total	State mental hospitals	General with psychiatric facilities	Private and V.A. hospitals	Outpatient clinics
Males	48.2	8.8	22.2	4.8	12.7
White					
Metrop.	54.9	8.5	27.6	6.1	12.7
Nonmetrop.	41.7	9.4	15.9	3.5	12.9
Nonwhite					
Metrop.	29.4	8.8	8.3	(0.1)	12.2
Females	95.6	14.0	48.9	10.1	22.7
White					
Metrop.	106.6	13.3	59.0	14.1	20.2
Nonmetrop.	79.3	14.6	35.9	4.9	23.9
Nonwhite					
Metrop.	80.7	17.8	23.9	(0.5)	38.5
Total					
Metrop.	79.0	11.2	41.0	9.2	17.6
Nonmetrop.	60.1	12.0	25.6	4.2	18.3

( ) Indicates less than 10 admissions per year.

Admission rates for women with a diagnosis of psychoneurosis were about twice as high as those for men, regardless of color, residence, or age (Tables 5.28 and 5.29). It is also seen that nonwhites have lower admission rates for psychoneurosis than whites. This was the reverse of what was found with respect to the other diagnoses. In the public facilities (that is, the state mental hospitals and the outpatient clinics) the admission rates were higher for nonwhite women than for white women and at about equal magnitude for white and nonwhite men. Admission rates for nonwhites by age peaked slightly in advance of their white counterparts – with 63 percent of the first admissions for nonwhites occurring in the age groups 35 years or younger. Among whites, 40 percent were admitted before their 35th birthday. For men, regardless of race, peak ages of admission occurred later than for women.

Table 5.29 Average annual first admission rates per 100,000 population to psychiatric facilities for psychoneurosis, by age, sex, color, and residence: Ohio, 1958-61

Sex, color, & residence	Total[a]	10-19	20-24	25-29	30-34	35-39	40-44	45-54	55-64	65 & over
Males										
White										
Metrop.	54.9	24.1	58.9	67.7	78.7	79.5	69.1	68.2	55.9	26.9
Nonmetrop.	41.7	14.5	28.4	48.8	73.2	73.0	69.3	53.8	45.8	18.8
Nonwhite										
Metrop.	29.4	20.9	30.4	52.8	46.2	41.2	31.4	21.3	19.1	11.6
Females										
White										
Metrop.	106.6	29.2	131.9	189.8	175.6	148.7	127.7	112.2	112.4	53.9
Nonmetrop.	79.3	20.8	96.1	142.0	147.2	126.3	102.4	88.5	91.7	29.5
Nonwhite										
Metrop.	80.7	41.8	145.5	145.6	142.4	90.4	81.4	60.1	34.6	10.9
Ratio: M/F										
White										
Metrop.	.5	.8	.4	.4	.4	.5	.5	.6	.5	.5
Nonmetrop.	.5	.7	.3	.3	.5	.6	.7	.6	.5	.6
Nonwhite										
Metrop.	.4	.5	.2	.4	.3	.5	.4	.4	.6	1.1

[a] Rates based on Ohio population 10 years of age and older.

Marital Status

Highest admission rates for psychoneurosis occurred among the divorced and separated, who comprised only 4 percent of the Ohio population 14-64 years of age but represented 8 percent of the first admissions in this age group. Among women, there was little difference in the age-adjusted admission rates for widowed and married, and single women had the lowest rates up to ages 45 and over (Table 5.30). Married and single men exhibited similar overall rates but considerable variation with respect to age-specific rates.

Occupation

Among women admitted for psychoneurosis, only 17 percent were employed, compared to 29 percent employed in the general population. Although rates for females classed as laborers were excessively high, this did not affect the overall rate for working

Table 5.30 Average annual first admission rates per 100,000 population to psychiatric facilities for psychoneurosis, by age, sex, marital status, and residence: Ohio, July 1, 1958 - December 31, 1961:

Sex, residence, and age	Single	Married	Widowed	Divorced and separated
Males				
Metropolitan				
Total	47.9	63.4	92.5	129.2
Adjusted[a]	65.7	61.1	133.3	139.4
14-24	35.5	51.2	(218.1)	(160.3)
25-34	87.0	67.1	(138.7)	174.1
35-44	78.5	68.6	(78.0)	179.5
45-54	84.4	62.0	(131.3)	93.3
55-64	(38.5)	55.2	(72.9)	(45.7)
Nonmetropolitan				
Total	25.9	49.5	88.1	102.2
Adjusted[a]	41.9	44.8	54.7	107.6
14-24	18.9	22.3	-	(99.3)
25-34	50.0	55.2	-	(124.6)
35-44	(51.2)	58.5	(71.5)	191.9
45-54	(61.0)	46.7	(160.0)	(57.0)
55-64	(28.4)	(42.5)	(65.6)	(25.4)
Females				
Metropolitan				
Total	79.9	133.4	124.6	206.3
Adjusted[a]	116.4	131.1	131.7	223.5
14-24	57.2	128.0	(93.8)	298.7
25-34	156.8	176.0	(169.0)	309.1
35-44	130.1	132.4	154.4	203.5
45-54	124.1	102.9	117.7	147.3
55-64	122.2	101.9	120.0	96.4
Nonmetropolitan				
Total	46.8	104.4	95.4	151.9
Adjusted[a]	77.0	100.5	132.6	165.7
14-24	35.8	80.5	(218.1)	(208.2)
25-34	88.2	138.5	(112.7)	261.1
35-44	101.3	108.2	(111.9)	132.5
45-54	90.8	80.0	108.7	118.4
55-64	(72.2)	90.7	83.4	(62.7)

[a] Adjusted rate based on total Ohio population 14-64 years of age.

( ) Indicates less than 10 admissions per year.

women, since laborers represent less than 1 percent of the employed females admitted. Over 40 percent of the females admitted for psychoneurosis worked in clerical occupations, which approximates the proportion of women in clerical employment in the state. It is suspected that housewives may have had higher rates than employed females, since the admission rates by occupation, with one exception, were lower than the overall rates for women. Men employed as operatives and craftsmen had the lowest admission rates for psychoneurosis, although they constituted almost 50 percent of the employed males in the state. With the exception of the laborer category, males and females employed in the white collar and professional occupation groups generally had higher rates.

Table 5.31 Average annual first admission rates per 100,000 population aged 15-64 years to psychiatric facilities for psychoneurosis, by sex, residence, and occupation: Ohio, 1958-61

Occupation	Males		Females	
	Metrop.	Nonmetrop.	Metrop.	Nonmetrop.
Professional, technical, and kindred workers	79.7	82.0	104.9	99.6
Managers, officials and proprietors	96.0	84.6	--	--
Clerical and kindred workers	58.2	53.8	81.6	74.5
Sales and kindred workers	77.4	58.1	--	--
Service workers except private household	71.2	42.6	82.2	48.9
Domestics (private household workers)	--	--	69.0	56.0
Farmers, farm laborers, farm managers	(75.7)	42.2	--	--
Craftsmen, foremen and kindred workers	54.1	40.4	--	--
Operatives and kindred workers	32.3	25.5	28.1	17.0
Laborers except farm and mine	102.8	118.3	704.3	640.1

( ) Indicates less than 10 admissions per year.

Education

Information on years of school completed was available only from state mental hospital records. Interpretation of the distribution shown in Table 5.32 requires considerable caution, as the state mental hospital admissions represent less than 19 percent of all psychoneurotic first admissions (Table 5.3). However, another 29 percent of the psychoneurotic patients used the outpatient psychiatric clinics, and their educational distributions are probably similar to those admitted to the state mental hospitals. To the extent that occupational groupings may be interpreted to reflect educational level, data by occupation suggest that the state mental hospital admissions were concentrated among the blue collar workers – over 64 percent of the males and 53 percent of the working women admitted were in the service, household, craftsmen, operatives, and laboring groups, compared to 50 percent among all males admitted and 37 percent among all females admitted. Facilities other than the state mental hospital furnished proportionately larger numbers of admissions in the professional, managerial, and white collar employment groups. If comparable data could be obtained, the presumption is that higher educational levels would be included, resulting in either a positive correlation between increased schooling and psychoneurosis or no relationship between education and psychoneurosis. Within the state mental hospitals the median years of schooling completed for patients admitted for psychoneurosis (11.5) was higher than the median for all patients admitted to state hospitals (9.9) and also higher than the median education for the general population of the state (10.9).

Table 5.32 Average annual age-adjusted[a] first admission rates per 100,000 population aged 25-64 to state mental hospitals for psychoneurosis, by residence, sex, and years of school completed: Ohio, 1958-61

Years of school completed	Metropolitan		Nonmetropolitan	
	Male	Female	Male	Female
Elementary (0-8)	11.1	16.8	12.6	21.1
High school (9-12)	13.1	19.4	12.7	18.2
College (1 or more)	8.4	13.0	8.3	12.1

[a] Adjusted rates based on total Ohio population 25-64 years of age.

Migration

Data on admissions for psychoneurosis by place of birth were also available only for the state mental hospitals and are subject to the same limitations discussed in the previous section on education. Among foreign-born men, less than 10 admissions a year occurred. Based on these admissions, however, an overall age-adjusted rate of 7.3 for the foreign-born men contrasts with 10.9 for white native-born. Among white females admitted to the state mental hospitals the rate was 17.2 for native-born versus 14.2 for foreign-born. Thus, foreign-born are seen to have lower rates of admission for psychoneurosis than the native-born. Among those born in the United States it was seen that white migrants to Ohio, both male and female, had slightly higher age-adjusted admission rates than did native Ohioans (Table 5.33). Among the nonwhites of both sexes, however, native Ohioans had higher admission rates than did in-migrating nonwhites.

Table 5.33 Average age-adjusted[a] first admission rates per 100,000 population to state mental hospitals for psychoneurosis, by sex, color, and nativity of native-born 10 years of age and over: Ohio, 1958-61

Color and place of birth	Male	Female
White		
Born in Ohio	10.6	16.6
Born in other states	12.4	20.0
Nonwhite		
Born in Ohio	16.0	22.6
Born in other states	8.1	19.9

[a] Rates based on Ohio population 10 years of age and older.

Discussion

The 1950 data indicated that the psychoneurotic patients represented less than 5 percent of state hospital first admissions, 13 percent of private mental hospital admissions, and more than 10 percent of general hospital psychiatric admissions. By 1960 the proportion of admissions had doubled. Since 1950 the numbers of general hospitals with psychiatric facilities had doubled, and there had been a phenomenal increase of outpatient psychiatric clinics. During this decade also, new therapeutic drugs were developed. The question that comes to mind is whether the times produce such undue stress that neuroses result or the availability of community resources, such as outpatient clinics, new facilities within general hospitals, and increased community awareness of current developments in psychiatry, allow such patients to seek relief hitherto thought to be unavailable. The increase in first admissions to state mental hospitals for psychoneurosis has been accompanied, interestingly enough, by a sharp decrease in admissions for the affective psychoses.

The almost equal rate of utilization of both outpatient and inpatient services by psychoneurotic patients, their numerical preponderance in the community-oriented facilities, and indications that these patients may not seek treatment when resources are remote, suggests that they are particularly amenable to the community concept of mental health.

6 / Patterns of Use of Psychiatric Facilities in Louisiana and Maryland, 1960

The emphasis of the data presented in this chapter is on the rates of use of psychiatric facilities according to socioeconomic and family relationship variables. To obtain the data required for such an analysis, a study was carried out in cooperation with the Louisiana State Department of Hospitals and the Maryland Department of Mental Hygiene. The primary purpose of this study was to obtain data on admissions to a complete range of psychiatric facilities in order to relate them to the detailed socioeconomic and family relationship data which were made available in the 1960 census.

Although the methodology of this study has been described in some detail elsewhere (Pollack et al., 1964; Pollack, 1965; Pollock et al., 1968), a brief description of some of its aspects will help to place the data which follow in perspective. Items of identifying information were obtained on all patients admitted to state mental hospitals, private mental hospitals, psychiatric services of general hospitals, Veterans Administration hospitals and outpatient psychiatric clinics in each of the two states during the year immediately following the 1960 census. This information was given to the Bureau of the Census for purposes of locating the corresponding 1960 census schedules for these individuals. The detailed socioeconomic and family relationship data on these individuals as reported to the Bureau of the Census made it possible to classify these patients according to socioeconomic and family relationship variables in the same way in which these individuals were classified in the general population data. The basic question this study attempted to answer was: Given the population as it existed on April 1, 1960, what is the probability of admission to a psychiatric faciltiy during the year following the census?

In the process of matching patient data to census records it was not possible to locate approximately one-third of the patients in the census records. A discussion of this problem and a formulation of it allowing for the extent of undercounts in both numerators and denominators of rates were presented in an earlier paper (Pollack, 1965). The numerators of all of the rates presented in this chapter are composites of two elements–the number of matched cases and an estimate of the number of nonmatched cases with the specific characteristics under consideration. The latter was obtained from the nonmatched portion of a 10 percent sample of all admissions in which more detailed census information was obtained directly from patients at time of admission. Another complicating aspect of this study was the number of cases available for analysis and the size of the sampling variation in the rates. The problems resulting from sample size and sampling variation are discussed briefly in Appendix E.

The method for computing rates in this chapter differs conceptually from that used for the rates presented in the preceding chapters. Those in the preceding chapters were obtained by dividing the number of admissions during the year by the population at the midpoint of the year in question. When rates for a three-year period were presented, the average annual number of admissions was divided by the population at the middle of the three-year period. In this study, on the other hand, the rates computed represent the probability of admission to a psychiatric facility during the year among those presumed to be in the population at the beginning of the year. This is a true probability, as compared with the usual "central rate." If it were possible to compute rates for a given area according to both of these methods, the resulting differences would be negligible, since the denominator for the central rate would be simply the population as of six months after the census.

DISTRIBUTION BY TYPE OF FACILITY

During the study year, there were 15,836 admissions to the Louisiana psychiatric facilities included in the study and 16,235 to those in Maryland. Because of the fact that persons admitted more than once during the study year were counted each time, these totals represented 13,634 and 14,427 separate individuals, respectively, in the two states. Thus, 9 percent of the admissions in Louisiana and 11 percent of those in Maryland represented repeated admissions of the same individuals during the study year. In Louisiana 59 percent of the persons admitted were experiencing their first contact with a psychiatric facility; the corresponding percentage for Maryland was 65.

The number of admissions, the number of individuals admitted, and the number of first admissions to each of the types of facilities included in the study for each state are given in Table 6.1. There was a considerable difference between the two states in the distribution of admissions among the various types of facilities. Maryland had a much higher proportion of outpatient clinic admissions, while Louisiana had a much higher proportion of general hospital admissions. These differences were undoubtedly due to differential availability of facilities. Maryland had more than twice as many outpatient psychiatric clinics as Louisiana, while Louisiana had seven general hospitals with psychiatric services compared to four for Maryland. One of the Louisiana hospitals was Charity Hospital in New Orleans, which maintained three inpatient psychiatric units and was affiliated with two medical schools. No comparable general hospital facility existed in Maryland.

There is evidence of difference between the two states in the extent of prior psychiatric experience of those admitted during the

Table 6.1 Numbers of admissions, persons admitted and first admissions to psychiatric facilities by type of facility: Louisiana and Maryland, 1960-61

Type of facility	Number of admissions	Number of persons admitted	Number of first admissions
Louisiana			
All facilities	15,836[a]	13,634[b]	7,983[a]
State & county mental hospitals	4,600	4,506	2,346
V.A. hospitals	757	705	180
Private mental hospitals	629	603	274
General hospitals	3,401	2,841	1,503
Outpatient psychiatric clinics	6,434	6,198	3,678
Maryland			
All facilities	16,235[a]	14,427[b]	9,350[a]
State & county mental hospitals	4,994	4,781	2,334
V.A. hospitals	366	357	79
Private mental hospitals	1,304	1,248	748
General hospitals	986	734	538
Outpatient psychiatric clinics	8,558	8,272	5,632

[a] The individual facility numbers add to slightly less than the total for all facilities since the small number of female V.A. hospital admissions were included in the total, but excluded from the V.A. hospital counts.

[b] The numbers for the individual facilities add to more than the total for all facilities since some persons were admitted to more than one type of facility during the year.

study year. Among the 8,272 persons admitted to outpatient psychiatric clinics in Maryland, 68 percent (5,632) were being admitted to a psychiatric facility for the first time, compared with ony 59 percent (3,678) of the 6,198 outpatient clinic admissions in Louisiana. Similarly, 60 percent of the persons admitted to private mental hospitals in Maryland were being admitted for the first time compared with 46 percent in Louisiana, and 60 percent of the persons admitted to general hospitals in Maryland were being admitted for the first time compared with only 53 percent in Louisiana.

To understand more fully the way in which psychiatric facilities are used by the populations they serve, it may be helpful to examine the distribution of admissions to the various types of psychiatric facilities according to specific patient characteristics. If the entire range of psychiatric facilities is considered to constitute a system, then these data show the extent to which specific groups in the population tend to use a particular type of facility as a point of first entry into the system. Data showing the percentage distribution of first admissions by type of admitting facility are presented in detail in Figures 6.1 through 6.12. Some of the striking patterns which emerge from these data are as follows:

1. Persons under 18 used outpatient psychiatric clinics predominately as a point of first entry, while those 65 years and over were first admitted primarily to inpatient facilities. Between these two extremes, there was an increasing proportion of inpatient first admissions with increasing age.

2. There was a greater proportion of general hospital first admissions in Louisiana and a greater proportion of private mental hospital first admissions in Maryland. Maryland also showed a greater proportion of outpatient first admissions than did Louisiana, and this was particularly pronounced among the nonwhites.

3. Of all the marital status groups, single persons had the greatest proportion of outpatient first admissions, but when these patterns are examined specific for age, it becomes apparent that this was due to the large proportion of single persons who were under 18 years of age. Among the other age groups, widowed persons, except those 65 and over, tended to have the highest proportion of outpatient first admissions, with married persons also having high proportions.

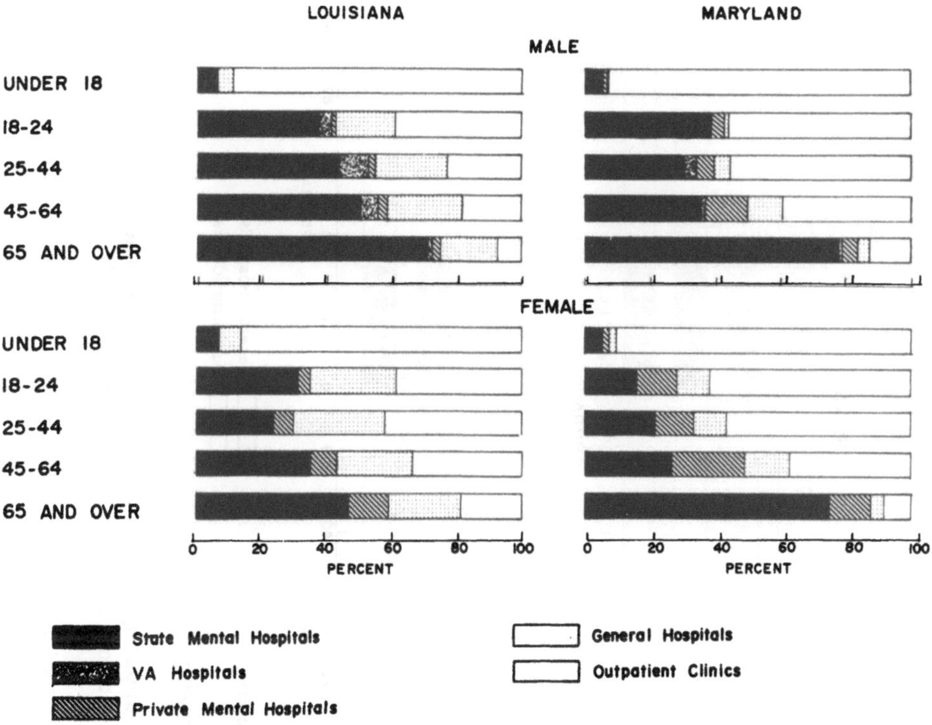

Fig. 6.1. Percentage distribution by type of facility of first admissions to psychiatric facilities. by age and sex: Louisiana and Maryland, 1960-61.

Source: Earl S. Pollack, "Monitoring a Comprehensive Mental Health Program: Methodology and Data Requirements," in Roberts, Greenfield, and Miller, eds., *Comprehensive Mental Health: The Challenge of Evaluation*, Madison, University of Wisconsin Press (copyright 1968 by the Regents of the University of Wisconsin), pp. 137-167.

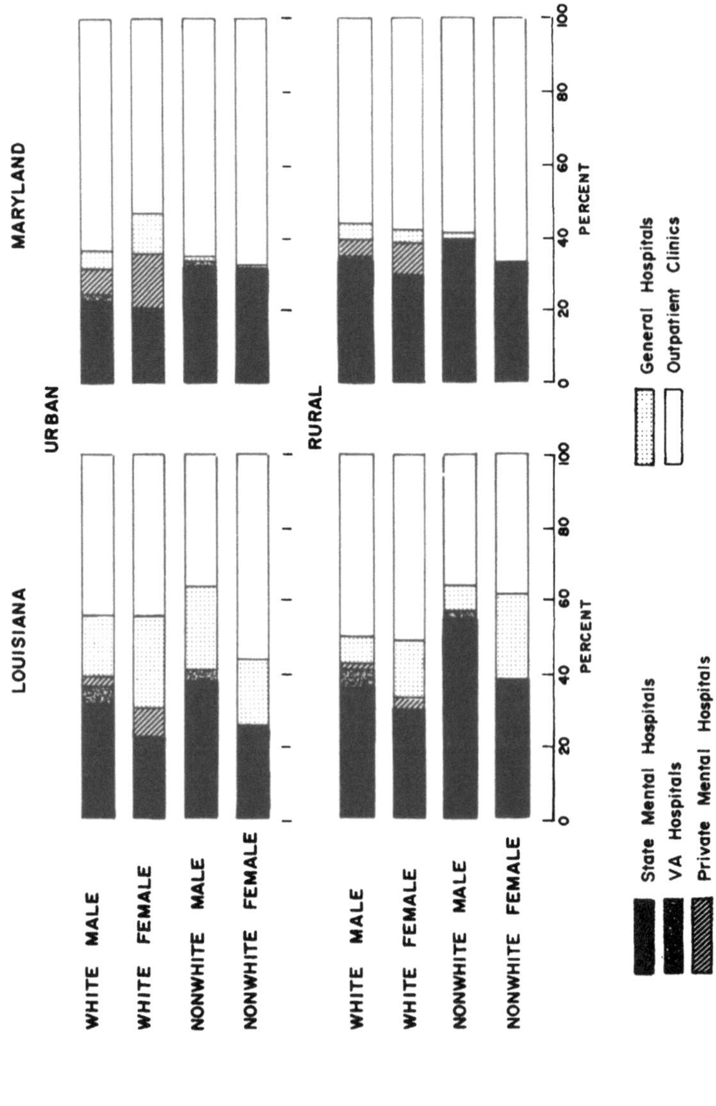

Fig. 6.2. Percentage distribution by type of facility of first admissions to psychiatric facilities, by sex, color, and residence: Louisiana and Maryland, 1960-61.

Source: Pollack, "Monitoring a Comprehensive Mental Health Program."

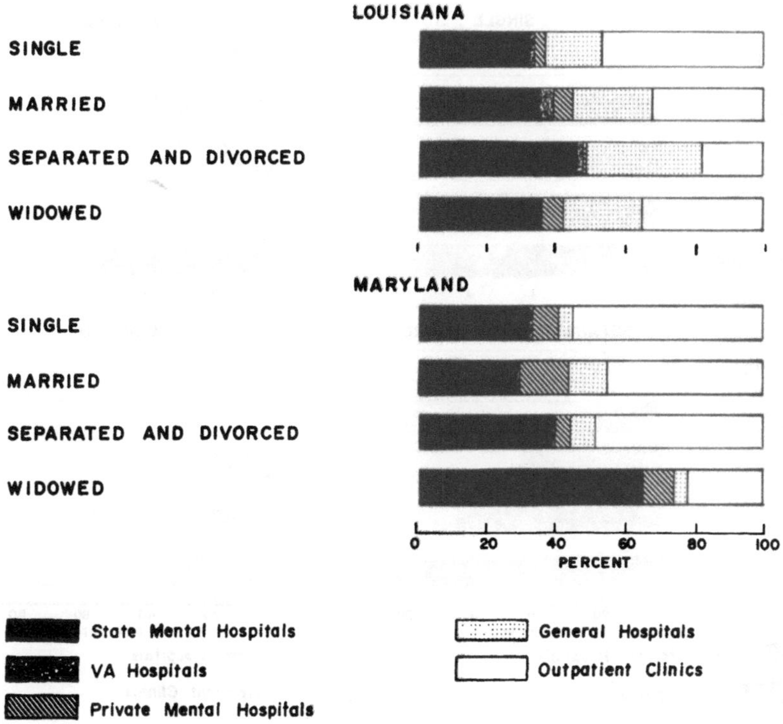

Fig. 6.3. Percentage distribution by type of facility of first admissions to psychiatric facilities, by marital status: Louisiana and Maryland, 1960-61.
Source: Pollack, "Monitoring a Comprehensive Mental Health Program."

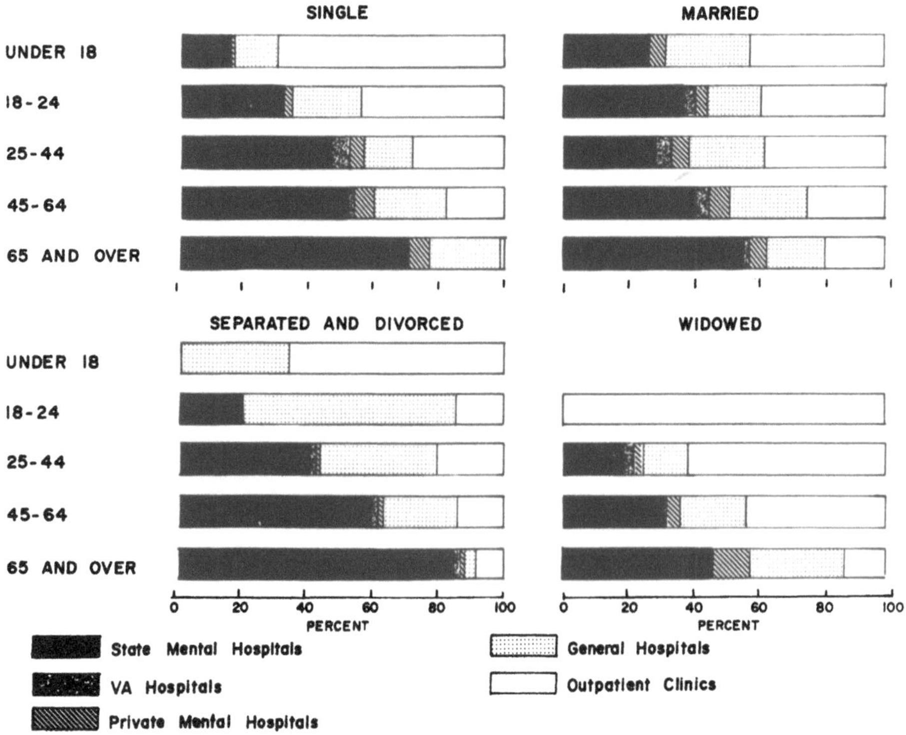

Fig. 6.4. Percentage distribution by type of facility of first admissions to psychiatric facilities, by age and marital status: Louisiana, 1960-61.

Source: Pollack, "Monitoring a Comprehensive Mental Health Program."

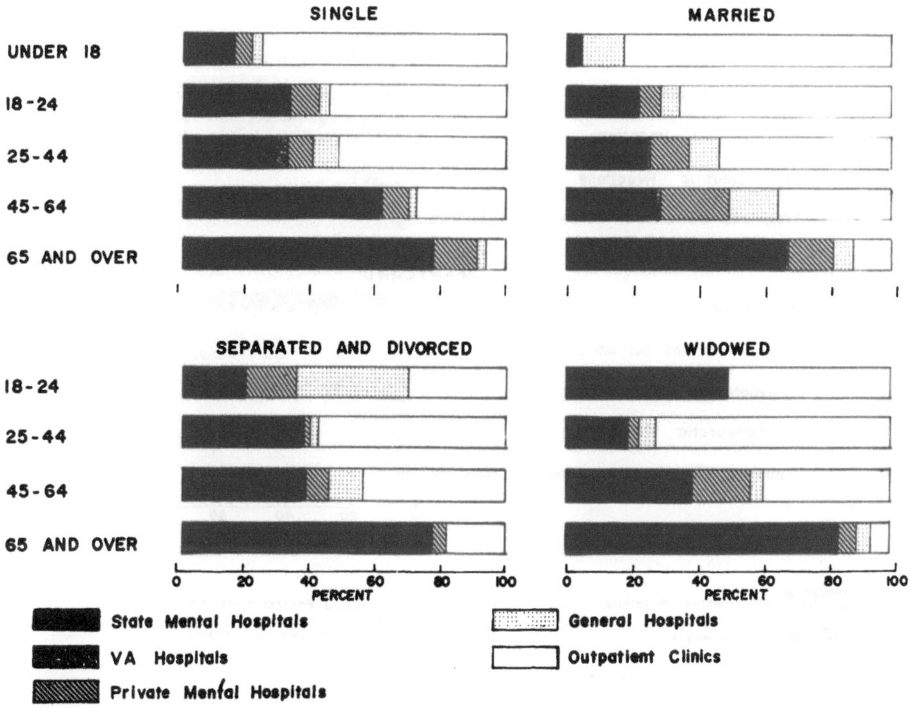

Fig. 6.5. Percentage distribution by type of facility of first admissions to psychiatric facilities, by age and marital status: Maryland, 1960-61.

Source: Pollack, "Monitoring a Comprehensive Mental Health Program."

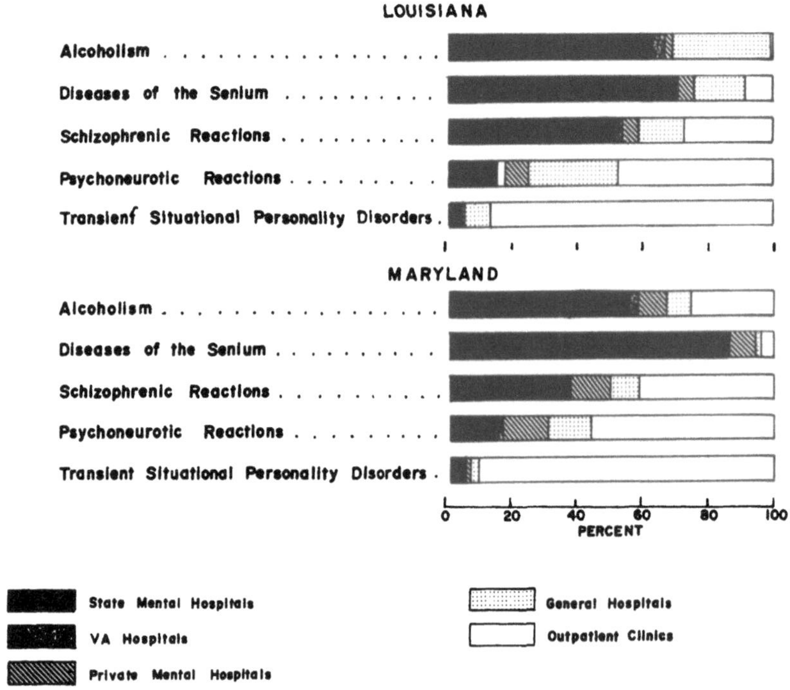

Fig. 6.6. Percentage distribution by type of facility of first admissions to psychiatric facilities, by diagnosis: Louisiana and Maryland, 1960-61.

Source: Pollack, "Monitoring a Comprehensive Mental Health Program."

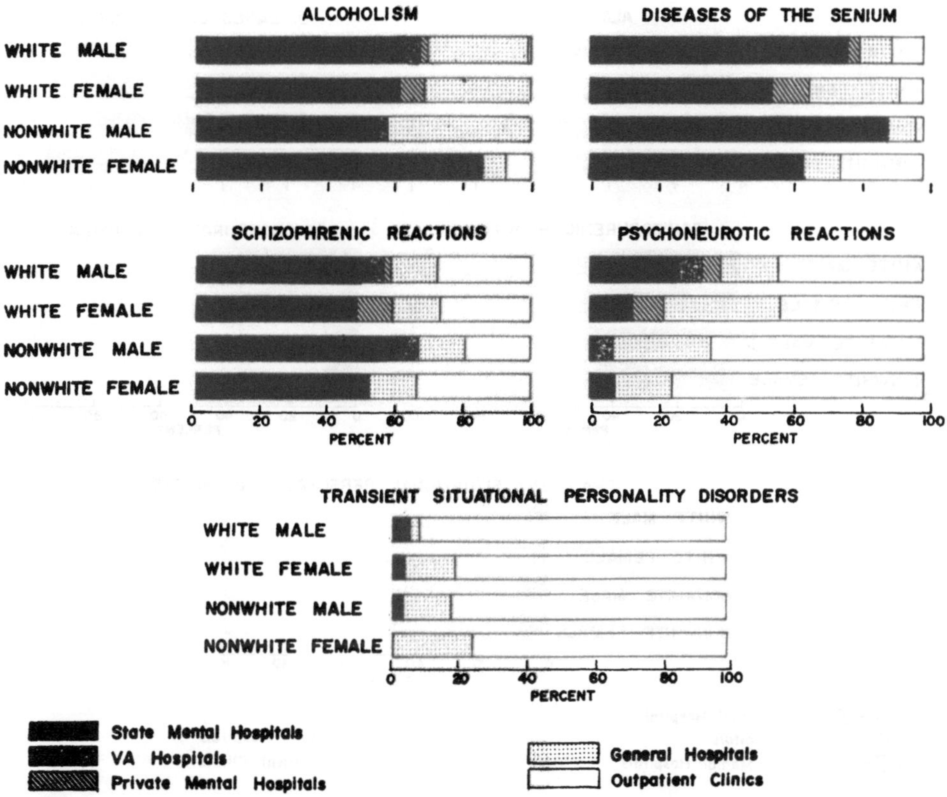

Fig. 6.7. Percentage distribution by type of facility of first admissions to psychiatric facilities, by diagnosis, color, and sex: Louisiana, 1960-61.
Source: Pollack, "Monitoring a Comprehensive Mental Health Program."

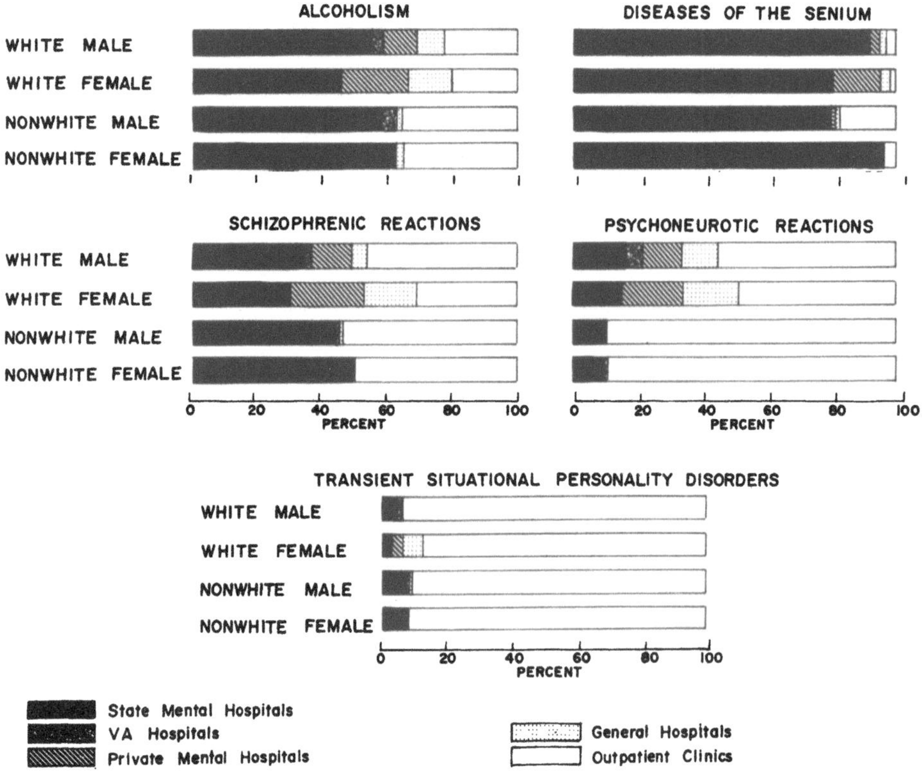

Fig. 6.8. Percentage distribution by type of facility of first admissions to psychiatric facilities, by diagnosis, color, and sex: Maryland, 1960-61.

Source: Pollack, "Monitoring a Comprehensive Mental Health Program."

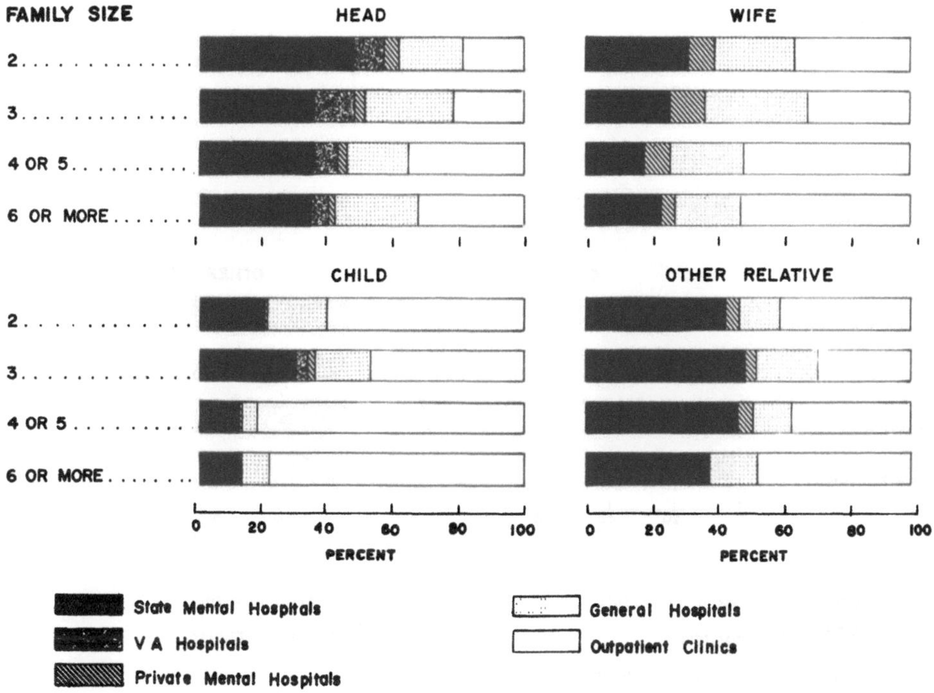

Fig. 6.9. Percentage distribution by type of facility of first admissions to psychiatric facilities, by family relationship and size: Louisiana, 1960-61.
Source: Pollack, "Monitoring a Comprehensive Mental Health Program."

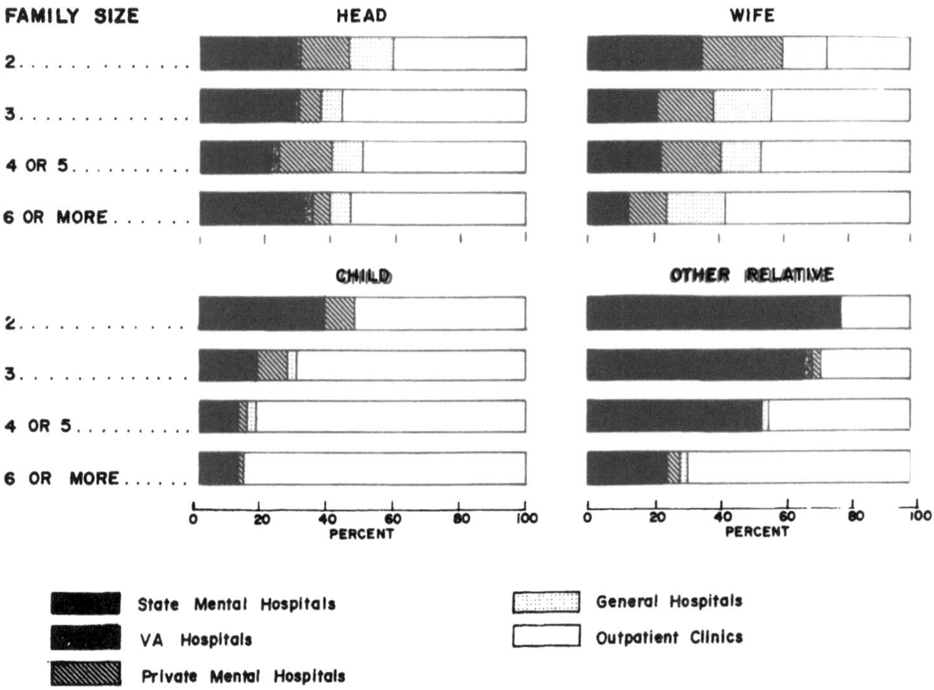

Fig. 6.10. Percentage distribution by type of facility of first admissions to psychiatric facilities, by family relationship and size: Maryland, 1960-61.
Source: Pollack, "Monitoring a Comprehensive Mental Health Program."

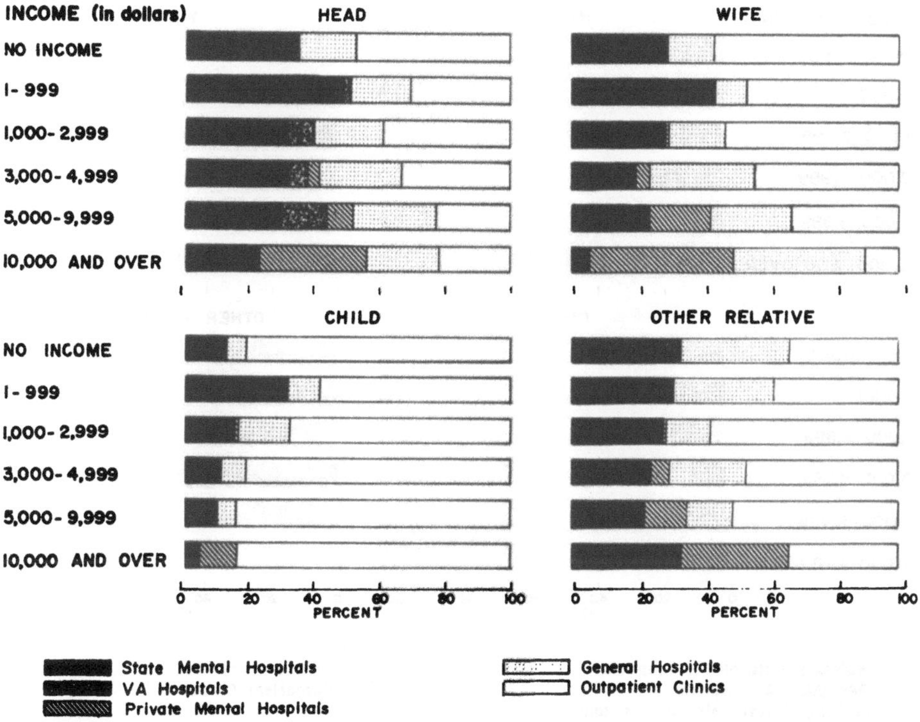

Fig. 6.11. Percentage distribution by type of facility of first admissions to psychiatric facilities, by family relationship and income of family head: Louisiana, 1960-61.

Source: Pollack, "Monitoring a Comprehensive Mental Health Program."

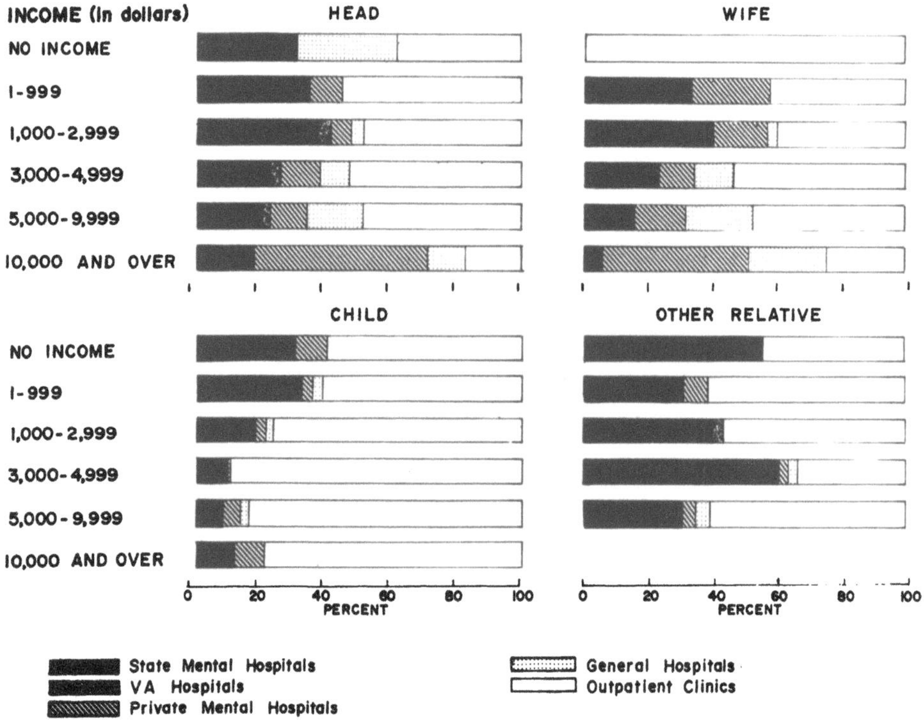

Fig. 6.12. Percentage distribution by type of facility of first admissions to psychiatric facilities, by family relationship and income of family head: Maryland, 1960-61.

Source: Pollack, "Monitoring a Comprehensive Mental Health Program."

4. Among psychoneurotics, the proportion of outpatient first admissions was greater among nonwhites than among whites. This was true for both Louisiana and Maryland.

5. There was a general tendency for decreasing proportions of inpatient first admissions with increasing family size. This was more pronounced for Maryland than for Louisiana.

6. For family heads, wives, and children, there were decreasing proportions of state mental hospital first admissions with increasing income of family head.

7. Family heads and wives of family heads whose income was $10,000 or more had high proportions of first admissions to private mental hospitals. However, this was not true for children whose fathers were in that income category. Over 80 percent of them were first admitted to outpatient clinics. Among children whose fathers earned less than $1,000, on the other hand, approximately 30 percent were first admitted to state mental hospitals.

Some of these findings were certainly to be expected, such as the high proportion of private mental hospital first admissions among persons in high-income families. Some of the differences in patterns between the two states can be explained on the basis of existing knowledge about the differential availability of facilities. For example, the higher proportion of private mental hospital admissions in Maryland can be accounted for by the fact that Louisiana had only one private mental hospital compared with 11 in Maryland. Similarly, Louisiana's higher proportion of general hospital admissions was due, in part, to the existence of seven general hospital psychiatric units in Louisiana compared with only four in Maryland. As indicated above, the existence of the psychiatric units in Charity Hospital in New Orleans undoubtedly played a large role in this regard.

FIRST ADMISSION RATES

Sex, Color, and Residence

Age-specific and age-adjusted first admission rates by sex, color, and urban versus rural residence are given for Louisiana in Table 6.2 and for Maryland in Table 6.3. The age-adjusted rates reveal that rates were higher among males than among females and higher among urban residents than among rural residents in both states. In

Louisiana the age-adjusted rate for whites was higher than that for nonwhites, while in Maryland the reverse was true.

While age-adjusted rates permit the comparison of rates among groups, eliminating insofar as possible the effect of age on these comparisons, they are nevertheless weighted averages of the age-specific rates. Therefore, they cannot present the complete picture when comparing two groups. Thus, there are some notable exceptions to the above generalizations. In all categories in both states, female rates were greater than those for males in the age group 18-24. In Louisiana rates were also higher among white females than

Table 6.2 Age-adjusted and age-specific first admission rates per 100,000 population to all psychiatric facilities by sex, color, and residence status: Louisiana, 1960-61.

Sex, color, and residence	Number of first admissions	Age-adjusted	Crude	<15	15-17	18-24	25-34	35-44	45-54	55-64
Total	7,983	250.6	245.1	146.6	293.4	301.9	397.8	335.2	270.1	242.5
Male	4,129	262.8	259.3	191.7	304.5	255.9	328.1	345.8	293.5	284.8
Female	3,854	233.5	231.5	100.2	282.2	343.6	427.4	325.3	247.6	203.3
White male	3,319	303.9	304.4	261.2	360.7	254.6	359.9	389.3	311.6	318.7
White female	2,974	262.6	265.2	137.9	271.0	356.4	490.9	343.6	260.6	228.4
Non white male	810	175.0	161.4	71.0	200.7	258.4	237.0	215.1	244.2	199.5
Non white female	880	172.6	162.0	36.9	302.9	317.9	274.5	278.5	215.8	141.8
Urban male	3,192	324.3	322.4	246.8	432.5	313.3	394.9	414.2	340.8	339.2
Urban female	3,057	283.1	285.6	129.2	413.2	407.9	486.6	381.5	314.3	230.4
Rural male	937	160.6	155.6	106.1	144.9	156.0	196.0	210.0	212.8	196.8
Rural female	797	141.8	134.1	54.3	102.2	206.6	303.3	208.8	119.6	152.9

Table 6.3 Age-adjusted and age-specific first admission rates per 100,000 population to all psychiatric facilities by sex, color, and residence status: Maryland, 1960-61

Sex, color, and residence	Number of first admissions	Age-adjusted	Crude	<15	15-17	18-24	25-34	35-44	45-54	55-64
Total	9,350	299.5	301.5	236.0	331.7	313.7	387.5	350.2	306.7	256.5
Male	5,160	334.9	336.3	306.9	391.6	284.5	343.5	401.2	377.8	300.6
Female	4,190	262.8	267.3	162.5	271.0	342.7	429.7	300.7	234.4	214.6
White male	4,113	321.7	322.7	315.0	384.6	255.9	301.8	355.5	376.9	291.2
White female	3,382	254.7	260.1	167.1	237.7	318.0	405.9	297.2	241.3	189.4
Non white male	1,047	407.1	403.1	272.8	423.7	420.0	553.5	656.4	382.4	352.5
Non white female	808	306.5	302.6	144.5	423.2	448.9	539.6	320.0	194.9	372.8
Urban male	4,119	373.2	375.9	307.7	456.9	406.5	417.2	450.7	449.4	301.7
Urban female	3,441	290.2	296.9	166.6	252.1	410.8	492.5	344.0	269.6	238.8
Rural male	1,041	242.1	237.4	304.7	253.9	79.3	141.0	258.3	180.1	297.7
Rural female	749	180.8	183.4	151.7	316.5	146.2	244.1	166.9	124.5	141.0

among white males in the age group 25-34 years and higher among nonwhite females than nonwhite males in the entire age range 15-44 years. The exceptions to male-female rate differences in Maryland were irregular, but female rates were consistently higher than male rates in the age group 65 and over. In Louisiana, where rates for whites were greater than those for nonwhites, the reverse was true for males age 18-24 years and among females age 15-17 years. In Maryland, where nonwhite rates were greater than those for whites, the reverse was true for those less than 15 years of age and for females aged 45-54.

Diagnosis

Tables 6.4 and 6.5 present first admission rates by psychiatric diagnosis for specific color-sex groups and residence-sex groups for Louisiana and Maryland, respectively. There is considerable similarity in the direction of male-female differences in the two states. The male rates for alcoholism were many times higher than those for females. Males also had higher rates for diseases of the senium, personality disorders, and transient situational personality disorders. Females had higher rates for schizophrenic reactions, all other psychotic disorders, and psychoneurotic disorders. The rates for white males are comparable in the two states, with the exception of alcoholism, where the Louisiana rate is about 40 percent higher than that for Maryland and personality disorders, where the Maryland rate is about 70 percent higher than that for Louisiana. There appears to be even greater similarity in the rates for white females in the two states. The major difference is in the psychoneurotic disorders group, where the Louisiana rate is about 50 percent higher than that for Maryland.

The greatest difference in rates between the two states occurred among the nonwhites, where the Maryland rates were considerably higher than those for Louisiana. Among nonwhite males the Maryland rates were consistently higher for every diagnostic category, for alcoholism they were five times higher, and for diseases of the senium and schizophrenic reactions more than twice as high. Similarly, the rates for nonwhite females in Maryland were consistently higher than those for Louisiana. The outstanding differences in this group occurred in the personality disorder and transient situational personality disorder categories, with rates of

28.6 and 22.5, respectively, for Maryland compared with 4.3 and 5.2 for Louisiana.

Marital Status

Most studies which have presented rates of admission to psychiatric facilities by marital status have indicated lowest rates among married persons, high rates among separated and divorced persons, and intermediate rates among single and widowed persons (Jaco, 1960; Malzberg, 1940; Locke et al., 1960). Similar patterns appeared for the 13 Model Reporting Area states in 1960, as indicated in Chapter 3. The present study also follows this general pattern, with one notable exception. In Louisiana the rate for married females was slightly higher than that for single females (Table 6.6). The reason for this deviation from the usual pattern is not readily apparent, but it may be accounted for by one or more specific diagnostic groups. Data in this detail were not tabulated by diagnosis. Further investigation revealed that this difference occurred in every age group and in every type of facility, with the exception of outpatient psychiatric clinics, where the rate for single persons was higher than that for married. Another deviation from the general pattern was the low rate among nonwhite divorced females in Louisiana.

Family Size and Type

This study places considerable emphasis on data related to the patient's family. Using the Census Bureau definition, the family includes the patient and any persons living with him who are related by blood, marriage, or adoption. By using the data on the families in which the patients were living made available through the census matching procedure, it was possible to produce tabulations which classify the patient not only according to his own characteristics but also according to his relationship to the family head, the characteristics of the family itself, and the characteristics of the family head. Similar data on the characteristics of individuals in the general population of the two states in specific types of families were made available by the Census Bureau to permit the computation of rates of admissions to psychiatric facilities according to these characteristics. No such person-in-family tabulations of the population had been available in census publications prior to 1960.

Table 6.4 Age-adjusted first admission rates per 100,000 population to all psychiatric facilities by psychiatric diagnosis, sex and color, sex, and residence status: Louisiana, 1960-61

Psychiatric diagnosis	All males	All females	White male	White female	Non white male	Non white female	Urban male	Urban female	Rural male	Rural female
All diagnoses	262.8	233.5	303.9	262.6	175.0	172.6	324.3	283.1	160.6	141.8
Alcoholism	43.7	5.2	53.4	4.8	16.1	5.8	55.9	7.0	21.5	1.7
Diseases of the senium	14.3	9.7	13.3	11.1	16.5	6.7	18.7	12.2	8.2	5.3
Schizophrenic reactions	37.3	41.6	38.5	39.2	33.5	47.6	42.3	50.7	27.9	24.8
All other psychotic disorders	8.6	17.1	10.9	19.4	2.8	11.5	9.8	17.9	6.5	15.6
Psychoneurotic reactions	33.8	76.2	40.7	90.4	17.6	41.9	40.3	91.0	22.3	47.5
Personality disorders	28.0	17.7	35.7	24.1	11.7	4.3	33.3	22.1	19.9	9.4
Transient situational personality disorders	30.0	19.4	43.4	27.4	6.0	5.2	38.8	26.0	16.5	8.8
All other mental disorders	35.3	21.8	32.2	21.3	44.8	23.0	43.1	24.8	23.0	16.8
Without mental disorder	10.2	8.2	7.9	5.0	16.4	16.7	13.1	11.1	5.1	2.5
Undiagnosed	21.6	16.5	27.9	19.8	9.4	9.9	29.1	20.4	9.6	9.3

Table 6.5 Age-adjusted first admission rates per 100,000 population to all psychiatric facilities by psychiatric diagnosis, sex and color, sex, and residence status: Maryland, 1960-61

Psychiatric diagnosis	All males	All females	White male	White female	Non white male	Non white female	Urban male	Urban female	Rural male	Rural female
All diagnoses	334.9	262.8	321.7	254.7	407.1	306.5	373.2	290.2	242.1	180.8
Alcoholism	45.9	8.3	39.1	6.9	80.6	14.1	53.2	9.8	27.2	3.7
Diseases of the senium	21.0	19.8	17.9	18.6	39.0	29.6	21.1	19.7	20.7	20.0
Schizophrenic reactions	42.5	47.2	36.4	40.7	73.7	76.7	50.3	53.3	24.7	29.0
All other psychotic disorders	12.0	15.0	13.5	14.8	3.3	15.9	13.2	17.0	8.9	9.3
Psychoneurotic reactions	40.9	60.0	43.5	62.8	28.8	46.2	47.0	70.3	25.9	29.8
Personality disorders	56.8	27.3	60.8	27.2	37.6	28.6	64.9	29.2	39.3	21.5
Transient situational personality disorders	40.2	27.7	42.4	29.0	30.9	22.5	42.0	28.7	35.9	24.7
All other mental disorders	35.5	26.6	29.1	24.0	65.2	39.0	36.2	26.0	34.2	27.9
Without mental disorder	5.2	6.1	5.4	7.1	4.2	2.3	3.3	6.5	10.2	5.0
Undiagnosed	34.8	24.7	33.6	23.6	43.8	31.6	42.0	29.7	15.3	9.9

Table 6.6 Age-adjusted first admission rates per 100,000 population to all psychiatric facilities by sex, color, and marital status: Louisiana and Maryland, 1960-61

Marital status	All males	All females	White Males	White Females	Nonwhite Males	Nonwhite Females
Louisiana						
Total	301.6	297.7	328.6	322.6	230.2	238.2
Single	521.7	255.7	596.5	279.1	370.7	210.5
Married	225.1	278.1	237.1	302.4	190.4	212.8
Separated	1018.5	546.1	1913.8	923.4	492.2	357.3
Widowed	364.8	300.7	285.2	264.4	445.2	330.2
Divorced	1812.2	589.7	2279.7	818.4	318.0	178.6
Maryland						
Total	350.5	312.3	326.2	298.5	478.6	382.8
Single	527.0	329.3	491.1	329.7	597.2	359.9
Married	333.7	267.3	352.7	263.6	302.4	302.3
Separated	862.2	694.4	1133.8	720.9	540.6	738.8
Widowed	359.1	488.0	444.0	424.7	240.8	606.4
Divorced	907.4	517.3	866.7	563.0	1118.8	344.0

Age-adjusted first admission rates to psychiatric facilities specific for three variables – type of family, size of family, and relationship to family head – were analyzed in an attempt to determine whether these variables might assist in identifying segments of the population having high risk of admission to psychiatric facilities. These rates were computed for each of the two states specific for color, residence, and selected diagnostic groups. To analyze these detailed data in some systematic fashion, differences in rates were examined by family type and family size for each relationship group.

Figures 6.13 - 6.17 show the age-adjusted first admission rates for family heads, wives, and children of family heads by type and size of family and by race and residence for each state. These charts do not show the rates for "other male head" families, nor those for other relatives of the family head because of the small number of cases in these categories.

The highlights resulting from the analysis of the first admission rates can be summarized briefly as follows:

1. The rates for heads of families headed by a female are generally higher than for those of husband-wife families, regardless of the size of the family (Figures 6.13 and 6.14).

2. The lowest rates for heads of husband-wife families are generally in families of size 3 (Figures 6.13 and 6.14).

3. For whites, female family heads living with only one other person have the lowest admission rates, and those in families of six or more have the highest rates (Figures 6.13 and 6.14).

4. For whites, wives in families of six or more members have higher rates than wives in smaller families (Figure 6.15).

5. With the exception of urban-nonwhite persons in Maryland, the highest rates for children in husband-wife families are for those living in families of size 3 (Figures 6.16 and 6.17).

6. Among other relatives in husband-wife families, the rates are unusually high in families of size 3.

Several studies of psychiatric admission rates have focused primarily on family variables. However, none were conducted in such a way as to permit a direct comparison of results with those of the present study. For example, in an analysis of family data on patients admitted to a Canadian mental hospital, Gregory (1959) used family of origin rather than family members living together at time of admission.

In a study of admission rates to psychiatric hospitals in Australia, Lindsay (1964) found that the rates decreased with increasing family size. Although this study employed a similar definition of family, rates were not computed specifically according to relationship to family head. Ferber and his associates (1966) found that persons in intact families were underrepresented and those from nonintact families or from nonfamily households were overrepresented among admissions to a large psychiatric emergency service in a general hospital. This is consistent with the finding in the present study that, regardless of relationship to the head, rates are higher for persons in families with a female head than those in husband-wife families. In spite of the fact that Ferber's study included patients admitted to only one specific type of psychiatric service, these results present further evidence that members of broken families are subject to high risk of coming under psychiatric care and that this group warrants further study to identify factors related to the etiology of mental disorders.

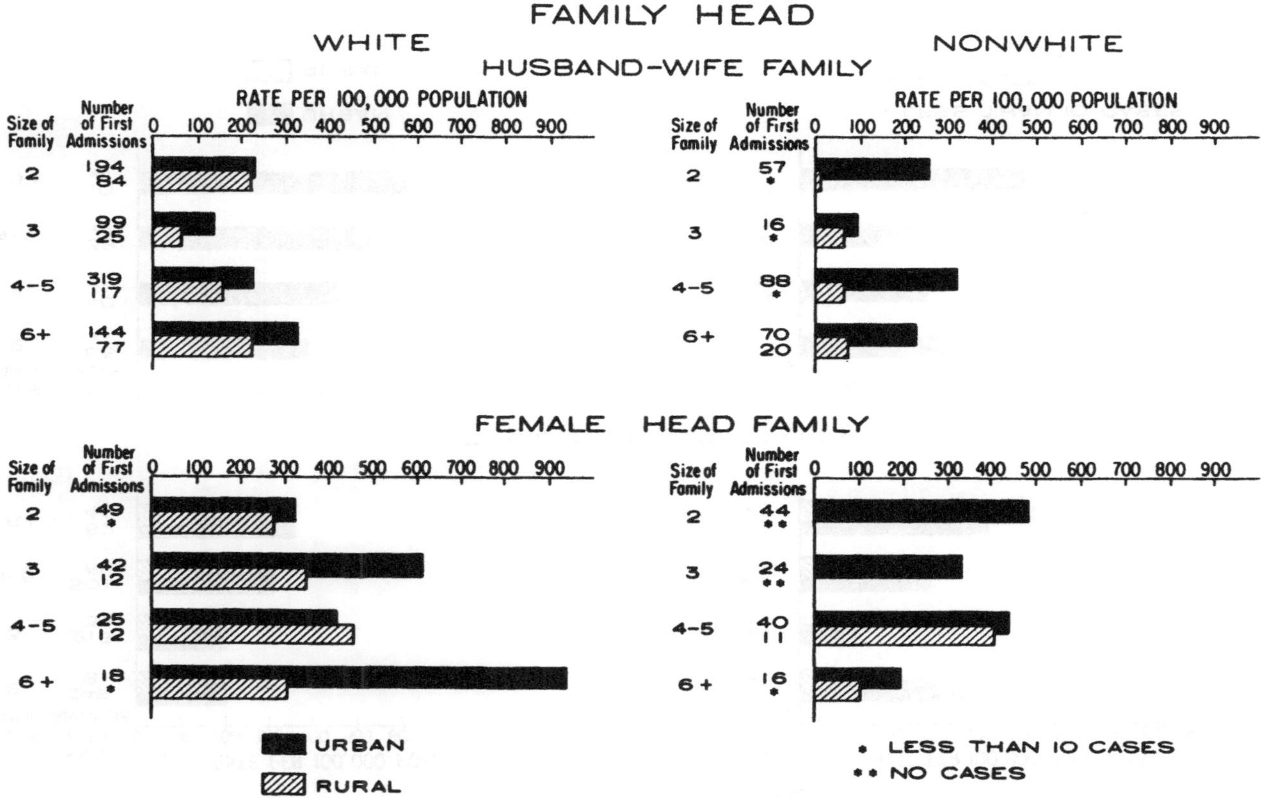

Fig. 6.13. Age-adjusted first admission rates per 100,000 population to psychiatric facilities for family heads, by family size, type of family, color, and residence: Louisiana, 1960-61.

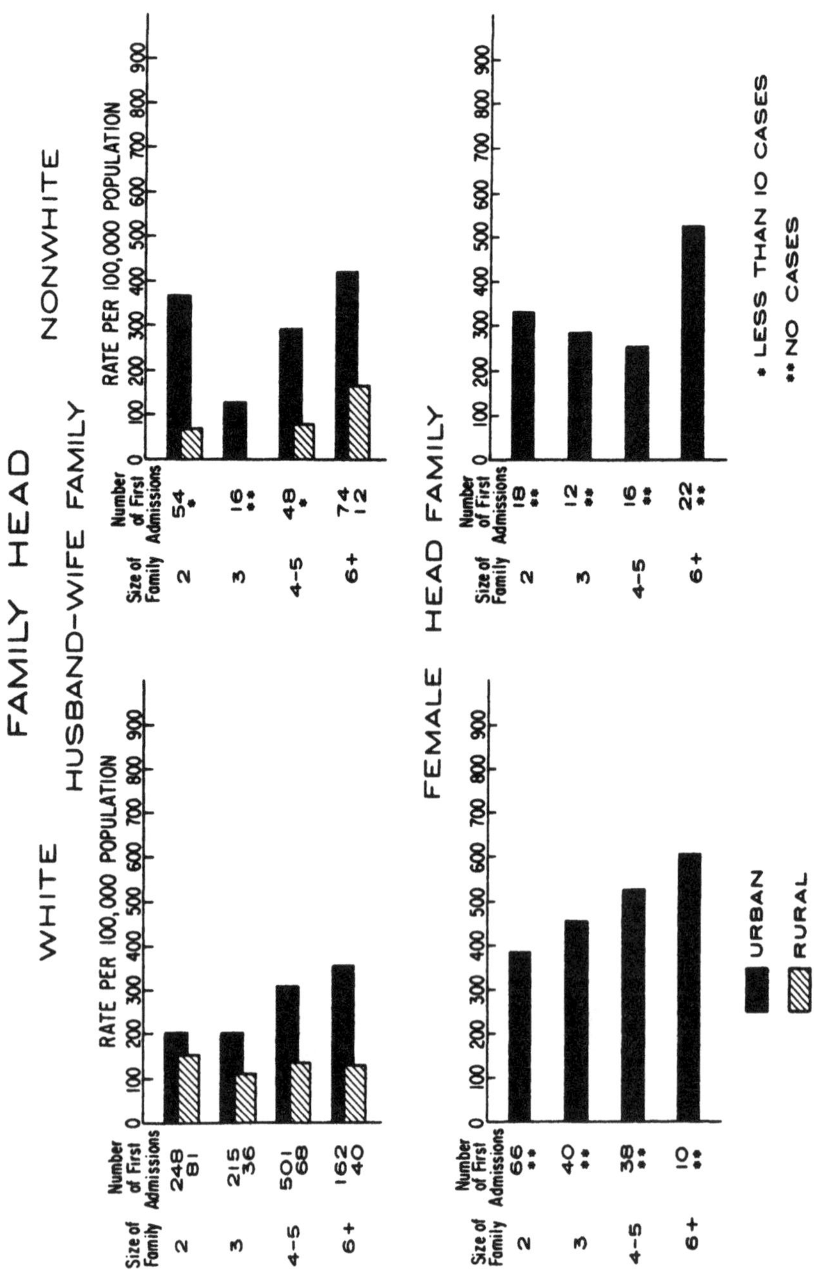
FAMILY HEAD
WHITE
NONWHITE
HUSBAND-WIFE FAMILY
FEMALE HEAD FAMILY
Size of Family
Number of First Admissions
RATE PER 100,000 POPULATION
0 100 200 300 400 500 600 700 800 900
2 248 81
3 215 36
4-5 501 68
6+ 162 40
2 54 *
3 16 **
4-5 48 *
6+ 74 12
2 66 **
3 40 **
4-5 38 **
6+ 10 **
2 18 **
3 12 **
4-5 16 **
6+ 22 **
URBAN
RURAL
* LESS THAN 10 CASES
** NO CASES

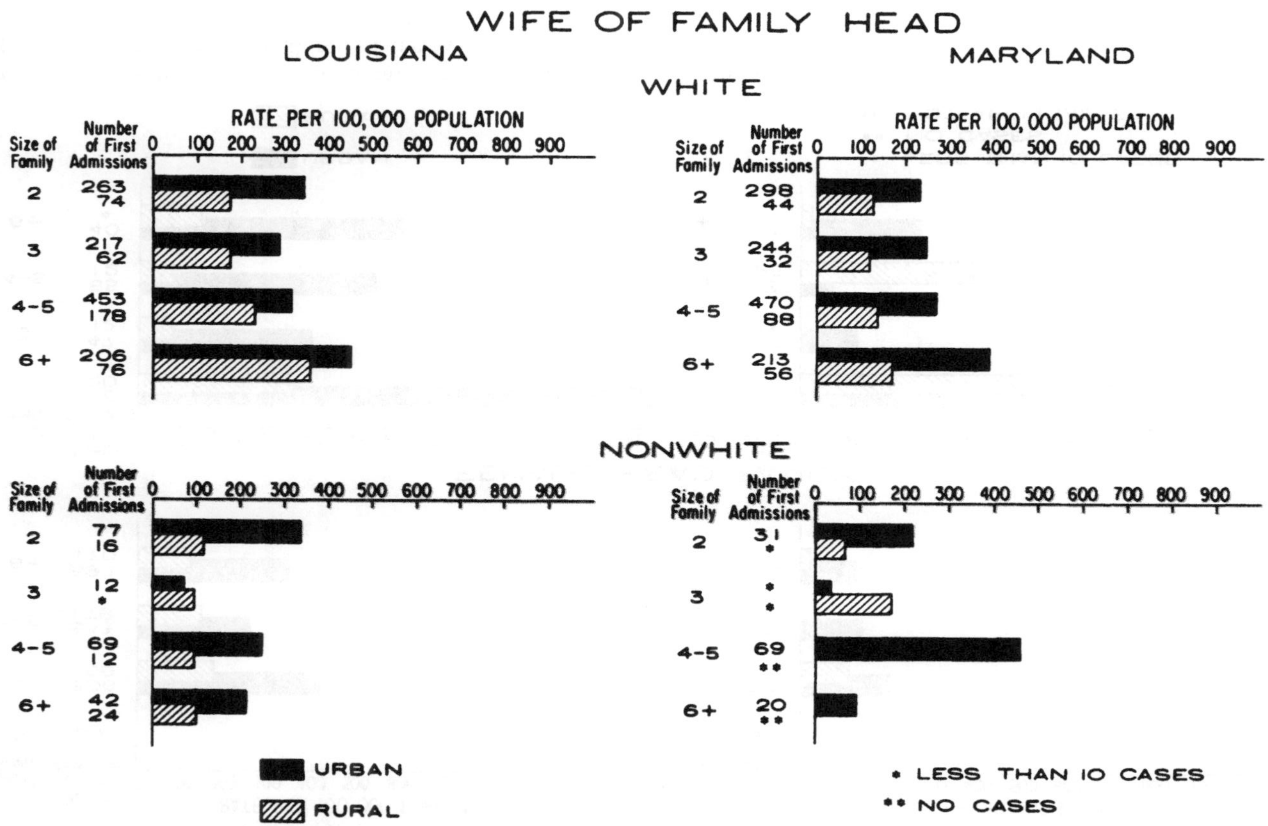

Fig. 6.15. Age-adjusted first admission rates per 100,000 population to psychiatric facilities for wives of family heads, by family size, color, and residence, Maryland and Louisiana, 1960-61.

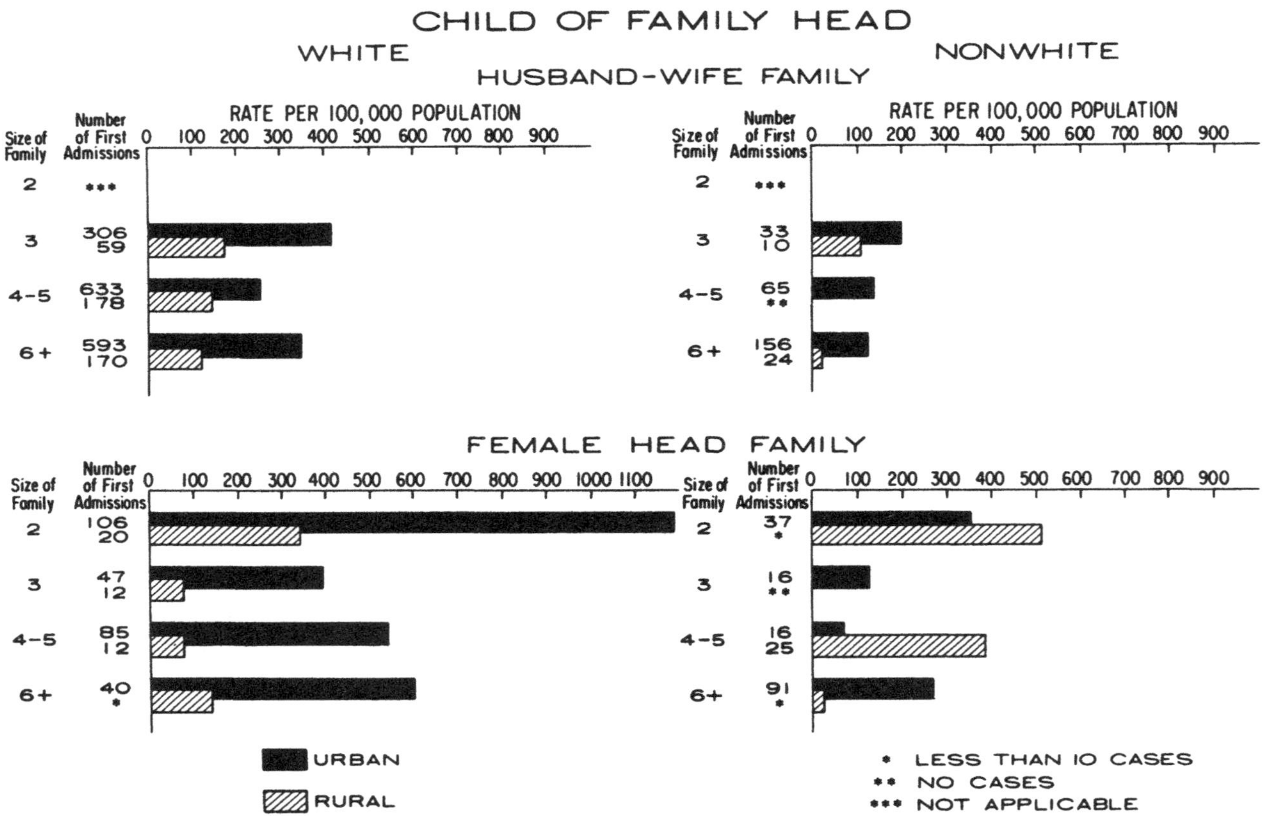

Fig. 6.16. Age-adjusted first admission rates per 100,000 population to psychiatric facilities for children of family heads, by family size, type of family, color, and residence: Louisiana, 1960-61.

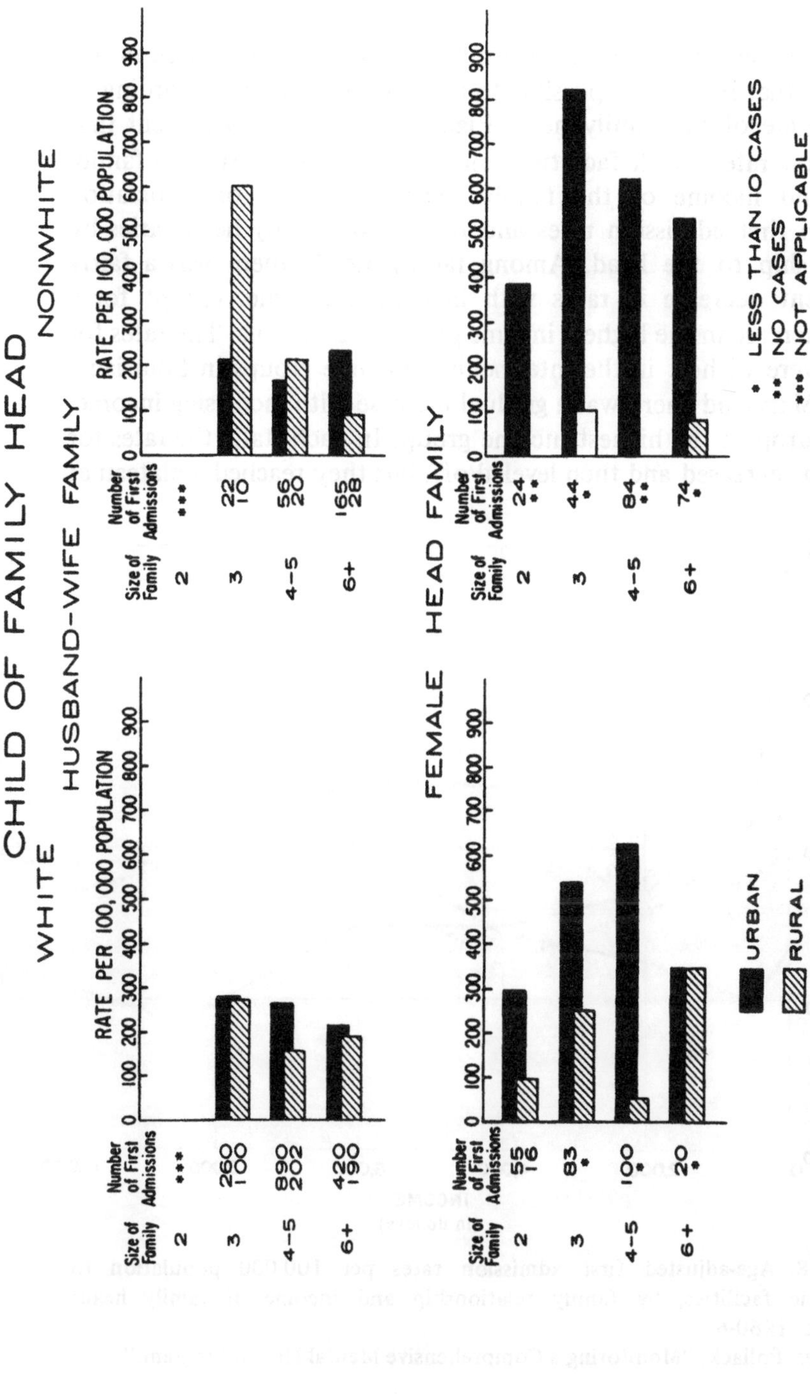

Fig. 6.17. Age-adjusted first admission rates per 100,000 population to psychiatric facilities for children of family heads, by family size, type of family, color, and residence: Maryland, 1960-61.

Income

One of the advantages of the census matching procedure used in this study is that it makes it possible to classify each patient according to the income of the family head. Figures 6.18 and 6.19 present first admission rates to all facilities combined by relationship to family head and income of the family head. The kind of association between first admission rates and income of family head varies by relationship to the head. Among family heads there was a fairly consistent decrease in rates with increasing income, except for a slight increase in the highest income group in Louisiana. The rates for wives were highest in the intermediate income groups in Louisiana, but in Maryland there was a gradual increase with increasing income, with a drop at the highest income group. In each state, the rates for children increased and then leveled off, but they reached a plateau at

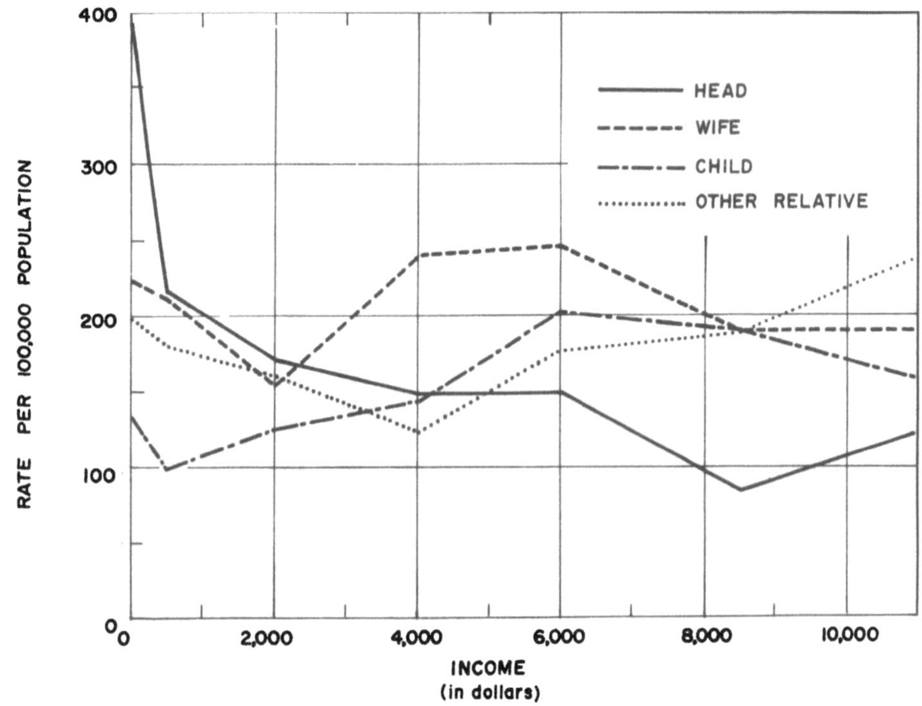

Fig. 6.18. Age-adjusted first admission rates per 100,000 population to psychiatric facilities, by family relationship and income of family head: Louisiana, 1960-61.

Source: Pollack, "Monitoring a Comprehensive Mental Health Program."

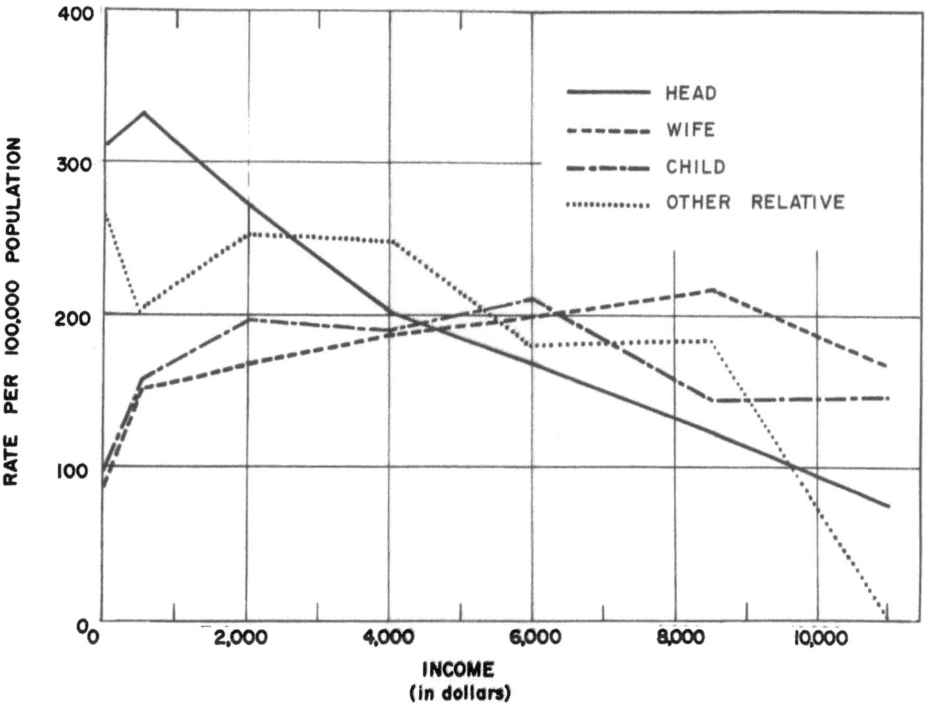

Fig. 6.19. Age-adjusted first admission rates per 100,000 population to psychiatric facilities, by family relationship and income of family head: Maryland, 1960-61.

Source: Pollack, "Monitoring a Comprehensive Mental Health Program."

a much lower income level in Maryland. Among other relatives, the Louisiana rates declined to a low at the $4,000 group, after which they increased consistently. In Maryland, on the other hand, the rates for other relatives showed a generally decreasing trend with increasing income.

Patients were also classified according to total family income, which included all of the income earned by members of the family in which the patient was living. Figures 6.20 and 6.21 present age-adjusted first admission rates to psychiatric facilities for Louisiana and Maryland, respectively, by family income, according to the relationship to family head. In general, the patterns according to family income are quite similar to those according to income of family head. The most notable exceptions to this were in Maryland, where the rates for family heads peaked in the $6,000-$7,999 group and the rates for wives peaked in the $4,000-$5,999 group.

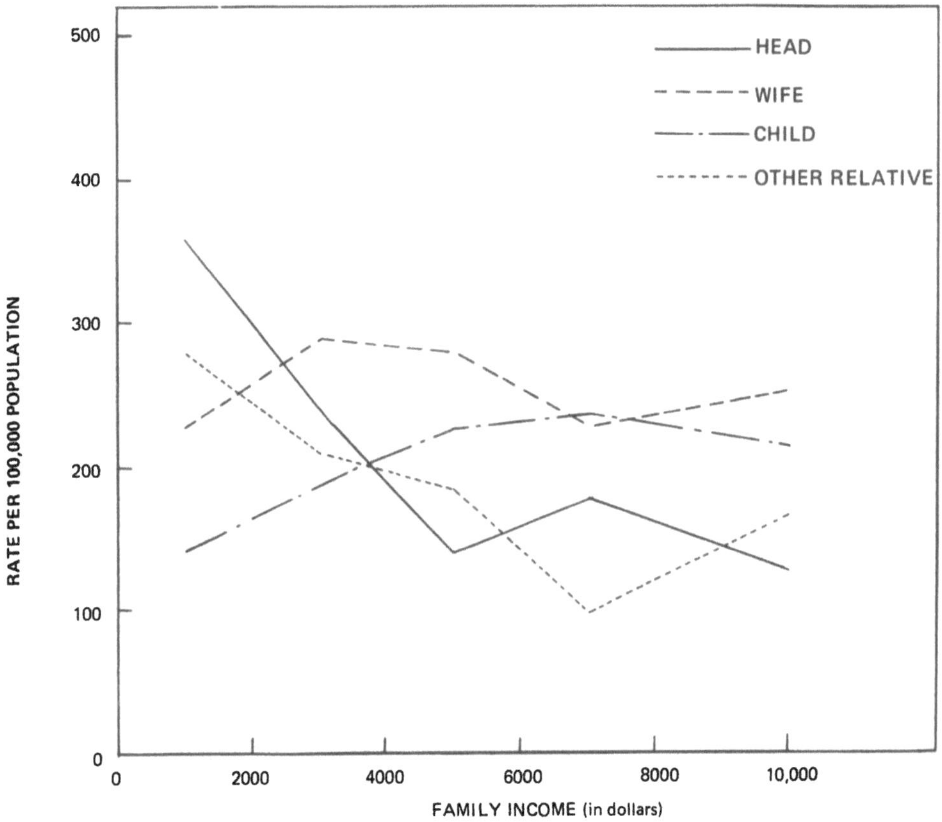

Fig. 6.20. Age-adjusted first admission rates per 100,000 population to psychiatric facilities, by family relationship and family income: Louisiana, 1960-61.

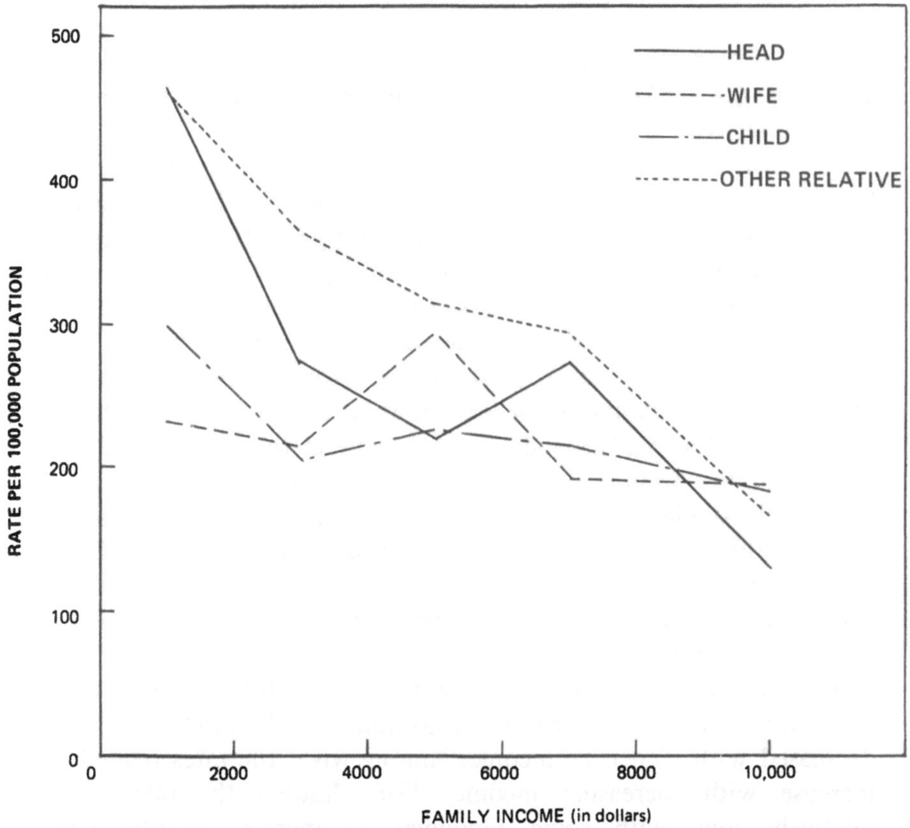

Fig. 6.21. Age-adjusted first admission rates per 100,000 population to psychiatric facilities, by family relationship and family income: Maryland, 1960-61.

Some more striking patterns of first admission rates by family income became apparent when the data were examined according to selected diagnostic groups, as indicated in Table 6.7 for Louisiana and Table 6.8 for Maryland. Some of the more prominent features of these patterns are as follows:

1. *Diseases of the senium* In both states, the first admission rates for "other relatives" were highest of all of the family relationship groups, and in each state these rates dropped off in the highest income categories. This group is undoubtedly heavily weighted with elderly parents of the family heads or of their spouses.

2. *Schizophrenic reactions* The rates for family heads were highest in the less than $2,000 income group in both states and dropped off to a minimum in the $8,000 and over category. Among wives, the rates in Maryland were very low in the less than $2,000 group and the $8,000 and over group, while in Louisiana the rates were fairly stable over the entire range (ranging between 32 and 53 per 100,000). Among children, the Louisiana rates were fairly constant but dropped off in the $8,000 and over group, while in Maryland the rate was high in the less than $2,000 group and fairly constant thereafter.

3. *Psychoneurotic reactions* The patterns in first admission rates were quite similar in both states. Among family heads, the rates decreased with increasing income. Among wives the rates tended to increase with increasing income. For children the rates were relatively low, with some tendency to increase slightly with increasing income, but in Louisiana the rate dropped in the $8,000 and over group.

4. *Personality disorders* Among family heads the Maryland rates decreased consistently with increasing income, while in Louisiana the rates were highest in the lower income categories and consistently low in the higher income categories. For wives the Louisiana rates showed a peak in the middle of the income range, whereas in Maryland the rate was highest in the less than $2,000 category. Among children the Louisiana rates tended to increase with increasing income, while this trend was not as pronounced in Maryland.

The interpretations which could be made of the differentials in first admission rates according to income for the various relationship groups are not at all clear. Very little data can be found in the literature on the "incidence" of treated mental illness according to

Table 6.7 Age-adjusted first admission rates per 100,000 population to all psychiatric facilities by diagnosis, relationship to family head, and income of family head: Louisiana, 1960-61

Diagnosis and relationship to family head	Total		Income of family head				
	Number	Rate	Under $2000	$2000-3999	$4000-5999	$6000-7999	$8000 and over
Alcoholism							
Head	256	32.9	35.8	32.5	34.5	29.3	28.2
Wife	33	5.5	9.2	2.8	3.5	4.2	4.1
Child	39	3.1	1.7	1.4	3.2	12.8	1.8
Other	16	7.1	22.3	0.0	0.0	0.0	13.4
Senium							
Head	76	10.4	17.8	8.5	5.7	0.0	6.1
Wife	49	8.8	10.2	11.2	7.1	0.0	8.2
Child	4	a	a	a	a	a	a
Other	55	34.4	28.9	40.1	77.2	9.1	12.8
Schizophrenia							
Head	262	33.4	88.8	37.3	18.2	22.0	6.9
Wife	294	43.1	50.3	43.8	53.6	35.8	32.0
Child	352	26.4	26.0	34.8	26.0	27.5	14.7
Other	119	51.8	114.4	52.5	24.4	13.6	48.6
Psychoneurosis							
Head	440	56.5	98.8	64.6	39.7	49.5	44.7
Wife	742	110.4	66.9	108.5	117.8	122.4	136.8
Child	242	18.1	13.1	18.9	21.6	21.9	15.8
Other	40	18.0	0.0	7.3	29.0	24.8	34.4
Personality disorder							
Head	202	25.1	35.4	37.0	14.4	14.0	15.7
Wife	142	20.6	17.0	34.2	20.4	11.8	10.0
Child	330	24.2	11.5	11.5	34.2	26.2	44.4
Other	38	12.5	20.1	22.3	0.0	12.4	0.0

[a] Rates were not computed when the total number of cases was less than ten.

Table 6.8 Age-adjusted first admission rates per 100,000 population to all psychiatric facilities by diagnosis, relationship to family head, and income of family head: Maryland, 1960-61

Diagnosis and relationship to family head	Total		Income of family head				
	Number	Rate	Under $2000	$2000-3999	$4000-5999	$6000 7999	$8000 and over
Alcoholism							
Head	272	34.4	22.5	54.6	32.7	49.5	20.3
Wife	87	13.0	18.9	24.5	12.8	8.2	11.9
Child	94	7.7	8.8	10.8	8.5	5.6	7.3
Other	70	30.4	27.9	31.9	21.1	54.8	24.3
Senium							
Head	110	17.8	51.4	23.6	11.9	10.9	4.6
Wife	33	6.8	12.2	3.2	0.0	0.0	14.0
Child	8	a	a	a	a	a	a
Other	168	85.4	182.7	108.5	137.1	73.5	45.9
Schizophrenia							
Head	226	27.9	80.9	29.2	30.1	29.6	15.2
Wife	289	41.2	3.0	51.6	65.3	55.5	17.5
Child	340	28.0	67.5	21.7	27.3	33.1	21.6
Other	87	38.5	36.2	56.7	66.9	36.8	22.2
Psychoneurosis							
Head	465	59.1	123.5	53.4	54.2	77.1	41.7
Wife	548	80.0	17.8	60.0	119.5	72.9	75.4
Child	239	19.8	9.4	9.9	15.9	21.3	25.5
Other	28	12.2	0.0	0.0	30.9	0.0	15.2
Personality disorder							
Head	281	35.4	80.9	55.0	34.9	30.0	12.4
Wife	135	19.1	68.2	20.6	8.2	11.4	23.7
Child	502	41.6	29.2	39.4	50.5	29.4	45.2
Other	50	22.4	53.0	55.4	32.7	0.0	18.4

[a] Rates were not computed when the total number of cases was less than ten.

income or socioeconomic status. Hollingshead and Redlich (1958) presented such rates for specific social classes. Lowest income individuals were found in Class V and highest income persons in Class I. The "incidence" rate for these socioeconomic classes occurred in the following order: Class V (139 per 100,000), Class III (114), Class I – II (97), and Class IV (89). Thus, no clearcut trend existed in the relationship between the "incidence" rate and social class. Some more definite relationship may have emerged had it been possible to compute "incidence" rates for specific subgroups within each social class.

The fact that conclusions may be altered by examining rates in more detail may be illustrated by considering the patterns mentioned above in rates of first admission for diseases of the senium, according to family income, among other relatives of the family head. While the age-adjusted rates indicated similar patterns for the two states, with the Maryland rates higher than those for Louisiana, examination of rates specific for sex among those 65 and over revealed that females had higher rates in Louisiana, whereas in Maryland the reverse was true. Futhermore, upon examining these specific rates for individual income categories, it was found that the two states differed in the income category in which the highest rates occurred. This suggests that, while elderly relatives of family heads were admitted to psychiatric facilities at higher rates than other family members with diseases of the senium in both states, there were differences in the two states in the way psychiatric facilities were used by these individuals. This is undoubtedly a reflection of the differential availability of nursing home facilities between the two states, accounting for the lower rates in Louisiana.

Educational Level

The age-adjusted first admission rates to psychiatric facilities according to educational level of family head are shown by relationship to family head and type of family for Louisiana and Maryland in Tables 6.9 and 6.10 respectively. While no consistent patterns are evident across all relationship groups and between states, the following facts seem to emerge:

1. Among family heads, the rates were lowest among those with four or more years of college, for each state and regardless of type of family.

Table 6.9 Age-adjusted first admission rates per 100,000 population to all psychiatric facilities according to educational level of family head by type of family and relationship to family head: Louisiana, 1960-61

Type of family and relationship to family head	Total		Elementary		High school		College	
	Number	Rate	Less than 8 yrs.	8 years	1-3 years	4 years	1-3 years	4 years or more
All families								
Head	1707	219.6	241.1	239.2	247.0	167.1	326.9	109.4
Wife	1713	257.6	216.6	258.4	292.2	327.0	208.7	196.7
Child	2751	202.8	182.6	218.5	240.2	196.1	246.4	142.7
Other relation	498	220.0	229.1	113.4	243.6	228.7	236.0	393.8
Husband-wife families								
Head	1327	198.0	208.3	212.2	199.8	172.5	320.1	108.9
Wife	1713	257.6	216.6	258.4	292.2	327.0	208.7	196.7
Child	2192	193.0	179.7	207.1	223.9	171.4	247.2	108.7
Other relation	258	197.3	153.9	111.6	282.4	226.9	275.9	436.0
Other male head families								
Head	74	353.6	482.4	252.8	469.1	176.0	0.0	0.0
Child	63	210.5	178.9	524.4	42.9	194.9	736.4	0.0
Other relation	52	203.2	214.4	135.7	401.9	97.2	0.0	247.5
Female head families								
Head	306	372.8	405.4	436.8	577.3	125.9	525.0	104.7
Child	496	271.6	203.0	291.1	302.0	431.6	294.5	706.1
Other relation	188	268.4	371.7	98.5	144.3	258.0	208.5	243.3

Table 6.10 Age-adjusted first admission rates per 100,000 population to all psychiatric facilities according to educational level of family head by type of family and relationship to family head: Maryland, 1960-61

Type of family and relationship to family head	Total		Elementary		High school		College	
	Number	Rate	Less than 8 yrs.	8 years	1-3 years	4 years	1-3 years	4 years or more
All families								
Head	1868	240.3	245.7	323.3	242.3	259.8	235.1	159.6
Wife	1509	224.4	207.2	233.4	251.7	205.8	225.4	227.7
Child	2714	225.0	266.7	253.7	208.3	208.9	296.2	167.9
Other relation	617	285.2	311.7	260.2	278.6	373.8	227.7	108.3
Husband-wife families								
Head	1526	224.3	220.5	311.2	219.2	236.6	225.5	150.3
Wife	1509	224.4	207.2	233.4	251.7	205.8	225.4	227.7
Child	2241	214.5	255.5	230.3	192.5	207.3	299.7	154.6
Other relation	332	253.0	225.7	300.9	203.3	466.4	312.7	29.6
Other male head families								
Head	120	601.8	685.3	246.0	1093.2	277.4	0.0	815.0
Child	40	181.0	177.9	266.6	32.5	0.0	801.8	520.5
Other relation	94	319.1	450.2	0.0	488.4	122.9	0.0	0.0
Female head families								
Heads	222	350.1	318.1	547.4	323.3	395.7	424.0	0.0
Child	433	359.3	397.7	519.2	325.9	257.5	302.1	542.6
Other relation	191	327.5	422.5	288.7	330.1	257.6	87.3	392.7

2. Among wives of family heads, rates were lowest among those whose husbands had four or more years of college in Louisiana, while for Maryland, the rates were amazingly stable across all educational levels.

3. Among children in each state, rates were lowest for those in husband-wife families in which the father had four or more years of college. Children of female heads with four or more years of college, on the other hand, had the highest rates among children in each state.

The finding of low rates of admission to psychiatric facilities among those with high educational level appears quite consistently in the literature. In a study in Monroe County, New York, Bodian et al. (1963) showed that among census tracts with high median educational level over half had low rates of admission of schizophrenics to psychiatric facilities and only 3 percent of these tracts had high rates. For each of the diagnostic groups studied by Locke in Ohio, the results of which are presented in Chapter 5, the lowest rates occurred among those with college education. In Jaco's study (1959) in Texas, on the other hand, admission rates for psychosis were found to be highest among those with no education and next highest among those with some college. However, educational level was very incompletely reported, particularly among Anglo-Americans.

It is indeed difficult to generalize on the basis of comparisons of the findings of the various studies. Educational level was measured in different ways, the universe of psychiatric facilities varied, different diagnostic groupings were used, and the way in which results were reported mitigated against truly valid comparisons.

DISCUSSION

In Chapter 4 it was pointed out that patterns of use of psychiatric facilities are a function of many complex variables and that the way in which these variables operate is influenced by demographic and socioeconomic characteristics of the patients and the populations from which they come. The rates at which patients were admitted to psychiatric facilities according to some demographic and socioeconomic variables were presented in this chapter for Louisiana and Maryland. Because most of the data were based on a 25 percent sample, however, it was not feasible to present rates for detailed cross-classifications of the variables, such as for specific types of psychiatric facilities or for specific psychiatric diagnoses. Nevertheless, the data presented above have provided some indication of demographic and socioeconomic factors associated with high risk of coming under psychiatric care.

In spite of the fact that the rates presented in this chapter pertain to only two states, it is tempting to generalize from them to all states. Some of the problems in doing so may be illustrated by a particular example. The age-specific first admission rates to the various types of psychiatric facilities are presented for each of the two states in Figure 6.22. The top line in the graph for each state represents the rate of first admission to all facilities combined. The shape and level of these two lines are remarkably similar for the two states. with two notable exceptions – the adolescent group and those aged 65 and over.

On the one hand, these two exceptions illustrate the value of interstate comparisons, but on the other, they indicate the problems in generalizing from rates based on only one state. It is only by comparing data for the two states that it became apparent that admission rates were unusually low in the adolescent group and in the age group 65 and over in Louisiana. The greater availability of outpatient psychiatric clinics in Maryland with their greater orientation toward services to children compared with other facilities undoubtedly accounted for the higher rate in the adolescent group.

The unusually low first admission rate to state mental hospitals in the age group 65 and over was undoubtedly influenced by extensive public assistance for the aged in Louisiana. At the time of this study, a state could receive federal Old Age Assistance funds for payment to aged individuals who were mentally ill only if they were placed in private, nonmedical nursing homes or if they remained at home. A study of trends in hospitalization of the aged mentally ill revealed that the greater the recipient rate for Old Age Assistance in a state, the lower the rate of first admissions to a state mental hospital (H.E.W., 1961). This is due perhaps to a greater use of nursing homes as an alternative for care or greater willingness on the part of families in states with high recipient rates to maintain the senile psychotic at home. Since the recipient rate in 1961 in Louisiana was 12 times that in Maryland (508 per 1,000 persons 65 years of age and over in Louisiana, compared with 41 in Maryland), this factor could account for Louisiana's low mental hospital first admission rate in that age

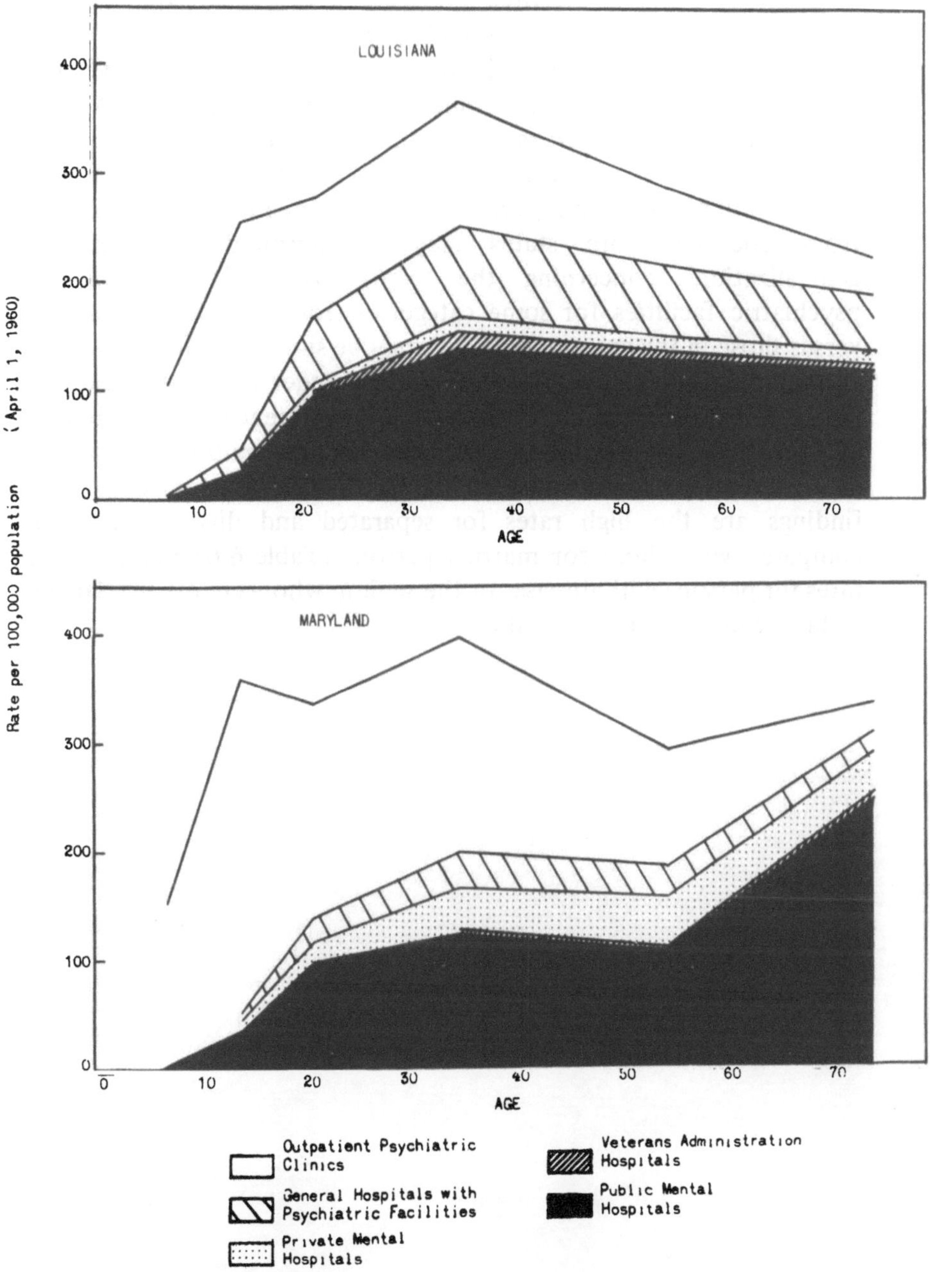

Fig. 6.22. First admissions per 100,000 population to psychiatric facilities, by type of facility and age: Louisiana and Maryland, 1960-61.

group. The evidence presented above seems to indicate that at least for certain age groups of the population the availability of facilities for the care of the mentally ill and the existence of alternatives for care, such as nursing homes and boarding homes, may exert a considerable influence on rates of admission to psychiatric facilities. To the extent that such availability of facilities varies among states, generalizations concerning *levels* of admission rates based on data from one or more states may be unsound. Furthermore, generalizations concerning the *relative risk* of admission to psychiatric facilities for some categories (for example, adolescents versus those in the age group 25-34) may be similarly affected.

Some of the relative risks of coming under psychiatric care as indicated by the study do not appear to be influenced by differences in availability of psychiatric facilities and generalizations can be made, therefore, with considerable confidence. Examples of such findings are the high rates for separated and divorced persons compared with those for married persons (Table 6.6) and the high rates for persons with diseases of the senium who were other relatives of family heads (Tables 6.7 and 6.8).

7 / Suicide

Suicide ranked twelfth among the leading causes of death in the United States in 1967. It was pointed out in Chapter 1 that there were 21,325 deaths from suicide during that year, but this number was probably underreported by one-fourth to one-third (Dublin, 1963). In addition, it has been estimated that each year there are between 175,000 and 200,000 persons who attempt suicide (Schneidman and Farberow, 1961). These estimates of attempted suicides and underreporting of completed suicides indicate the serious magnitude of this problem.

The suicide problem is further compounded by the fact that. unlike death from an organic disease, for which the intermediate processes and primary causes leading to death are more or less traceable, death by suicide is a psychological act which can be analyzed only with great difficulty. Thus, Rosenbaum (1967) points out that "although almost all persons who attempt or commit suicide are ill (94 percent psychiatrically ill and 4 percent physically ill, according to one survey). it by no means follows that suicide or its attempt can be considered to be a clinical entity. The clinical entity comprising the highest incidence of suicide is psychotic depression, incorporating the manic-depressive, involutional, and late-life depressions," but, he continues, "when the depression is 'masked' by physical symptoms, its recognition becomes more difficult."

Grinker (1967), presenting a similar viewpoint, states that "there are a variety of clinical entities, of situations. and of personality characteristics associated with suicide. This act is a final common pathway of several, if not many, dynamic processes which can be explained by no simple stereotype. Specific economic and structural characteristics may be essential precursors, but the dynamics culminating in the final act are probably diverse. This makes it all the more difficult to determine the mental mechanisms directly involved in suicide." In view of these difficulties and as a means of trying to overcome them, various efforts have been made over the years to develop theoretical approaches to the study of suicide which have utilized either separately or in combination social and/or psychological factors as causative explanations for the act of suicide. Illustrative of some of these varying approaches are the contributions of Durkheim, Freud, and Henry and Short.

A first major effort in approaching the problem of suicide from a sociological point of view was made by Durkheim (1951) at the end of the last century. His primary interest was not in the internal forces which motivate individuals but in the forces of society which affect the individual's actions. This led him to classify suicides into three social categories, which, briefly described, are: (1) *egoistic suicide,* resulting when the individual is not strongly integrated into his society; (2) *altruistic suicide,* wherein there is excessive integration of the individual with society and he sacrifices himself, such as the soldier in battle; and (3) *anomic suicide,* in which the individual's adjustment to or integration with society is disrupted or unbalanced, as might occur, for example, in times of economic depression. The essence of Durkheim's contribution was to introduce the social dimension into the problem of suicide. "He showed," as Hendin (1965) points out, "that suicide, like crime, neurosis and alcoholism, is a factor that measures social pressure and tension."

Many of the subsequent sociological investigators of the phenomenon extended and refined Durkheim's original contribution, concentrating on studies of the ecologic distribution of suicide and on the relationship between suicide and the business cycle (Cavan, 1928; Sainsbury, 1955; Schmid, 1928). Whereas Durkheim exhibited neither interest in nor orientation toward the psychological aspects of suicide. Freud displayed a similar disregard for the social aspects and presented the first important psychological insight into the phenomenon. In his publication "Mourning and Melancholia." Freud (1916) posited that the self-hatred seen in depression originated in anger toward a love object which the individual then turned back upon himself. Suicide was regarded as the ultimate form of this phenomenon – a kind of inverted murder. Freud viewed instincts as having no societal boundaries, a frame of reference which precluded any concern with the psychological impact of the social institutions of particular cultures or with such questions as to why suicide rates varied from country to country (Hendin, 1965). The latter was of concern to Durkheim, who theorized that "social facts," as for example suicide, were a function of social institutions, which, in turn, were a function of a particular society or culture (Hendin, 1965).

Although both Durkheim's and Freud's theoretical concepts must be regarded as major contributions to the problem of understanding the complex phenomenon of suicide, Hendin (1965) indicates that "neither approach by itself is adequate. A sociological approach provides no way of evaluating the relative impact of different social pressures and tends to be blind or at best weak in seeing how social forces are integrated by the individual personality. On the other hand, psychiatric thinking that starts with the individual and never leaves the individual can be equally blind in understanding the specific psychosocial attitudes within the culture and the role they play in shaping the individual personality."

One attempt to synthesize the various sociological and psychological theories about suicide within a single conceptual framework has been made by Henry and Short (1957), who said: "sociologic evidence suggests that suicide is a form of aggression against the self aroused by some frustration, the cause of which is perceived by the person as lying within the self." As with the theories of Durkheim and Freud, the theoretical concepts advanced by Henry and Short have undergone close examination, creating both adherents as well as critics, from whom a considerable body of additional studies on the nature and circumstances of suicide has developed. It is not possible within the confines and purposes of this chapter to review all of this literature, but reference will be made to various of these studies as they may relate to the materials to be presented. It is apparent, however, that serious problems in classifying suicides and suicidal behavior exist and that mortality data provide only a partial picture of the problem.

Since the general purpose of this monograph series is to serve as a source of morbidity and mortality data which will reflect in some detail the health status of the population, the discussion of suicide in this chapter will be oriented largely toward a description of the incidence of this phenomenon among population groups defined by various demographic and socioeconomic variables, as well as an examination of the national trends in suicide over time and some reference to international differences in suicide rates. The census year 1960 will serve as the base time period for which data will be presented. The source of these data are special detailed tabulations on suicide made available for this monograph by the National Center for Health Statistics (N.C.H.S.) for the three-year period 1959-1961. These data will be supplemented with more recent as well as earlier suicide data from various N.C.H.S. publications and from studies carried out by other investigators.

DEMOGRAPHIC VARIABLES AND SUICIDE

Age, Sex, and Color

Data in Table 7.1, some of which are illustrated in Figure 7.1, show the striking variations in suicide rates for the different sex-color groups by age in the three-year period around 1960. Male rates exceeded female rates, and rates for the white population exceeded those for nonwhites at all ages, except under 15 years, where the rates were negligible. When broken down into sex-color groups, rates for nonwhite males are seen to almost approximate those for white males up through age group 25-34. They then taper off, however, and fluctuate only between 12 and 18 per 100,000 in subsequent age groups, whereas the rates for white males continue a pattern of steady, rapid increase in almost every succeeding age group. The age pattern of rates for white females, unlike that for white males, exhibits only a gradual increase up through age group 45-54, a leveling off in the 55-64 age group, and a gradual decline from that point on. Rates for nonwhite females are seen to be lowest and show little or no fluctuation by age, varying only between 3 and 4 per 100,000 for the age groups over 25 years.

In attempting to explain the striking difference noted between male and female suicide rates. attention is usually focussed on the difference between the male and the female roles in society. For

Table 7.1 Suicide rates per 100,000 population by age, color, and sex: United States, 1959-61

Age	All persons			White			Nonwhite		
	Total	Male	Female	Total	Male	Female	Total	Male	Female
All ages									
Crude	10.5	16.4	4.8	11.3	17.5	5.2	4.6	7.5	1.9
Age-adj.	10.5	16.6	4.9	11.0	17.3	5.2	5.5	9.1	2.3
Under 15	0.2	0.3	0.0	0.2	0.3	0.0	0.1	0.1	0.1
15-24	5.1	8.0	2.2	5.2	8.2	2.3	4.1	6.5	1.9
25-34	10.0	14.6	5.6	10.2	14.6	5.8	8.6	14.4	3.6
35-44	14.0	20.9	7.5	14.8	21.9	8.0	7.5	12.1	3.5
45-54	20.3	31.2	9.7	21.6	33.1	10.4	8.1	13.6	2.9
55-64	23.7	38.4	10.0	25.1	40.7	10.6	9.6	15.8	3.6
65-74	23.2	39.9	8.8	24.5	42.2	9.2	8.0	13.6	2.9
75-84	27.5	52.8	7.9	28.8	55.6	8.2	9.9	17.6	3.0
85 & over	25.6	58.1	4.9	27.1	62.4	4.0	7.9	12.8	4.1

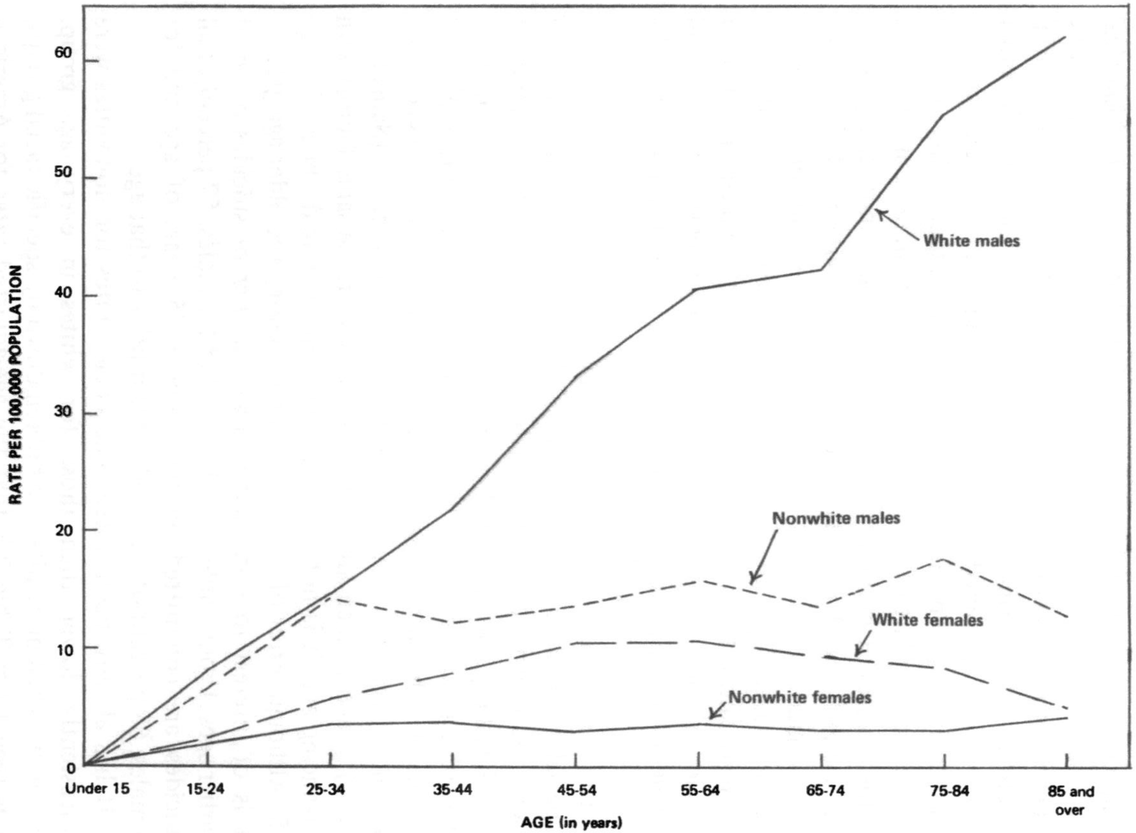

Fig. 7.1. Deaths from suicide per 100,000 population, by age, sex, and color: United States, 1959-61.

example, Sainsbury (1955) has pointed out that "when the biological and social roles of the two sexes are compared, the female role appears more precisely defined, and her biological and social functions more harmonized. That of the urban male, on the other hand, is less restricted by social conformity; in fact, an agressive individualism is encouraged in him. The responsibility for the support and welfare of his family devolves on him; he is more subject to the stresses of mobility and change. The male's more independent and arduous social role, as indicated by the marked liability of the male suicide rate in social and economic stresses and the frequency among males of causes of suicide related to problems of social readjustment, affords a likely explanation of the excess of male over female suicides." Some of these distinctions between male and female social roles are now becoming less clear-cut, and it may be necessary to look elsewhere for explanations.

The exceedingly high suicide rates in the older age groups, especially noted for white males, can be attributed to a number of social and individual factors which are most prevalent at this time of life. Sainsbury has indicated such social factors as social isolation, lack of employment and loss of status in society, and individual factors which encompass the higher incidence of depression and organic psychosis, physical illness, and bereavement (Sainsbury, 1962). Since women are exposed to some of these same factors with advancing age, it is not clear why their suicide rate declines after age 55. Although *rates* of suicide are higher among the older age groups, it is of interest to note that a larger *number* of suicides occur at earlier ages. From Table 7.2 it is seen that for males, 57 percent of all suicides are committed by those under 55 years of age and for females, 65 percent of all suicides occur prior to that age.

It has already been noted that suicide rates for nonwhites were consistently lower than those for whites in every age group. However, when nonwhites are broken down by specific racial groups, it is seen from Table 7.3 that the age-adjusted rates for American Indians and Chinese are higher than those for the white population whereas the rates for Japanese, Negroes, and other nonwhites are about the same as or lower than those for the white rate. This same pattern generally holds with respect to age-specific rates (see Table 7.3 and also Figure 7.2) with two major exceptions: (1) rates for Indians drop substantially below the white rates after age 55, and (2) the rates for Japanese 65 years and over are considerably higher than the white rates for this age group.

A comparison of the age-specific rates for the four nonwhite groups indicates the Negro rates were, in general, consistently the lowest and exhibited very little variation by age. The rates for Chinese and Japanese increased gradually up to age 55 and then rose precipitously from that age on. The Chinese rates were higher than the Japanese rates at every age level except 15-24 years. The rates for American Indians exceeded those of the other races in the 15-44 age span but then declined to about the level of the Negro rates after age 55.

Table 7.2 Percent distribution and cumulative percentage of suicides by age and sex: United States, 1959-61

Age (in years)	Percent distribution			Cumulative percent distribution		
	Total	Male	Female	Total	Male	Female
All ages	100.0	100.0	100.0	-	-	-
Under 15	0.5	0.5	0.3	0.5	0.5	0.3
15-24	6.4	6.5	6.1	6.9	7.0	6.4
25-34	12.1	11.3	14.7	19.0	18.3	21.1
35-44	17.9	17.0	20.9	36.9	35.3	42.0
45-54	22.0	21.8	22.8	58.9	57.1	64.8
55-64	19.6	20.0	18.2	78.5	77.1	83.0
65-74	13.5	14.1	11.7	92.0	91.2	94.7
75 & over	8.0	8.8	5.3	100.0	100.0	100.0

Table 7.3 Age-adjusted rates for suicide per 100,000 population for specific race groups by age: United States, 1959-61

Age (in years)	Nonwhite						White
	Total	Negro	American Indian	Japanese	Chinese	Other	
All ages	5.5	4.8	14.6	11.8	21.3	9.3	11.0
Under 15	0.1	0.1	0.0	0.0	0.0	0.2	0.2
15-24	4.1	3.5	17.9	7.4	7.3	7.8	5.2
25-34	8.6	7.9	30.6	7.5	16.5	10.3	10.2
35-44	7.6	6.8	23.4	10.7	21.4	9.8	14.8
45-54	8.1	7.4	15.7	14.5	30.7	13.4	21.6
55-64	9.4	8.4	6.9	27.7	48.2	13.8	25.1
65 & over	8.5	6.1	10.4	60.4	96.7	27.9	26.2

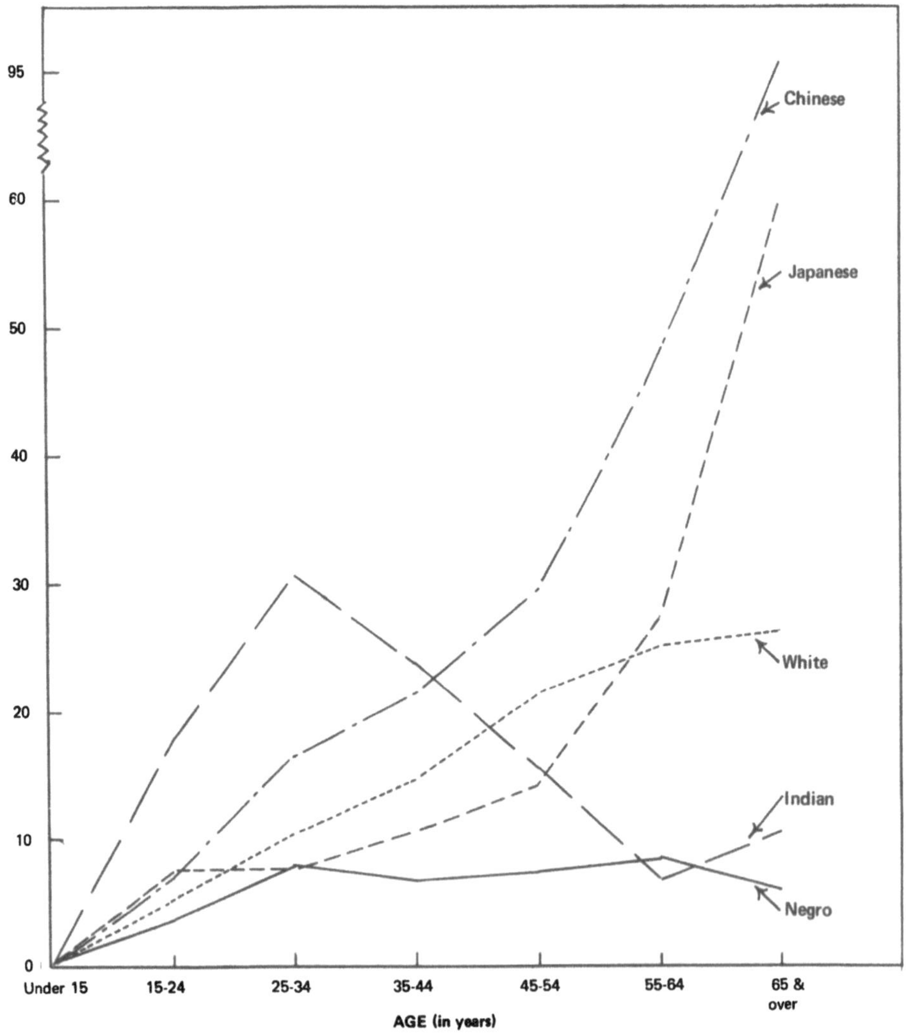

Fig. 7.2. Deaths from suicide per 100,000 population for selected race groups, by age: United States, 1959-61.

Dublin (1963), noting the variations in suicide rates among the different racial groups, states that "these differences do not suggest that the tendency to suicide is a heritable trait. It seems more probable that national and racial proclivities are the result of cultural factors." In another study, MacMahon and his associates (1963), using suicide data for the period 1948-1952, examined white and Negro rates for regions of the North and South as a means of offering some possible explanation for differences in these rates. They observed that "in the two southern regions (South Atlantic and East South Central combined), in which nonwhite population is almost exclusively Negro, rates for whites were between 2 and 4 times as high as those for Negroes at all ages for both sexes. However, in two northern regions (Middle Atlantic and East North Central combined), which also have substantial and almost exclusively Negro nonwhite populations, rates for nonwhites up to age 35 are as high as those for whites and the differences after that age are not as great as in the south. Negro males show a somewhat greater tendency to approach rates of suicides in whites than do Negro females" (see Figure 7.3). Suicide rates computed for these same regional groupings from the 1959-1961 data, presented in Table 7.4 and Figure 7.4 show that the patterns of age-sex-race differentials in rates between the two areas are somewhat similar to those reported by MacMahon for the earilier period.

As a possible explanation for these observations. MacMahon et al. (1963) note that "they may relate to differences in the social and economic pressures experienced by Negroes in the North compared with those in the South, or they may be interpretable in terms of the known higher rates of suicide among migrants, in general, since a large proportion of the northern Negro population has migrated within a lifetime. However, whatever the specific explanation, the findings indicate that the difference between rates of suicide in Negroes and whites depends, at least in part, on environmental factors and not on any innate personal characteristics."

Nativity

The crude suicide rate for the foreign-born population in the United States in the period 1959-1961 was almost twice as high as that for the native-born population (Table 7.5). This was also true of the male and female rates for the two populations. However, when

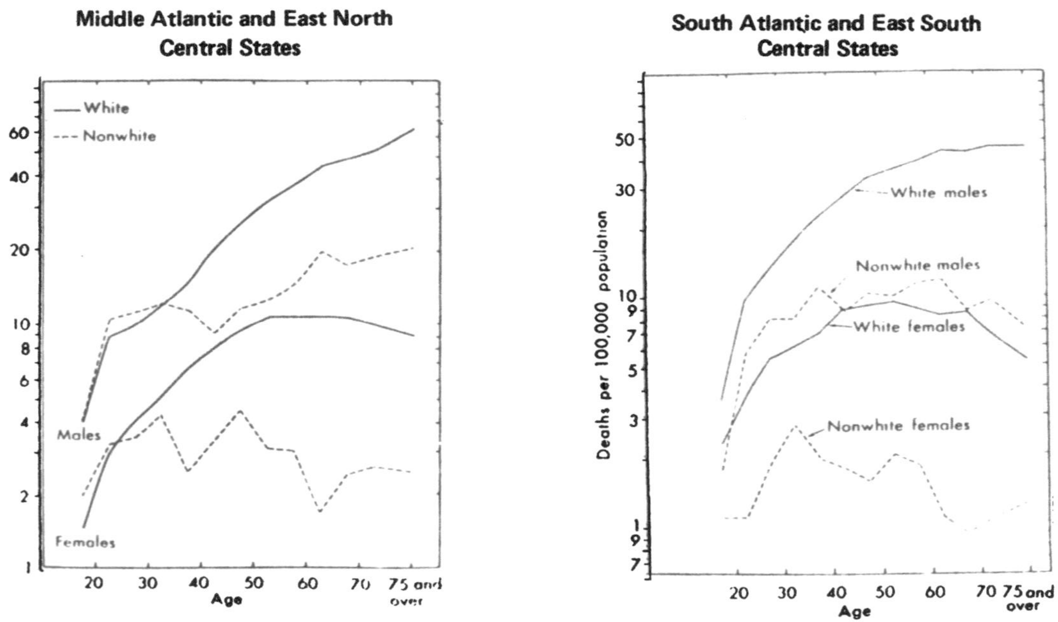

Fig. 7.3. Deaths from suicide per 100,000 population, by age, sex, and color: Middle Atlantic and East North Central states combined and South Atlantic and East South Central states combined, 1948-52.

Source: MacMahon, Brian, Johnson, Samuel, and Pugh. Thomas. *Relationship of Suicide to Social Conditions.* Public Health Reports, vol 78, no. 4, April 1963, figures 4 and 5.

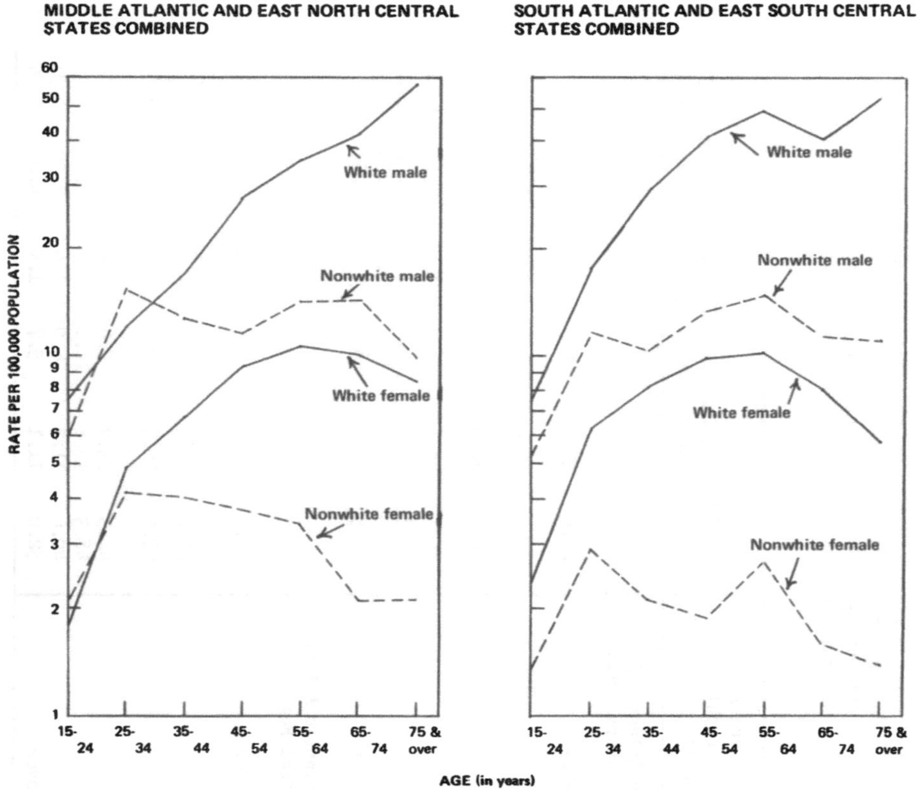

Fig. 7.4. Deaths from suicide per 100,000 population by age, sex, and color: Middle Atlantic and East North Central states combined and South Atlantic and East South Central states combined, 1959-61.

Table 7.4 Suicide rates per 100,000 population by age, color, and sex and ratios of white rates to nonwhite rates: Middle Atlantic and East North Central Regions combined and South Atlantic and East South Central Regions combined, 1959-61

Age in years and geographic areas	Male		Female		Ratio white to nonwhite	
	White	Nonwhite	White	Nonwhite	Male	Female
Middle Atlantic & E.N.Central Regions						
15 & over	22.6	11.9	6.9	3.4	1.89	2.03
15-24	7.5	6.0	1.8	2.1	1.25	.86
25-34	12.1	15.1	4.8	4.1	.80	1.17
35-44	16.8	12.8	6.8	4.0	1.31	1.70
45-54	27.4	11.3	9.2	3.7	2.42	2.49
55-64	35.3	14.0	10.6	3.4	2.52	3.12
65-74	41.9	14.2	10.1	2.1	2.95	4.81
75 & over	57.5	9.7	8.4	2.1	5.93	4.00
So. Atlantic & E.S. Central Regions						
15 & over	28.2	10.3	6.9	2.0	2.74	3.45
15-24	7.5	5.3	2.4	1.4	1.42	1.71
25-34	17.7	11.7	6.3	2.9	1.51	2.17
35-44	29.0	10.3	8.2	2.1	2.82	3.90
45-54	41.3	13.3	9.8	1.9	3.11	5.16
55-64	48.3	14.8	10.1	2.7	3.26	3.74
65-74	40.6	11.3	6.9	1.6	3.59	4.31
75 & over	52.0	11.1	5.7	1.4	4.68	4.07

Table 7.5 Suicide rates per 100,000 population by nativity, age, and sex for white persons: United States, 1959-61

Age in years	Native-born			Foreign-born		
	Both Sexes	Male	Female	Both Sexes	Male	Female
All ages						
Crude	10.5	16.3	4.9	21.7	34.3	9.8
Age-adjusted	10.8	17.2	5.0	11.1	16.6	6.0
Under 15	0.2	0.3	0.0	0.4	0.7	0.0
15-24	5.1	8.0	2.2	6.2	9.8	3.1
25-34	10.0	14.3	5.7	10.7	15.2	7.3
35-44	14.7	21.9	7.8	12.7	17.3	8.8
45-54	21.4	32.9	10.2	19.3	28.5	10.6
55-64	24.8	40.8	10.2	23.8	35.5	12.2
65-74	23.4	41.3	8.8	29.2	46.5	11.2
75 & over	26.7	55.4	6.8	38.7	66.3	11.6

account is taken of the fact that the foreign-born were concentrated in the older age groups, where high suicide rates prevailed, and when adjustment is made for age, it is then seen that the rates for the foreign-born population almost approximated those for the native-born population. Examination of the age-specific rates for the two populations in Figure 7.5 shows that the rates for foreign-born males were somewhat higher than those for native-born males for ages under 35 years and 65 years and over but were lower for the intervening ages. Foreign-born females, on the other hand, had slightly higher rates than native-born females in every age group.

When country of birth of the foreign-born population is considered, it is seen from Table 7.6 that among those nativity groups which proportionately have sizeable representations among foreign-born whites, those born in Britian, Ireland, Norway, Italy, Canada, and Mexico had rates which, in general, were lower than the overall rate for foreign-born whites, whereas the rates for persons born in the other countries listed were higher. The highest rates, particularly for males, occurred among those born in Sweden, Czechoslovakia, Austria, Hungary, and Yugoslavia. Of the foreign-born groups shown, all but those of Mexican birth had rates higher than that of the native-born white population.

It should be pointed out that since age-specific rates were not available for each country of birth, it was not possible to compute

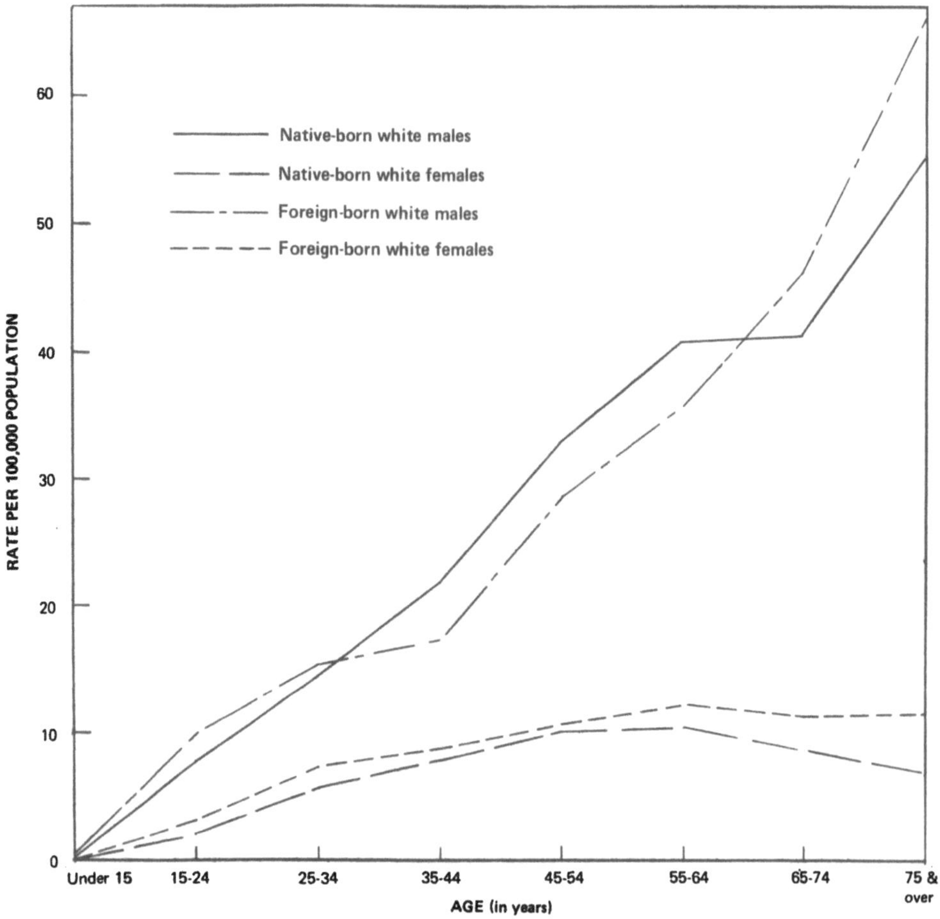

Fig. 7.5. Deaths from suicide per 100,000 population among white persons by nativity, age, and sex: United States, 1959-61.

Table 7.6 Suicide rates per 100,000 population for native-born whites and foreign-born whites by country of birth and sex: United States, 1959-61

Place of birth	Rates per 100,000 population[a]		
	Total	Male	Female
Native-born whites	10.5	16.3	4.9
Foreign-born whites	21.7	34.3	9.8
United Kingdom	15.4	25.8	7.8
Ireland	14.2	22.1	8.9
Norway	21.4	35.1	6.0
Sweden	33.1	52.6	12.0
Germany	25.5	42.5	11.9
Poland	24.1	37.5	11.1
Czechoslavakia	28.9	49.7	10.9
Austria	33.8	57.2	13.9
Hungary	32.9	52.2	15.3
Yugoslavia	34.6	54.5	10.7
U.S.S.R.	27.1	40.9	13.5
Italy	17.4	27.5	5.4
Canada	20.2	32.6	10.8
Mexico	8.7	13.8	3.0

[a]Crude Rate

age-adjusted rates. In view of the effect which age-adjustment had on the native-born versus foreign-born comparison in Table 7.5, serious question can be raised about the validity of the comparisons of the rate for the various foreign-born groups against that for native-born whites presented in Table 7.6. Age distributions were available for each of the foreign-born populations, however, thus making it possible to adjust the rates for age by the indirect method, using the U.S. native-born, white age-specific rates as the standard. The resulting age-adjusted rates left the ranking by country of birth virtually unchanged.

Marital Status

In studies carried out as early as the end of the nineteenth century, differences in suicide rates were found among various marital status groups which, in general, still hold. For example, Durkheim (1951), observing data from various countries of the world in this early period, found a smaller incidence of suicide among married persons than among those who were single, widowed, or divorced. Today, this same pattern is in evidence from the 1959-1961 U.S. data on suicide by marital status. Table 7.7 shows that for each sex-color group the age-adjusted rate for married persons was lowest, followed by that for single persons. The highest rates are found among the widowed except for white females, where the rate for divorced persons was highest.

Table 7.7 Age-adjusted suicide rates per 100,000 population 15 years of age and over by sex, color, and marital status: United States, 1959-61

Color and sex	Total	Single	Married	Widowed	Divorced
Both colors					
Male	22.1	33.2	18.0	78.4	69.4
Female	6.5	7.7	5.5	10.7	18.4
White					
Male	23.1	35.2	18.7	90.6	75.7
Female	6.9	8.2	5.8	12.0	20.6
Nonwhite					
Male	12.2	17.0	9.9	39.5	21.3
Female	3.0	2.5	2.4	6.0	4.3

Similar differences in rates between the marital status groups generally prevail when age-sex specific rates are examined. In Figures 7.6 and 7.7, it is seen that except for the age group 15-19, married males and females had the lowest rate in each age group. The rates for single persons were next in order of magnitude. For females, the highest rate at every age interval except 20-24 years occurred among the divorced, whereas for males the highest rate occurred among the widowed for the age groups under 40 years and among the divorced for the age group 40 years and over. A further breakdown of the data by race in Table 7.8 shows that the patterns of rates by marital status were essentially similar for each sex-color-age group, with the exception of nonwhite females. where little or no pattern is evidenced because of the small magnitude of the rates.

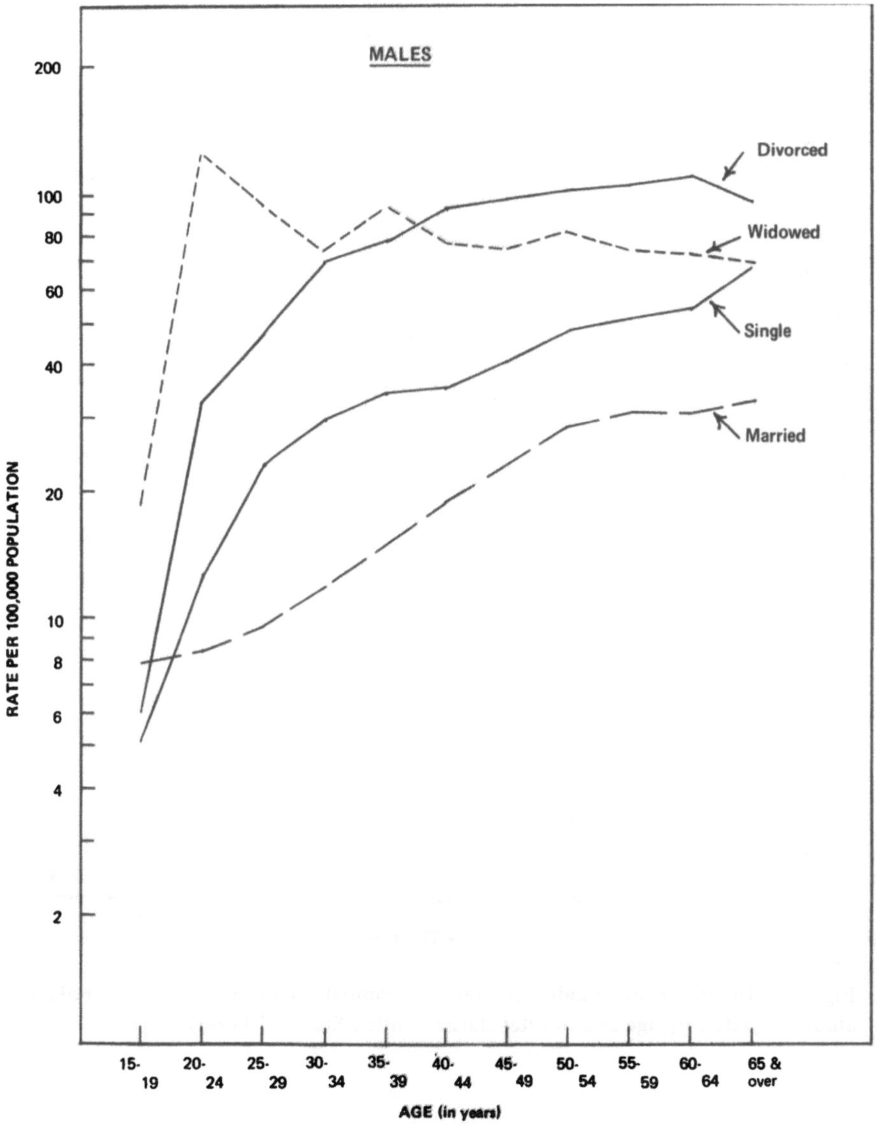

Fig. 7.6. Deaths from suicide per 100,000 population 15 years of age and older among males, by age and marital status: United States 1959-61.

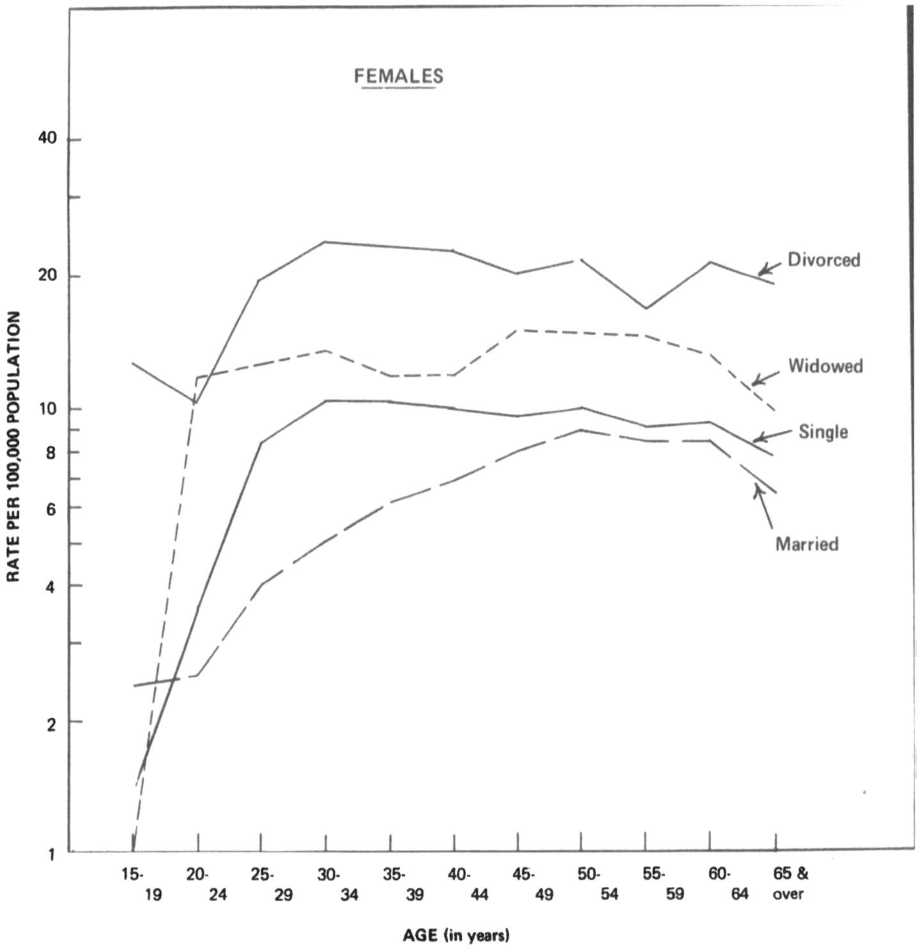

Fig. 7.7. Deaths from suicide per 100,000 population 15 years of age and older among females, by age and marital status: United States, 1959-61.

Table 7.8 Suicide rates per 100,000 population 15 years and over, by age, sex, color, and marital status: United States, 1959-61

Age	Total	Single	Married	Widowed	Divorced
Male white					
15 & over	23.1	35.2	18.7	90.6	75.7
15-19	5.6	5.4	8.3	26.0	6.8
20-24	11.4	13.1	8.4	142.3	34.1
25-34	14.6	26.7	10.8	87.9	65.6
35-44	21.9	37.1	17.9	103.6	96.3
45-54	33.0	48.0	27.6	97.1	108.9
55-64	40.5	56.6	33.1	84.8	118.4
65-74	43.0	67.0	32.7	75.9	98.9
75 & over	59.2	84.5	40.0	81.8	121.0
Male nonwhite					
15 & over	12.2	17.0	9.9	39.5	21.3
15-19	3.4	3.3	4.5	0.0	0.0
20-24	10.4	11.0	8.7	79.0	15.7
25-34	14.5	20.8	11.5	68.2	23.5
35-44	12.1	20.8	9.3	35.9	24.8
45-54	13.7	17.1	11.4	21.3	31.9
55-64	15.6	20.7	12.8	23.9	22.5
65-74	13.7	17.6	10.4	20.2	21.2
75 & over	17.2	37.2	11.1	21.3	28.6
Female white					
15 & over	6.9	8.2	5.8	12.0	20.6
15-19	1.6	1.3	2.4	0.0	13.8
20-24	3.1	3.8	2.5	10.9	10.8
25-34	5.8	10.0	4.7	15.6	25.2
35-44	8.0	11.1	6.8	13.2	25.4
45-54	10.3	10.3	9.0	16.8	23.1
55-64	10.5	9.6	8.7	14.9	19.6
65-74	9.3	9.2	7.3	11.0	18.6
75 & over	7.9	5.1	5.7	8.5	24.2
Female nonwhite					
15 & over	3.0	2.5	2.4	6.0	4.3
15-19	1.5	1.4	1.8	0.0	0.0
20-24	2.5	2.6	2.1	13.2	5.6
25-34	3.6	5.2	3.0	5.5	5.5
35-44	3.5	2.9	2.8	7.7	8.0
45-54	2.9	2.2	2.4	4.8	2.9
55-64	3.5	0.8	2.7	4.4	4.7
65-74	2.9	0.0	1.1	4.6	0.0
75 & over	3.2	0.0	0.9	4.1	0.0

Examination of the age-adjusted suicide rates by marital status for geographic regions in Appendix Table 10 reveals that in every region the white male rates were lowest among married persons and next lowest among single persons. In some regions, white male rates were highest among the widowed, while in others they were highest among the divorced. For white females, on the other hand, the identical pattern appeared for every region – lowest among the married, next lowest among the single, and highest among the divorced.

The patterns of rates by marital status were not as clear among the nonwhites. For nonwhite males, identical patterns appeared in five regions, the Middle Atlantic, the three Southern regions, and the Pacific. The pattern was: lowest rate among the married, next lowest among the single, and highest among the widowed. In the remaining four regions, the patterns were variable, undoubtedly due to the fact that these comprise the northern and mountain states where the number of nonwhites is relatively small. The rates for nonwhite females by region were too small to establish any consistent pattern by marital status.

When the suicide rates by marital status for the United States are compared to those for other countries for which such data are available, it is seen (Table 7.9) that, with few exceptions, the pattern of rates in other countries was fairly consistent with that for the United States, that is, the lowest rates occurring among the married and the highest rates among the widowed and divorced. The exceptions occurred in the male rates for France, Italy, and Scotland and the female rates for Canada, France, the Netherlands, England Scotland, Australia, and New Zealand, where rates for single persons were slightly lower than those for married persons. However, it is quite possible that adjustments made for age might alter this pattern in these countries. Data were not available to permit such adjustment.

In commenting on the relationships between marital status and suicide, Dublin (1963) states that "the evaluation of this relationship must start with the recognition of psychological differences which doubtless prevail among the various conjugal groups. Psychological factors commonly determine whether a given person ever marries and they are likewise important in determining whether or not a marriage will be a success or failure. Hence, it may well be that it is not marriage per se that influences the suicide rate but rather, to a large degree, marital status and the frequency of suicide are both influenced by the same psychological determinants."

Table 7.9 Suicide rates per 100,000 population 15 years and older, by sex and marital status: selected countries for the time periods indicated

Country	Year	Male				Female			
		Single	Married	Widowed	Divorced	Single	Married	Widowed	Divorced
United States	1959-61	33.2	18.0	78.4	69.4	7.7	5.5	10.7	18.4
Canada	1960-62	18.0	15.6	45.0		3.4	4.4	8.0	
Denmark	1959-61	32.8	26.5	90.1	163.7 1/	14.6	12.1	34.5	55.0 1/
Finland	1959-61	48.5	41.4	106.7	175.8	13.5	10.4	15.7	30.6
France	1961-63	23.5	29.6	124.9	65.7	7.8	8.1	20.1	15.6
West Germany	1961	29.2	28.9	90.0	146.7	14.6	13.6	24.5	41.9
Italy	1960-62	9.5	10.0	37.3	35.7 1/	4.8	3.6	7.2	61.2 1/
Netherlands	1959-61	10.6	9.9	64.7	54.0	5.4	6.2	18.3	22.1
Norway	1956-65	17.4	12.8	33.7	46.9	4.8	3.5	6.2	10.0
Sweden	1959-61	33.6	28.4	81.3	107.9	12.6	8.8	14.6	29.5
Switzerland	1959-61	37.8	28.3	115.8	128.7	14.6	10.3	19.8	35.0
England and Wales	1961	14.4	13.4	58.8	49.8	9.2	9.4	24.7	24.6
Scotland	1960-62	12.9	13.4	45.3	85.9	6.6	6.8	14.2	22.2
Australia	1960-62	24.3	20.5	54.0	90.6	7.7	9.3	16.6	37.7
New Zealand 2/	1960-62	21.6	16.4	53.7	23.3	5.4	6.6	16.4	12.0

Source: World Health Statistics Report, Vol. 21, No. 6, Table 3.2 (Geneva, Switz.: World Health Organization, 1968).

1/ Includes legally separated.

2/ Based on data for persons 16 years and over.

Residence

Data for 1959, obtained by Dublin from the National Center for Health Statistics and reproduced here in Table 7.10, show that the suicide rate for all urban areas combined was 10.7 per 100,000 while the rate for all rural areas was 10.0.* Dublin (1963) points out that "in 1929, in contrast, the cities in the Registration States recorded a rate of 17.4 per 100,000 and the rural part of these States only 11.0 per 100,000, an excess of 58 percent. Thus, the gap between the urban and rural areas of the country has greatly narrowed in recent years to only 7 percent. The shift has been accomplished through the persistent decline in suicide in the cities, while there has been very little change in the rural areas."

---

*Data on urban and rural suicide rates were not made available in the special 1959-1961 tabulations provided by the National Center for Health Statistics for the monograph.

Table 7.10 Death rates from suicide, by place of residence: United States, 1959.

Place of residence	Rate per 100,000[1/]
All urban areas combined	10.7
Places of 250,000 or more	11.5
" " 100,000-250,000	10.3
" " 50,000-100,000	10.7
" " 25,000-50,000	10.6
" " 10,000-25,000	10.0
" " 2,500-10,000	10.1
All rural areas combined	10.0

Source: Dublin, L.I. Suicide: A Sociological and Statistical Study, Table 11, p. 51.

1/ Population as of April 1960.

Speculating on the causes for this change in the suicide picture during the last three decades of increased urbanization, Dublin (1963) states: "unquestionably, the condition of the industrial population, which is largely urban in character, has greatly improved economically, with attendant improvement in their housing and health conditions generally. This improvement is shown by the much lower death rates from all causes. Working conditions have likewise greatly improved. On the other hand, the rural population has not fared so well. Standards of living are still relatively low over large rural areas and suicide rates in the predominately rural states are, with few exceptions, higher than average for the country. It may well be that these figures are a good index of the difficulties confronting the population on the farms of which farm surpluses and continued migration to the cities are symptoms of basic economic and social maladjustment."

When the small urban-rural difference in suicide rate for the United States is compared to that for certain European countries in Dublin's study, it is seen that in England and Wales, Denmark, Sweden, and Austria, urban rates are, in general, markedly higher than rural rates (Dublin 1963). In France, however, the higher urban rate is found only among males 65 years of age and over. For males under 65 years rural rates are higher and female rates are so low that no urban-rural differential is discernible.

In the 1959-1961 special tabulations on suicide a classification of residence is used to examine rates, which would appear to be an attempt to take into account the increased movement of urban population in recent years to suburban areas. According to this new classification, the data are broken down by metropolitan counties with and without central cities and nonmetropolitan counties.* The major limitation of this type of classification is that county boundaries are political boundaries and do not accurately reflect the characteristics of the area, such as the extent to which it contains urban and rural parts. For example, a metropolitan county without a central city, although basically metropolitan in character, may have portions of its area which are just as rural as sections of nonmetropolitan counties. Also, metropolitan counties with a central city, in some cases, include only the central city and in other cases

*Metropolitan counties are the counties which are included in the Standard Metropolitan Statistical Areas (referred to as "SMSA's").

include area beyond the limits of the central city. This classificatory scheme for counties, however, appears to be an attempt to rank them from the most urban to the least urban.

An examination of the suicide rates for the three classifications of counties in Table 7.11 shows that for the entire United States the rate of 10.9 per 100,000 population for nonmetropolitan counties was just slightly higher than the rate of 10.5 for metropolitan counties with central cities and that the metropolitan counties without central cities had the lowest rate – 9.5 per 100,000. Although these rate differentials are very small, the pattern of the slightly higher rate in the least urban of the three classifications is contrary to what might have been expected on the basis of the differences in urban-rural rates described above, where the urban rate was seen to be slightly higher than that for rural areas. Differences in the racial composition of the populations in these areas may have contributed to these variations.

If the suicide rates for the three residence classifications are further examined on a regional basis, it is seen (Table 7.11) that except for the eastern part of the country, where the nonmetropolitan rates were higher than the others, the rates for all three types of areas were remarkably similar to each other within a given region. The variation among regions in the level of the rates was much greater than the variation within individual regions.

Among the four sex-color groups shown in Table 7.11, the rates for white males for the United States were highest in the nonmetropolitan counties, whereas those for nonwhite males show little or no difference in terms of metropolitan or nonmetropolitan residence. Females, both white and nonwhite, are seen to have the highest rate in the metropolitan counties with central city Regionally, the pattern of rates varies considerably by this residence classification for all of the sex-color groups except the white female, which has consistently higher rates in the metropolitan counties with central city. These inconsistencies in the patterns of rates and the small differentials in the rates between metropolitan and nonmetropolitan areas, along with the negligible urban-rural differences noted in Dublin's study, would seem to indicate that it is not possible to categorize these types of areas as having high or low suicide rates.

Table 7.11 Age-adjusted suicide rates per 100,000 population, by sex and color, for metropolitan counties with and without central cities and non-metropolitan counties: United States and each geographic region, 1959-61

Region and residence area	Total	White		Nonwhite	
		Male	Female	Male	Female
United States	10.5	17.3	5.2	9.1	2.3
Metropolitan counties	10.3	16.6	5.6	9.1	2.5
With central city	10.5	17.0	5.8	9.2	2.6
Without central city	9.5	15.2	4.7	8.0	2.0
Non-metropolitan counties	10.9	18.6	4.4	9.1	1.8
New England	8.8	14.3	3.9	10.1	2.9
Metropolitan counties	8.0	12.6	4.0	8.4	2.8
With central city	8.1	12.7	4.1	8.3	2.8
Without central city	7.1	12.0	2.7	14.3	0.0
Non-metropolitan counties	11.6	19.6	3.9	26.3	4.3
Middle Atlantic	8.6	13.5	4.6	9.3	2.7
Metropolitan counties	8.2	12.6	4.6	9.3	2.7
With central city	8.3	12.6	4.8	9.7	2.8
Without central city	8.0	12.5	4.2	7.4	2.2
Non-metropolitan counties	10.6	17.3	4.4	9.8	1.5
East North Central	10.1	16.5	4.8	8.1	2.2
Metropolitan counties	9.5	15.5	4.8	7.9	2.2
With central city	9.5	15.5	4.9	8.1	2.2
Without central city	9.5	15.3	4.3	6.0	2.2
Non-metropolitan counties	11.1	18.1	4.6	9.3	2.8
West North Central	10.4	17.3	4.3	10.0	3.5
Metropolitan counties	10.6	18.2	4.5	8.0	3.7
With central city	11.0	19.1	4.7	8.3	4.2
Without central city	9.1	15.5	3.7	6.2	0.0
Non-metropolitan counties	10.4	16.7	4.1	15.7	2.7
South Atlantic	11.4	20.9	5.6	8.1	1.6
Metropolitan counties	11.3	19.8	6.4	8.1	2.0
With central city	11.5	20.8	6.8	7.8	2.4
Without central city	11.1	18.0	5.4	10.8	2.4
Non-metropolitan counties	11.4	22.1	4.7	8.1	1.3
East South Central	9.4	18.2	3.8	7.0	1.4
Metropolitan counties	9.3	17.9	4.3	7.8	1.8
With central city	9.2	17.9	4.4	7.9	1.8
Without central city	9.9	18.1	3.5	5.1	2.4
Non-metropolitan counties	9.5	18.4	3.5	6.4	1.2
West South Central	8.9	15.8	4.1	7.7	1.4
Metropolitan counties	9.6	17.0	4.5	7.9	1.5
With central city	9.7	17.2	4.6	8.1	1.6
Without central city	8.7	15.7	3.5	5.4	0.0
Non-metropolitan counties	8.1	14.4	3.6	7.7	1.4
Mountain	14.6	23.0	6.0	22.8	6.9
Metropolitan counties	15.3	24.9	6.8	10.7	4.7
With central city	15.5	25.2	6.9	10.5	4.8
Without central city	14.1	22.4	6 0	16.9	0.0
Non-metropolitan counties	13.9	21.3	5.2	31.9	8.3
Pacific	14.9	22.2	8.9	14.4	5.2
Metropolitan counties	15.1	22.3	9.5	14.2	4.6
With central city	15.3	22.6	9.7	14.5	4.6
Without central city	14.1	20.6	8.5	10.9	5.5
Non-metropolitan counties	13.9	21.6	6.2	14.8	8.4

When the 1959-1961 suicide rates for the twelve largest standard metropolitan areas and the total United States are compared (Table 7.12), it is seen that the total age-adjusted rates for all but two of the areas either approximate or are lower than the United States rate. Only Los Angeles and San Francisco have substantially higher rates. With a few exceptions, the same pattern generally prevails when the data are further broken into the various sex-color-nativity groups shown. The consistently higher rates for the two West Coast cities are not unexpected in view of the fact that among the geographic divisions of the country the highest suicide rates are found on the Pacific Coast and in the Mountain States (see Table 7.13). The lowest rates are seen generally to prevail in the New England, Middle Atlantic, and West South Central divisions. This pattern of low rates for these three divisions is not always consistent when the data are further broken down by such variables as race, marital status, and metropolitan–nonmetropolitan residence (see Table 7.11 and Appendix Table 11), but the rates for the two western divisions are almost invariably the highest no matter how detailed the breakdown of data.

Causal explanations for the persistently high incidence of suicide in the western United States are difficult to provide in the absence of more detailed information on the characteristics of those who commit suicide. A contributing factor may be the greater mobility of the population, as evidenced by the high proportion of migrants (persons who lived in different counties in 1955 and 1960) found in the two western divisions (28 percent in the Mountain and 25 percent in the Pacific) compared to that for the total United States (17 percent) in the 1960 census. The possible association between high suicide rates and high morbidity is discussed in some detail below. Also, in 1960, both western divisions had substantially higher proportions of persons born in a different state – 47 percent for the Mountain and 51 percent for the Pacific – compared to that for the total United States (26 percent). In addition, in both of these population groups – the migrants and those born in a different state – the proportions of those 65 years of age and over (for whom suicide rates are highest) was larger in the western region in 1960 than in the three major regions of the country (Northeast, North Central, and South). Another factor which may contribute to the higher suicide rates in the West is the proportionately larger number of Chinese and American Indian population in this region, all of whom have a high incidence of suicide.

Table 7.12 Age-adjusted suicide rates per 100,000 population, by sex, color, and nativity: selected Standard Metropolitan Areas, United States 1959-61

Color and sex	United States	Baltimore	Boston	Chicago	Cleveland	Detroit	Los Angeles	New York	Philadelphia	Pittsburgh	St. Louis	San Francisco	Washington
Both colors	10.5	9.9	7.2	8.2	10.0	10.2	15.9	8.1	8.8	8.2	9.6	17.2	10.7
Male	16.6	15.3	11.8	12.6	15.5	15.4	22.2	11.6	13.3	12.7	16.0	24.2	15.9
Female	4.9	5.2	3.1	4.2	5.1	5.3	10.4	5.1	4.7	4.0	4.1	10.6	5.9
Total white	11.0	11.0	7.2	8.6	10.6	11.0	16.5	8.2	9.2	8.4	10.2	18.1	12.2
Male	17.3	16.9	11.9	13.2	16.7	16.4	22.9	11.5	13.9	13.0	17.1	25.5	18.3
Female	5.2	5.8	3.1	4.4	5.2	5.8	10.9	5.2	5.1	4.2	4.3	11.4	7.0
Native white	10.8	10.5	7.0	7.8	10.2	10.4	16.5	7.6	8.7	8.0	10.0	18.0	12.0
Male	17.2	16.2	11.7	12.0	15.9	15.7	22.8	10.7	13.1	12.3	16.7	25.6	18.2
Female	5.0	5.5	3.0	4.0	5.3	5.4	11.1	5.0	4.9	4.2	4.3	11.4	6.5
Foreign-born white	11.1	13.5	5.8	10.0	9.2	11.6	14.4	8.5	11.8	10.0	6.5	16.5	14.9
Male	16.6	20.7	9.3	14.8	14.1	16.0	21.6	12.0	18.4	15.2	13.1	20.9	20.4
Female	6.0	7.3	3.0	5.4	4.4	7.3	8.0	5.4	6.2	5.1	0.5	11.9	11.2
Nonwhite	5.5	5.1	5.2	4.6	5.1	4.8	9.6	6.8	5.6	4.5	5.3	9.5	5.2
Male	9.1	7.9	6.9	6.8	7.1	7.9	14.4	10.9	8.9	8.6	8.0	14.4	8.2
Female	2.3	2.6	3.9	2.7	3.3	2.0	4.9	3.6	2.8	0.8	3.1	4.1	2.5

Table 7.13 Age-adjusted suicide rates per 100,000 population, by sex and race: United States and each geographic region, 1959-61

Region	Total	Male	Female	White	Nonwhite
United States	10.5	16.6	4.9	11.0	5.5
New England	8.8	14.2	3.9	8.8	6.4
Middle Atlantic	8.6	13.3	4.5	8.8	5.8
East North Central	10.1	15.9	4.6	10.4	5.1
West North Central	10.4	17.0	4.3	10.6	6.6
South Atlantic	11.4	18.5	4.8	13.0	4.7
East South Central	9.4	16.1	3.3	10.7	4.0
West South Central	8.9	14.6	3.7	9.7	4.4
Mountain	14.6	23.2	6.1	14.5	14.9
Pacific	14.9	21.5	8.5	15.3	10.1

Mobility and Suicide

Very little exploration has been made into the background of those committing suicide to determine what relationship may exist between the degree of physical mobility, in terms of changes in residence, and incidence of suicide. In the few studies which have examined the ecological aspects of suicide in large metropolitan areas, for example, Sainsbury (1955) in London, Schmid (1928) in Seattle and Minneapolis, and Cavan (1928) in Chicago, the areas within the cities studied which were characterized by considerable spatial mobility or transiency were generally found to have high rates of suicide. MacMahon and his associates (1963) indicated that since a sizeable proportion of the northern Negro population had migrated within their lifetime, their higher rates of suicide compared to Negroes living in the South may be interpreted in terms of known higher suicide rates among migrants in general. This latter explanation was also put forth in the foregoing section to possibly account for the fact that the western region of the United States, which has larger proportions of immigrants and mobile persons than the United States as a whole, also has a higher incidence of suicide.

Some additional evidence of a possible link between the migration factor and suicide may be shown in the data on state of birth versus state of residence of native-born persons committing suicide in the period 1959-61. A summarization of the data shown in Appendix Table 12 indicates that for total as well as for white population, suicide rates in 45 of the 50 states were higher among those born outside the state of residence than among those born within the state of residence. In the remaining five states, there was either little difference in rates between the two groups or the pattern was reversed. For the nonwhite population, the pattern of higher rates for those from outside the state was observed in only 32 states. In 15 of the remaining 18 states, nonwhite rates were higher among those born within the state and, in the other three states. there was little or no difference in rates. It should be noted that the pattern of rates for nonwhites may be influenced to some extent by the fact that the nonwhite populations in certain of the smaller, more distant (relative to migration distances from the South) states of the Northeast, Midwest, and Far West are proportionately very small.

A further examination of the suicide rates among the total population born outside the state of residence (Appendix Table 12) indicates that the rates for those born in contiguous states were higher than for those born in noncontiguous states in 32 of 48 states.* It was assumed that the rate might be higher among those who had migrated greater distances (noncontiguous states), but this seems to have been the case in only 13 of the 16 remaining states, mostly those in the Mountain and Pacific regions, where rates for those born in noncontiguous states were higher. In the three other states there was little or no rate differential. Suicide rates for white population born in contiguous and noncontiguous states follow much the same patterns as those for the total population in each state, but among nonwhites there was somewhat greater variation in the rates.

When the state of birth–state of residence data are combined into regional groupings, it is seen (Appendix Table 13) that with some few exceptions the suicide rate among native-born persons residing in their region of birth was generally lower than among those who were born outside their region of residence. Because the state of birth – state of residence data were not broken down by age, age-adjustment of suicide rates by the indirect method for all of the 50 states did not seem practicable. However, in order to provide some indication of what effect age differences between "migrants" and "nonmigrants" might have on the suicide rates of the two

---

*States are considered contiguous if their boundaries touch at any point. Alaska and Hawaii are excluded since there are no contiguous states.

groups, an age-adjustment of rates by the indirect method was carried out for the United States and for each of its four major geographic regions (Northeast, North Central, South, and West). As seen in Table 7.14, age-adjusting the rates reduced the magnitude of the difference between the rates for those born in the state of residence and those born outside the state of residence. Nevertheless, the rates for the latter group still remain somewhat higher, except in the North Central region, where age-adjustment produced a reversal of the pattern.

The data presented in this section offer, at best, only a very crude measure of migration and, therefore, are inadequate to provide any really significant clues concerning the possible relationship between the degree of mobility and the incidence of suicide. Factors such as the age, sex, and socioeconomic characteristics of the migrants, patterns of migration (e.g., number of times moved, distance moved, length of time between moves), and reasons for migration, represent the additional kinds of information that would be needed to more accurately assess such a relationship.

Table 7.14 Suicide rates per 100,000 population for persons born within and outside state of residence:[a] United States and each major region, 1959-61

Region	Crude		Age-adjusted	
	Born in state	Born outside state	Born in state	Born outside state
United States	8.4	14.4	9.9	11.7
Northeast Region	7.7	11.4	8.5	9.2
North Central Region	9.2	12.4	10.5	9.9
South Region	8.4	13.3	9.7	11.3
West Region	8.0	19.2	14.2	15.4

[a] Age-adjusted by the indirect method.

TRENDS IN SUICIDE IN THE U.S.

An analysis of the trend in suicides in the United States is somewhat complicated by the fact that the official death registration area, on which the data for trends are based, comprised only ten States and the District of Columbia in 1900.* The area gradually expanded over the years until 1933, when it included all states except Alaska and Hawaii, which were subsequently added when they achieved statehood. Dublin (1963) has pointed out that "as a result [of this continual expansion], the composition of the area by age, sex and color changed from year to year as additional States were admitted. Under these conditions, the best practice is to consider the figures for the Expanding Death Registration States. These will give the best approximation of complete national rates and permit comparisons to be made over a period of years."

In 1965, the age-adjusted suicide rate of 11.4 per 100,000 population for the United States was just slightly higher than the rate of 11.3 per 100,000 which prevailed at the beginning of the century. In the intervening years, the trend of the total age-adjusted rates as seen in Figure 7.8 and Appendix Table 14 showed that by 1908 the rate had increased to 18.6 and remained at or about this higher level until 1916, the year preceding the United States entry into World War I, when it declined somewhat sharply. A decrease in the rate continued through the war and immediate post-war years, returning to a low of 11.5 per 100,000 in 1920. By 1921 the rate had increased to 13.9, and it remained somewhere near that level until 1926 when it began to climb upward, reaching a peak of 18.6 per 100,000 in 1932, at the height of the depression years. Thereafter, the rate, with some fluctuation, declined to 9.6 per 100,000 in 1944 during World War II, the lowest rate observed up to that time. After that, the rate showed some slight increase in the post-war years but gradually declined to 9.6 again by 1957. The jump in rate between 1957 and 1958 can be mostly attributed to a classification change wherein certain accidental deaths were included under suicides, beginning in 1958. Since that time, the suicide rate has shown a tendency toward some slight increase despite minor fluctuations.

---

*The ten states were Maine, New Hampshire, Vermont, Massachusetts, Connecticut, Rhode Island, New York, New Jersey, Michigan, and Indiana.

The pattern of trends in male suicide rates is considerably different from that for females, as indicated in Figure 7.8. Since the male rates were so high compared with those for females, the trend for total rates follows exactly the same pattern as that for males, but at a lower level. The female rates, on the other hand, fluctuated within the narrow range of 4 to 9 per 100,000 over the years, and the peaks and troughs were much less severe than those for males. Since 1957 the rates for females have shown a more steady increase than those for males. When the trend data are further broken down into color-sex groupings (Figure 7.9) for the period 1910-65, it is seen that the suicide rates for white males predominate over those for the other groups during the entire time period and exhibit considerably greater fluctuations in response to the periods of economic depression and war than do the rates for nonwhite males and white females. Rates for nonwhite females are seen to have remained at or about the same low level over most of the time interval, with little or no fluctuation comparable to those of the other groups. Since 1958, both white and nonwhite female rates appear to have exhibited a slight upward trend, whereas the male rates did not give evidence of this. Nonwhite males, however, have shown a general tendency toward an increasing rate since the end of World War II. There is no immediate explanation for the unusually high rates observed for nonwhite males and females prior to 1916, since the source of these rates provided no numerator or denominator data or descriptive text.

An examination of the trends in age-specific suicide rates for males in Figure 7.10 indicates that the pattern of a higher rate for each succeeding older age group, noted previously with respect to the 1960 male suicide rates, was prevalent at almost every point in time between 1900 and 1965. Over this time span the rates for males at the older ages are seen to have experienced more pronounced fluctuations during the periods of economic instability or war than have the rates for males at the younger ages. This also appears to be true when trends in the rates for older and younger females are compared in Figure 7.11. The magnitude of the fluctuations in rates for the older females, however, were considerably less than those observed for the older males. Further examination of Figure 7.11 shows that suicide rates for females in the 45-64 age groups were for the most part consistently higher than the rates for other age groups throughout most of the period 1900-65.

Focussing on the trend of age-specific suicide rates in the most recent years (since 1958), it is seen in Figure 7.10 that male rates for the age groups under 45 years have been increasing, whereas rates for males in the older age groups were decreasing. Female rates, however, appear to have increased at all ages, including those groups not shown in Figure 7.11.

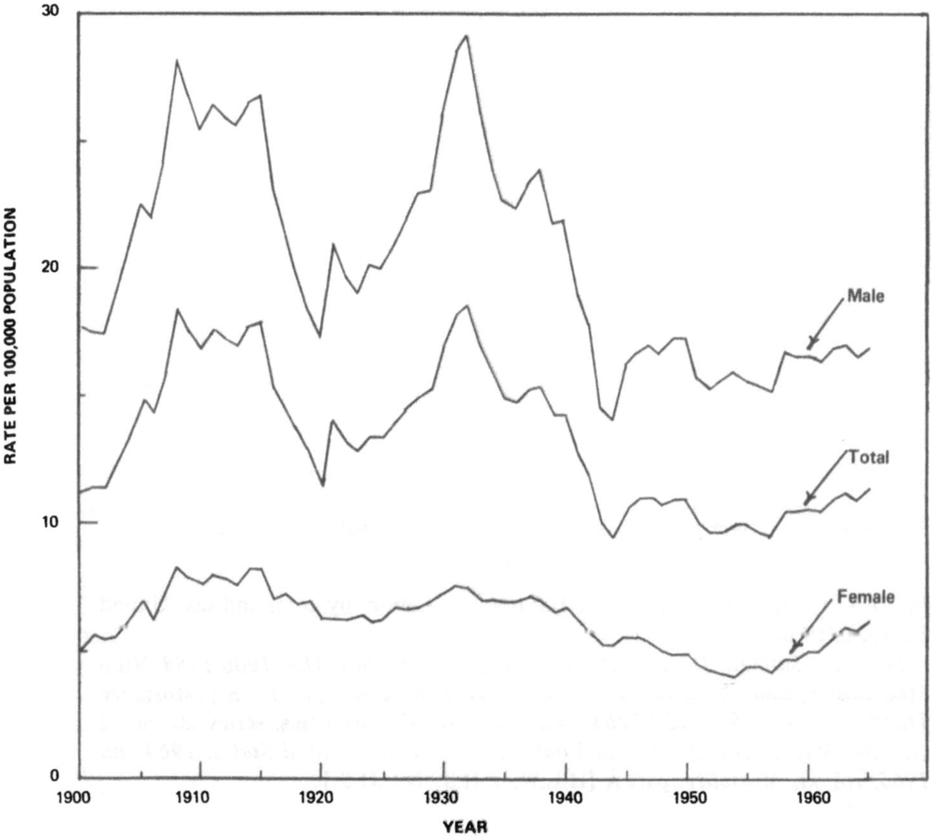

Fig. 7.8. Age-adjusted death rates from suicide per 100,000 population, by sex: United States, 1900-65.

Sources: Suicide: Death Rates by Age, Race, and Sex, U.S. 1900-1953. Vital Statistics–Special Reports, vol. 43, no. 30 [H.E.W., P.H.S., N.O.V.S.] ; *Mortality Trends in the U.S., 1954-1963.* Vital and Health Statistics, series 20, no. 2 [H.E.W., P.H.S., N.C.H.S.] ; and *Vital Statistics of the United States, 1964 and 1965,* vol. xi, *Mortality,* part A [H.E.W., P.H.S., N.C.H.S.] .

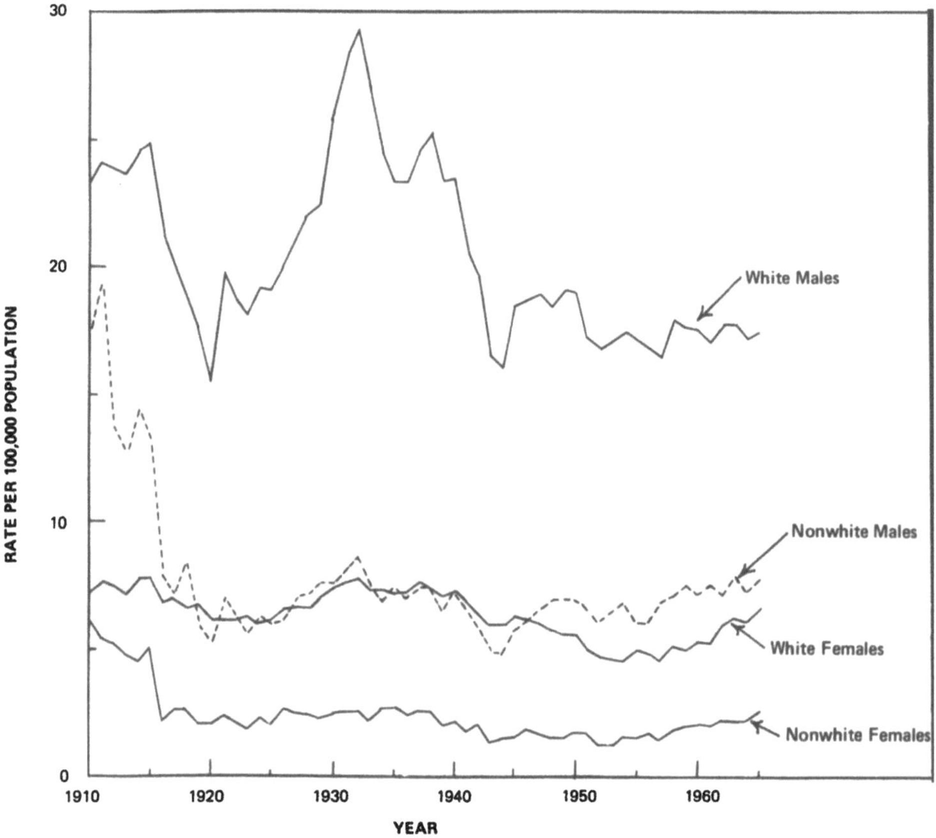

Fig. 7.9. Deaths from suicide per 100,000 population, by color and sex: United States, 1910-65.

Sources: Suicide: Death Rates by Age, Race, and Sex, U.S. 1900-1953. Vital Statistics–Special Reports, vol. 43, no. 30 [H.E.W., P.H.S., N.O.V.S.] ; *Mortality Trends in the U.S., 1954-1963.* Vital and Health Statistics, series 20, no. 2 [H.E.W., P.H.S., N.C.H.S.] ; and *Vital Statistics of the United States, 1964 and 1965,* vol. xi, *Mortality,* part A [H.E.W., P.H.S., N.C.H.S.] .

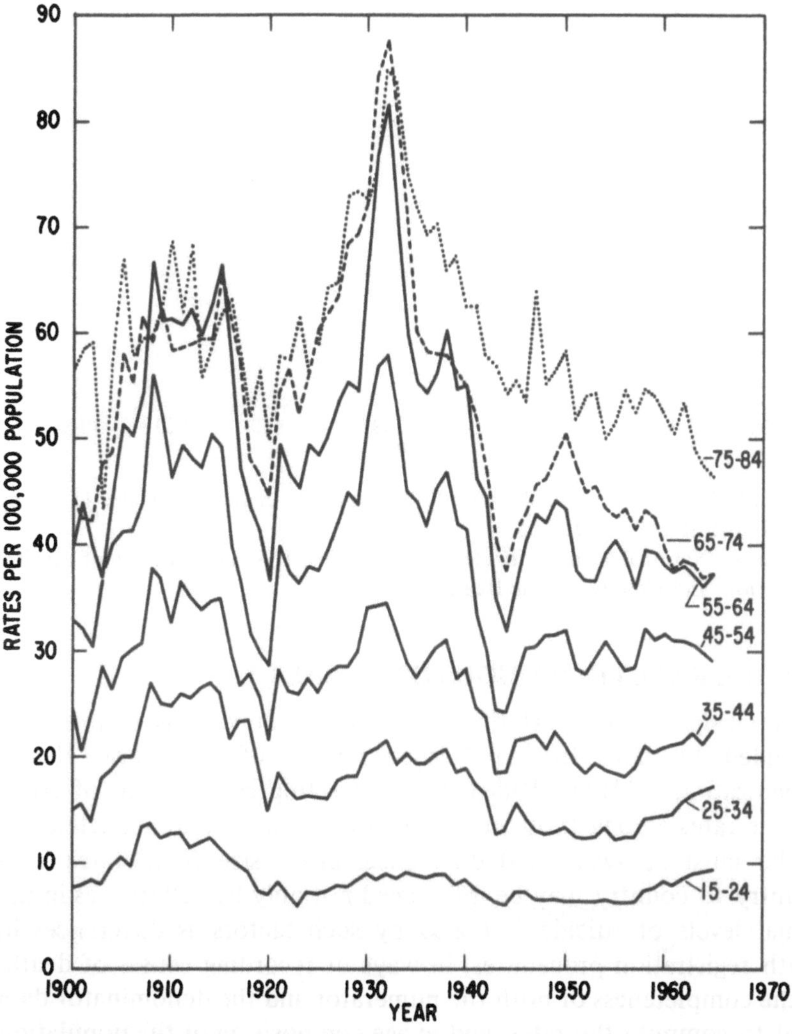

Fig. 7.10. Deaths from suicide per 100,000 population among males 15-84, by age: United States, 1900-1965.

Source: National Center for Health Statistics, U.S. Department of Health, Education, and Welfare, Public Health Serivce.

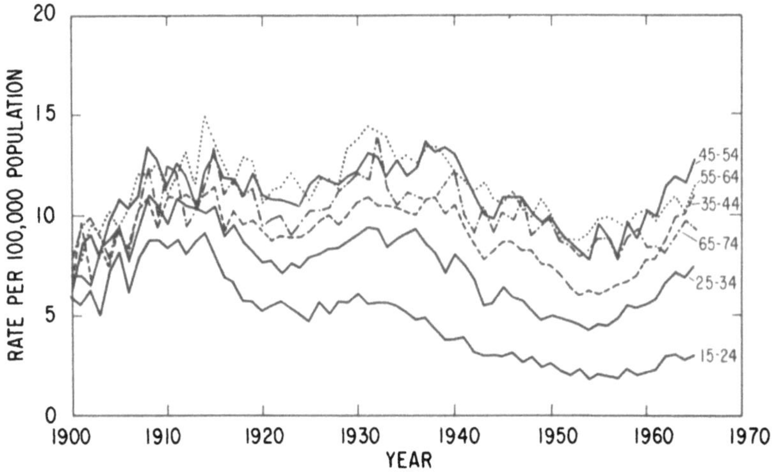

Fig. 7.11. Deaths from suicide per 100,000 population among females 15-84, by age: United States, 1900-1965.

Source: National Center for Health Statistics, U.S. Department of Health, Education, and Welfare, Public Health Service.

SUICIDE RATES IN VARIOUS COUNTRIES

Some insight into mortality from suicide in various countries is provided by data from published reports of the World Health Organization (W.H.O., 1968). In interpreting comparisons of crude suicide rates among those countries for which data are reported, the reader must be aware that differences in the size of the rates from country to country may be influenced not only by differences in the actual levels of suicide but also by such factors as differences in death registration procedures, in ways of recording causes of death, in the completeness of both the numerator and the denominator data used to compute the rates, and in age composition of the population and other factors. Of the suicide rates shown for 58 countries or territories in Table 7.15, almost one-third are based on estimated data or on data from civil registers which are incomplete or of unknown reliability. In addition, the rates for eleven of the countries are based on only part of the total population or on selected population groups as indicated.*

---

*These countries include South Africa, Southern Rhodesia, Egypt, Panama, Brazil, Peru, Venezuela, Burma, Philippines, Israel, and Turkey.

Table 7.15 Suicide rates per 100,000 population: countries reporting these data, 1960

Country	Rate
Africa	
Nigeria (Lagos-Federal Territory)	0.8*
Southern Rhodesia (European Population)	12.4
South Africa	
Asiatic population	8.2
Colored population	4.3
White population	14.2
United Arab Republic (Egypt)[a]	0.1*
Americas	
United States	10.6
Canada	7.6
Costa Rica	2.1
Dominican Republic	1.0*
El Salvador	11.3*
Guatemala	2.7
Mexico	1.9
Nicaragua	0.3*
Panama[b]	5.2*
Puerto Rico	9.7
British Guiana	5.1*
Brazil (State of Guanabara)	14.2*
Chile (1961)	7.7
Columbia	2.9*
Peru[c] (1959)	1.4*
Uruguay (1959)	12.2*
Venezuela[d]	5.0*
Asia	
Burma[e] (1959)	9.3*
Ceylon	9.9*
China (Taiwan)	15.6
Hong Kong	11.1
Israel (Jewish population)	6.4
Japan	21.6
Jordan	0.5*
Philippines[f]	0.7*
Singapore	8.6
Thailand	3.5
Turkey[g]	1.5
Europe	
Austria	23.1
Belgium	14.6
Bulgaria	17.7
Czechoslavakia (1961)	20.6
Denmark	20.3
Finland	20.5
France	15.9
West Germany	18.8
West Berlin	37.0
Greece	3.8*
Hungary	24.9
Iceland	8.0
Ireland	3.0
Italy	6.1
Luxembourg	10.2
Netherlands	6.6
Norway	6.4
Poland	8.0
Portugal	8.7
Spain	5.5
Sweden	17.4
Switzerland	19.0
United Kingdom	
England & Wales	11.2
Northern Ireland	4.4
Scotland	7.8
Oceania	
Australia	10.6
New Zealand	9.7

Source: United Nations Demographic Yearbook, 1961 (Table 17) and 1962 (Table 20); World Health Statistics Report, Vol. 21, No. 6, Table 1.2 (World Health Organization: Geneva, 1968).

* Data are unreliable or of unknown completeness.

[a] Deaths in Health Bureau localities comprise approximately 50 percent of total deaths.

[b] Excludes data for Canal Zone and tribal Indian population numbering 60,540 in 1960.

[c] Excludes Indian jungle population estimated at 100,830 in 1961.

[d] Data comprise approximately 90 percent of total deaths.

[e] Data are for a number of towns having a present population of approximately 2,000,000.

[f] Data are incomplete returns from only 88 percent of local civil registrars but rates are computed on total population.

[g] Data are for provincial capitals and district centers.

If it were possible to adjust for the deficiencies that may be present in the reported data, it is likely that differences in suicide rates observed among the countries shown in Table 7.15 might still prevail owing to the effect of cultural, social, psychological, economic, and political factors which influence the behavior of various national groups. While each of these factors may exert some influence on the level of the suicide rate, data are not available in sufficient detail to permit one to isolate the effect of each factor.

Of the 47 countries for which suicide data were available for the total population, 16 had higher suicide rates than the United States in 1960. These included 11 countries in Europe (Austria, Belgium, Czechoslovakia, Denmark, Finland, France, West Germany, Hungary, Sweden, Switzerland, and England and Wales); three in Asia (Taiwan, Japan, and the crown colony of Hong Kong); one in Central and one in South America (El Salvador and Uruguay), and Australia. The rates ranged from just slightly higher than the U.S. rate in El Salvador, Hong Kong, England and Wales, and Australia to double or more in Japan, Austria, Czechoslovakia, Denmark, Finland, and Hungary.

Among those European countries with somewhat comparable sociocultural backgrounds, such as the Scandinavian countries, or those existing under somewhat comparable sociopolitical conditions, such as the Iron Curtain countries, it is of interest that the variation in suicide rates within groups of countries was greater than might have been expected. Examples of this are the low rate for Norway compared to those for Sweden, Finland, and Denmark, and the low rates for Poland and Bulgaria compared to those for Czechoslovakia and Hungary. This tends to point out a significant characteristic of the phenomenon of suicide, namely, the high degree of variability in its incidence with respect to place. As Dublin (1963) points out, "this variability presents a major challenge and opportunity to all students of the subject – psychiatrists, psychologists, sociologists and statisticians – to unravel and evaluate the many causitive factors involved."

As noted earlier, the trend in the suicide rate in the United States over the 10-year period 1955-65 has been slightly upward despite some minor fluctuations. An examination of suicide rates over the same time period for 17 other countries (Figure 7.12) indicates that only 7 of these countries (Hungary, West Germany, Poland, Canada, Sweden, Australia, and the Netherlands) exhibited a similar trend in their rates. The pattern of these trends ranged from one of

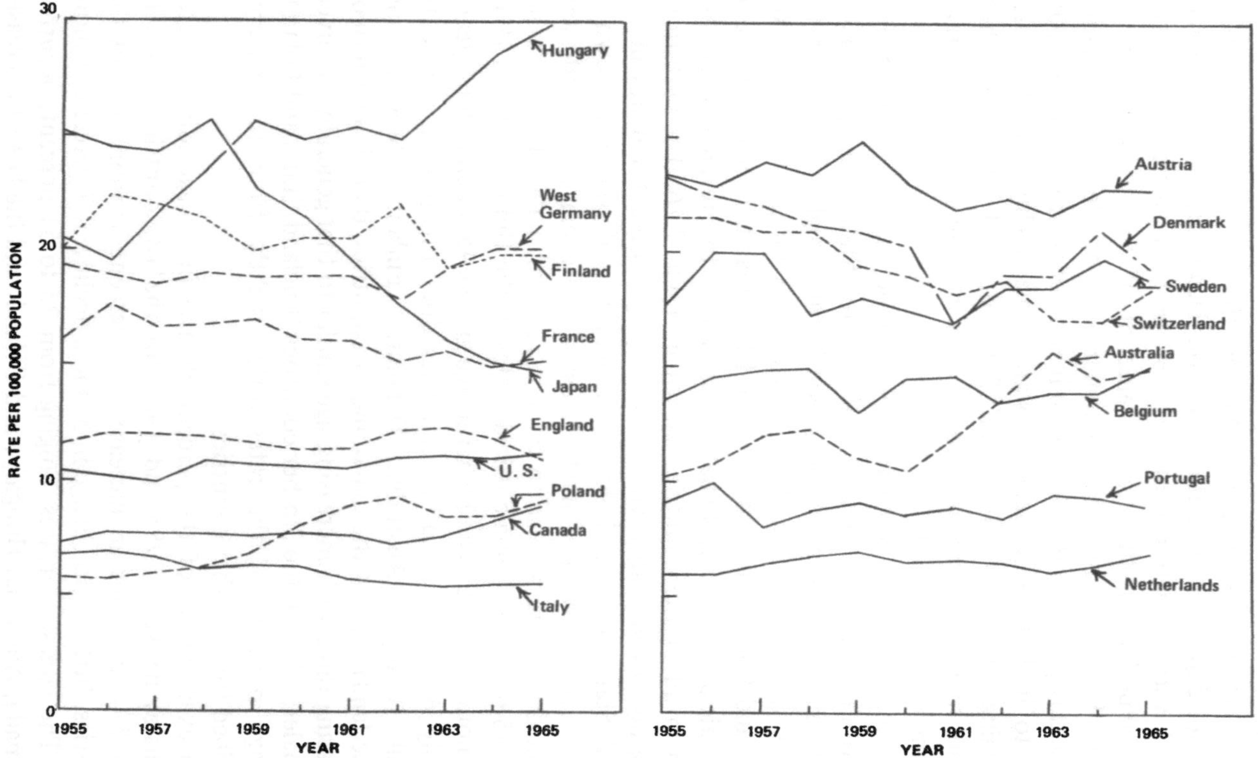

Fig. 7.12. Deaths from suicide per 100.000 population: Selected countries with 500 or more suicides per annum, 1955-65.

substantial increase in Hungary to that of a barely perceptible increase in the Netherlands. Among the other 10 countries, 7 (Finland, Japan, France, Italy, Austria, Denmark, and Switzerland) showed varying patterns of decrease in their suicide rates, with Japan experiencing the greatest amount of decline. The rates for Austria, Denmark, and Finland underwent considerable fluctuation during this period, but a close examination of their trend lines would seem to indicate a tendency toward some decline. For the three remaining countries – England, Belgium, and Portugal – there appears to be no clearcut pattern of an increase or decline in rates over the ten-year period.

In those countries reporting 500 or more suicides in 1965, it is seen from Table 7.16 that, as in the United States, the age-adjusted suicide rate among males was consistently higher than that for females. The ratios of male to female rates ranged from 1.5:1 for Japan and England to as high as 4.7:1 for Poland. This dominance of male suicide rates over female rates is seen to prevail in every age group in all of the countries shown in Table 7.16. The pattern of increasing suicide rates with increasing age noted for males in the United States seems to hold for the majority of countries shown in Table 7.16. Only in Canada, Australia, Denmark, Finland, and Poland does there appear to be a peaking of male rates in the age range 45-64 years. Female suicide rates in the United States in 1965 were noted to have been higher in age groups 45-54 and 55-64 years. In only 6 of the 17 other countries does this pattern appear to prevail (Canada, Australia, Denmark, Finland, Sweden, and Switzerland). In 8 of the remaining 11 countries, there is a pattern of increasing rates with increasing age similar to that generally observed for males, while in the 3 other countries (England, Italy, and Poland) the age patterns of the rates differ slightly from the patterns described for the other countries.

An examination of the percent changes in the age-adjusted rates for males between 1955 and 1965 for the 18 countries shown in Table 7.16 indicates an increase of 7 percent or more in 7 of the countries, little or no change in 5, and a decline of 7 percent or more in 6. The largest increases, ranging from 25 to 51 percent, occurred in Canada, Australia, Hungary, and Poland, and the largest decreases were observed in Denmark, Italy, and Japan. Among females, the age-adjusted rate rose in 9 of the countries, showed little or no change in 3, and decreased by 5 percent or more in 6. Substantial

Table 7.16a Suicide rates per 100,000 population for 1965 and percent change in rates 1955-1965, for males by age: selected countries[a]

Country	All ages: Age adjusted	All ages: Crude	15-24	25-34	35-44	45-54	55-64	65-74	75 & over
United States	16.9	16.1	9.4	17.3	22.6	29.1	37.3	37.4	47.7
Canada	14.3	12.9	9.0	15.1	19.9	25.8	32.0	28.5	23.2
Australia	19.6	18.8	10.6	23.2	30.2	36.6	34.0	42.9	31.2
England & Wales	11.3	12.7	6.3	10.6	15.5	18.5	25.6	28.8	31.2
Austria	29.7	32.0	18.7	29.5	41.7	53.9	66.1	53.8	70.3
Belgium	17.4	20.7	9.1	13.7	17.3	28.3	43.9	51.2	87.9
Denmark	22.5	24.0	10.4	21.3	37.3	47.0	48.1	36.1	42.1
Finland	34.1	32.2	14.7	38.1	59.2	56.2	73.0	69.3	57.1
France	20.7	23.0	6.2	16.2	26.3	40.6	55.4	51.4	77.8
West Germany	24.6	26.8	18.1	24.8	30.8	42.8	53.7	48.7	64.9
Hungary	39.9	42.6	30.3	44.3	56.1	59.9	72.7	76.5	141.2
Italy	7.2	7.8	3.3	4.8	8.6	12.8	19.0	21.7	27.7
Netherlands	8.2	8.5	4.2	6.3	8.4	12.5	20.8	24.7	46.7
Poland	16.3	14.9	12.3	21.1	25.6	28.8	26.3	25.0	19.5
Portugal	15.2	14.9	5.5	10.0	18.1	25.8	40.6	49.3	70.5
Sweden	24.1	27.7	10.9	27.0	36.3	47.7	44.4	50.5	54.1
Switzerland	25.6	27.5	17.6	21.3	35.4	43.4	54.4	65.0	68.6
Japan	18.3	17.3	15.3	20.9	15.6	22.2	37.0	55.0	86.3
				Percent change in rates 1955-1965					
United States	7.6	0.6	54.1	39.5	20.2	-2.0	-8.1	-16.0	-10.2
Canada	25.4	20.6	109.3	42.5	30.1	14.7	13.9	-1.4	-5.7
Australia	28.9	24.5	8.2	61.1	67.8	54.4	0.9	-9.3	-22.2
England & Wales	-7.3	-11.2	57.5	9.3	19.2	-13.1	-20.5	-31.8	-32.6
Austria	0.3	-3.3	-7.9	1.7	17.8	-6.4	-2.1	-9.6	13.6
Belgium	7.4	3.5	51.7	48.9	0.6	-2.4	3.8	-7.9	0.2
Denmark	-26.0	-25.0	-25.2	-32.6	-13.7	-22.8	-32.1	-38.6	-21.3
Finland	-3.1	-0.6	-23.4	-8.9	5.7	-15.5	5.8	19.1	-10.8
France	-4.2	-6.9	1.6	11.0	1.5	-10.8	1.7	-14.2	-15.3
West Germany	3.8	3.1	0.6	11.2	2.0	-2.7	7.8	9.4	-0.8
Hungary	42.5	49.0	36.5	62.3	106.3	46.8	32.7	4.8	-6.8
Italy	-23.4	-18.7	-31.2	-29.4	-14.0	-33.3	-20.5	-17.2	-6.4
Netherlands	10.8	13.3	50.0	40.0	23.5	-17.2	28.4	-47.7	15.0
Poland	50.9	55.2	46.4	77.3	62.0	44.0	32.8	56.3	-3.9
Portugal	-9.0	0.7	-25.7	11.1	6.5	-17.0	-7.7	-22.0	11.2
Sweden	2.6	1.8	38.0	29.2	13.3	1.3	-25.3	-10.3	-8.3
Switzerland	-12.0	-12.4	-12.4	-23.4	1.1	-15.6	-9.6	-9.1	-21.0
Japan	-48.6	-45.1	-74.6	-52.9	-35.3	-36.0	-27.5	-26.9	-25.2

Source: World Health Statistics Report, Vol. 21, No. 6, Table 1.2 (World Health Organization: Geneva, 1968).

[a] Countries with 500 or more suicides.

Table 7.16b Suicide rates per 100,000 population for 1965 and percent change in rates 1955-1965, for females by age: selected countries

Country	All ages: Age Adj.	All ages: Crude	15-24	25-34	35-44	45-54	55-64	65-74	75 & over	Ratio of male to female age-adj. rate
United States	6.2	5.9	3.0	7.4	10.1	12.7	11.4	9.4	7.5	2.73
Canada	5.0	4.5	2.3	6.0	7.9	10.1	10.4	8.1	4.9*	2.86
Australia	11.2	10.8	6.4	13.5	16.5	21.3	23.9	19.0	10.2	1.75
England & Wales	7.4	9.0	2.6	6.9	10.7	14.1	18.0	18.7	14.0	1.53
Austria	11.8	14.7	4.9	9.3	16.6	27.4	24.2	25.0	32.9	2.52
Belgium	7.7	9.6	3.9	6.9	8.9	14.1	16.9	22.2	24.6	2.26
Denmark	12.9	14.7	5.4	10.7	18.9	28.2	34.6	20.8	22.7	1.74
Finland	8.1	8.1	3.9*	10.2	13.8	15.0	16.2	12.9	4.1*	4.21
France	6.2	7.5	3.6	6.3	7.6	9.6	15.1	15.2	16.9	3.34
West Germany	11.2	13.8	6.7	9.8	13.8	23.0	24.4	25.9	27.2	2.20
Hungary	15.2	17.9	11.6	13.3	17.6	26.1	29.5	28.3	58.9	2.63
Italy	2.8	3.1	2.0	2.7	3.5	5.4	5.9	6.7	5.9	2.57
Netherlands	4.8	5.3	1.1*	4.0	5.2	9.4	11.9	16.2	18.4	1.71
Poland	3.5	3.4	3.6	3.6	3.9	6.2	6.7	5.8	6.4	4.66
Portugal	3.5	3.7	2.7	3.4	4.2	5.4	7.2	8.4	13.5	4.34
Sweden	9.1	10.1	5.2	11.8	14.8	16.7	17.6	13.0	8.1*	2.65
Switzerland	8.8	9.7	5.7	10.1	12.4	16.4	17.2	15.9	15.2	2.91
Japan	12.1	12.2	11.7	13.6	9.7	13.1	19.4	40.1	68.3	1.51
	Percent change in rates 1955-1965									
United States	37.8	28.3	50.0	60.9	65.6	33.7	16.3	2.2	-3.8	
Canada	38.9	32.4	43.8	36.4	38.6	53.0	18.2	52.8	11.4	
Australia	111.3	100.0	433.3	125.0	101.2	63.8	95.9	134.5	104.0	
England & Wales	13.8	7.1	100.0	53.3	42.7	-4.7	-5.3	-7.0	11.1	
Austria	-7.8	-2.6	-60.8	-24.4	-1.2	30.5	-0.8	4.6	1.9	
Belgium	40.0	31.5	160.0	165.4	64.8	25.9	-13.8	58.6	13.9	
Denmark	-5.8	-0.7	-23.9	-33.1	12.5	-5.1	34.1	-33.8	9.1	
Finland	-5.8	-4.7	-7.1	-1.9	5.3	-23.9	-1.8	1.6	141.2	
France	1.6	-3.8	9.1	50.0	26.7	-23.8	-1.9	-14.6	-13.3	
West Germany	0.0	6.2	-21.2	-3.9	-6.1	5.0	9.4	14.1	21.4	
Hungary	26.7	36.6	12.6	30.4	15.8	35.9	42.5	29.8	19.2	
Italy	-20.0	-16.2	-48.7	-15.6	-12.5	1.9	-21.3	-1.5	-26.2	
Netherlands	9.1	15.2	-26.7	66.7	18.2	13.3	-10.5	-4.7	64.3	
Poland	52.1	54.5	33.3	71.4	-2.5	100.0	48.9	87.1	100.0	
Portugal	-2.8	0.0	-43.7	21.4	16.7	17.4	4.3	-7.7	43.6	
Sweden	23.0	18.8	73.3	53.2	10.4	33.6	0.0	3.2	-33.1	
Switzerland	-19.3	-21.8	-12.3	20.2	-0.8	-43.8	-27.4	-18.5	-7.3	
Japan	-41.0	-35.8	-67.9	-41.9	-37.0	-25.1	-26.0	-16.1	-8.7	

Source: World Health Statistics Report, Vol. 21, No. 6, Table 1.2 (World Health Organization: Geneva, 1968).

* Less than 20 deaths.

[a] Countries with 500 or more suicides.

increases were observed for the United States, Canada, Australia, Belgium, Hungary, Poland, and Sweden, and the greatest amount of decline occurred in Italy, Switzerland, and Japan.

Further examination of Table 7.16 with respect to the percent change in age-specific rates for males between 1955 and 1965 indicates that in the 7 countries experiencing an upsurge in male suicides, the largest increases were registered in age groups under 45 years, whereas the rates for males 45 and over either showed increases of smaller magnitude or declined. This same general pattern was also observed in four countries (Austria, France, Germany, and Sweden) where the age-adjusted rates for males underwent little or no change over the ten-year period and in England and Wales, where there was a decline in the age-adjusted rate. For the remaining 6 countries, other patterns of change were observed in the male age-specific rates, with four of the countries (Denmark, Italy, Switzerland, and Japan) experiencing declines in every age group. In 6 countries where the overall suicide rates for females increased between 1955 and 1965 (United States, Australia, England, Belgium, Netherlands, and Sweden) and in France, where the rate remained about the same, the most substantial rise in age-specific rates occurred at ages under 45. Among the other countries, Canada, Austria, Denmark, Finland, Germany, Hungary, and Poland generally experienced higher rates of increase in the age group 45 and over, whereas in Italy, Switzerland, and Japan female rates declined at all ages.

METHODS OF SUICIDE

Of the various methods used to commit suicide in the United States, firearms were employed in almost half the cases during the years 1959-61 as well as in the later period 1964-66 (Table 7.17). Poisons and gases constituted the next most widely used means of suicide at both time periods, accounting for about one-quarter of the suicides, while hanging and strangulation ranked third in importance. Going back in time, it is seen from Table 7.17 that these methods have always been the primary means of suicide but that there have been notable shifts in the extent to which they were used. The proportion of suicides by firearms has increased steadily since the beginning of the century, from about 25 to almost 50 percent in 1964-66, whereas the number of suicides by poisoning or asphyxiation has

Table 7.17 Percent distribution of suicides, by specified method: U.S. registration area 1901-05, 1911-15; U.S. registration states 1926-30; and total U.S. 1950-52, 1959-61, and 1964-66

Method	1964-1966[b]	1959-1961[b]	1950-1952[b]	1926-1930[a]	1911-1915[a]	1901-1905[a]
Total	100.0	100.0	100.0	100.0	100.0	100.0
Poisons and gases	27.0	22.7	22.3	31.1	39.9	42.1
Hanging and strangulation	14.3	17.7	21.2	18.1	14.6	15.0
Drowning	2.6	3.4	4.1	5.2	5.6	5.1
Firearms and explosives	47.6	47.4	43.7	35.1	30.0	24.4
Cutting or piercing instruments	2.0	2.5	3.3	5.4	6.4	5.7
Jumping from high places	3.6	3.7	3.5	3.1	1.9	1.2
Other or unspecified	2.9	2.6	1.9	2.0	1.6	6.5

[a] Source: Dublin, Louis I., Suicide - A Sociological and Statistical Study, (New York: The Ronald Press, 1963) Table 7, p. 38.

[b] Source: U.S. Dept. of Health, Education and Welfare, Public Health Service, Vital Statistics of the United States, Volume II - Mortality (annual).

(Note: data from annual publications were combined to provide the three year averages shown.)

declined from about two-fifths to approximately one-quarter of all suicides. Suicide by hanging has ranked third almost consistently over the 65-year period, showing some increase in importance into the 1950s but a decline in the two later periods. Although the other methods of suicide constituted only small proportions of the total, it is seen in Table 7.17 that the percentage of suicides by drowning and use of cutting and piercing instruments has declined, while the proportion of suicides by jumping from a high place has remained almost constant since 1926-30.

A comparison of male and female suicides with respect to method used indicates that the most significant difference lies in the use of firearms by males and of poisons and gases by females. In every year shown in Table 7.18, more than one-half of the male suicides were by firearms, while that method was used by only one-quarter of the female suicides. The proportion of female suicides in which poison and gas were used was two or more times the corresponding proportion for males. Over the ten-year period 1955-65, there has been little change in the distribution of methods of suicide among males, except for a small increase in the use of poison and gases and a decrease in suicide by hanging. Among females, on the other hand, poison and gas have assumed greater importance over time as methods of suicide, while hanging has declined in importance.

Sex-race differences in methods of suicide shown in Table 7.19 for the period 1959-61 indicate that between white and nonwhite males there was virtually no difference in the proportion committing suicide by firearms. The percentage of white males using poison and gases. however, was almost twice that for nonwhite males, whereas the latter resorted to drowning and jumping from high places in proportionately greater numbers. Differences between white and nonwhite females in methods of suicide followed much the same pattern observed for thier male counterparts, that is. almost identical proportions using firearms but higher percentages of white females using poison and gases and of nonwhite females resorting to drowning or jumping from high places.

The distribution of male and female suicides according to the method used is shown in Table 7.20 for 16 other countries from which such data were available in 1960. For males it is seen that with the exception of Canada, Australia, and New Zealand, the use of firearms, so predominant in the United States, was not the primary means of suicide in the other countries. Hanging, which ranked second in the United States, was the method most used in ten of the other countries, accounting for more than half the suicides in Belgium, France, Germany, and Ireland. In Japan the largest proportion of male suicides were by poisoning, followed closely by hanging; and in England and Wales and Scotland almost half of the males committed suicide by asphyxiation.

Poisoning was the leading method of suicide among females not only in the United States but also in 7 other countries (Canada, Venezuela, Japan, Denmark, Sweden, Australia, and New Zealand). Hanging was the principal means of suicide among females in Belgium, France, Germany, and Italy; asphyxiation was most

Table 7.18 Percent distribution of suicides, by specified method and sex: United States, 1955-65

Method	1955	1956	1957	1958	1959	1960	1961	1962	1963	1964	1965
Male - Total suicide	100.0	100.0	100.0	100.0	100.0	100.0	100.0	100.0	100.0	100.0	100.0
Poisoning & gases	16.9	16.4	16.3	17.5	17.5	18.1	19.0	19.4	20.8	19.9	20.5
Hanging	20.8	20.7	20.7	18.8	18.9	17.7	16.8	16.3	15.5	15.3	15.8
Drowning	2.9	2.6	2.7	2.5	2.7	2.3	2.3	2.3	2.1	2.0	2.0
Firearms	52.5	53.2	53.4	54.3	53.7	54.2	54.6	54.5	54.0	55.7	54.6
Cutting or piercing instr.	2.8	2.8	2.7	2.2	2.5	2.7	2.3	2.3	2.1	2.0	1.9
Jumping from high places	2.6	2.8	2.7	3.3	3.1	3.2	3.3	3.4	3.3	3.2	3.1
other or unspecified means	1.5	1.4	1.4	1.5	1.6	1.7	1.7	1.8	2.1	1.9	2.0
Female - Total suicide	100.0	100.0	100.0	100.0	100.0	100.0	100.0	100.0	100.0	100.0	100.0
Poisoning & gases	32.7	33.1	33.6	35.1	36.2	37.7	38.9	42.8	46.8	46.2	46.8
Hanging	23.8	25.3	23.8	20.7	18.9	17.6	16.1	13.6	12.5	12.7	12.4
Drowning	7.2	6.6	7.7	7.3	6.7	6.4	6.2	5.6	4.5	4.4	4.3
Firearms	25.2	24.6	25.3	25.7	24.7	25.3	25.2	25.0	24.2	25.4	24.0
Cutting or piercing instr.	3.2	2.7	2.7	2.4	2.7	2.1	2.2	2.1	1.6	1.5	1.9
Jumping	5.0	5.1	4.4	6.1	5.8	5.1	5.5	5.6	5.1	5.0	4.8
other or unspecified means	3.1	2.6	2.6	2.6	4.8	5.9	6.0	5.2	5.0	4.8	5.9

Source: World Health Statistics Report (World Health Organization, Geneva, 1968), Vol. 21, No. 6, Table 2.

Table 7.19 Percent distribution of suicides by specified method, by sex and race: United States, 1959-61

Method	Total	White males	White female	Nonwhite males	Nonwhite females
Total	100.0	100.0	100.0	100.0	100.0
Poisons and gases	22.7	18.6	38.2	9.8	26.1
Hanging	17.7	17.9	17.6	16.9	14.8
Drowning	3.4	2.2	6.2	6.5	10.9
Firearms and explosives	47.4	54.3	25.1	53.3	24.6
Cutting and piercing instruments	2.5	2.5	2.3	2.9	2.8
Jumping from high places	3.7	2.9	5.1	8.2	2.9
Other and unspecified	2.6	1.6	5.5	2.4	7.9

[a] Source: U.S. Dept. of Health, Education, and Welfare, Public Health Service, Vital Statistics of the United States, Volume II - Mortality, (annual).

Note: data from annual publications were combined to provide the three year average shown.

predominant in Ireland, the Netherlands, England and Wales, and Scotland; and almost two-fifths of the female suicides in Norway were by drowning. Firearms, ranking second and accounting for about one-quarter of the female suicides in the United States, ranked a low third in Canada and Venezuela, and accounted for few if any suicides in most of the remaining countries.

SUICIDE AND RELIGION

Among the earlier investigators of the phenomenon of suicide, Durkheim (1912) was one of those who found that the incidence of suicide in those European countries for which such data were available was higher among persons of the Protestant faith than among Catholics or Jews. In explaining these differences Durkheim

Table 7.20 Percent distribution of suicides, by specified method and sex: selected countries, 1960

	Total suicide	Poisoning	Gases	Hanging	Drowning	Firearms & explosives	Cutting or piercing instr.	Jumping from high places	Other unspecified means
MALES									
United States	100.0	6.9	11.2	17.7	2.3	54.2	2.7	3.2	1.7
Canada	100.0	8.4	9.1	23.5	5.8	46.5	2.5	2.6	1.7
Venezuela	100.0	19.1	--	41.9	--	27.9	2.0	7.4	1.7
Japan	100.0	40.4	2.9	36.5	5.4	0.8	1.7	1.7	10.6
Belgium	100.0	3.8	9.1	63.1	10.4	4.5	0.6	2.5	6.0
Denmark	100.0	24.0	23.7	35.0	5.3	9.4	0.3	1.3	1.0
France	100.0	3.3	5.5	58.0	11.2	12.4	1.3	1.3	7.1
Germany	100.0	6.5	20.1	51.8	5.4	5.7	1.9	2.6	5.9
Ireland	100.0	5.1	11.9	50.8	15.3	8.5	3.4	--	5.1
Italy	100.0	6.1	5.8	37.4	13.1	16.8	2.7	11.1	6.9
Netherlands	100.0	6.7	19.0	44.0	18.2	3.0	1.9	1.9	5.3
Norway	100.0	10.7	1.6	39.2	8.6	31.2	3.2	3.8	1.6
Sweden	100.0	14.5	11.2	39.9	8.3	17.5	2.4	3.7	2.4
England & Wales	100.0	12.8	49.6	13.6	8.4	5.5	3.5	2.0	4.7
Scotland	100.0	6.1	47.2	17.1	9.1	8.4	5.3	2.3	4.6
Australia	100.0	19.8	16.8	15.8	4.0	34.2	3.6	3.3	2.6
New Zealand	100.0	12.7	24.2	17.0	10.9	27.9	3.0	2.4	1.8
FEMALES									
United States	100.0	30.1	7.6	17.6	6.4	25.3	2.1	5.1	5.9
Canada	100.0	30.4	6.0	21.8	13.9	17.7	2.6	3.8	3.8
Venezuela	100.0	48.3	--	28.0	--	10.2	1.7	5.9	5.9
Japan	100.0	40.4	5.8	27.3	16.3	0.1	1.0	1.0	8.1
Belgium	100.0	9.1	16.0	40.5	21.9	1.6	1.6	4.8	4.5
Denmark	100.0	41.6	23.6	18.2	11.5	0.3	1.0	2.9	1.0
France	100.0	8.9	13.6	38.1	26.1	2.5	1.2	3.3	6.3
Germany	100.0	12.3	28.7	32.6	12.3	0.4	1.8	7.0	5.1
Ireland	100.0	20.0	36.0	4.0	32.0	--	--	4.0	4.0
Italy	100.0	16.3	12.1	22.8	19.6	2.0	1.5	20.1	5.5
Netherlands	100.0	13.6	33.3	17.3	26.9	--	1.7	3.1	4.1
Norway	100.0	22.2	--	26.7	37.8	2.2	4.4	6.7	--
Sweden	100.0	31.5	9.2	27.5	20.1	1.2	1.5	4.3	4.6
England & Wales	100.0	26.8	52.9	6.0	8.9	0.4	0.9	2.1	1.9
Scotland	100.0	24.1	53.8	6.9	11.0	--	--	2.1	2.1
Australia	100.0	47.2	22.6	9.2	8.9	5.4	1.9	3.5	1.3
New Zealand	100.0	24.6	21.6	6.2	21.5	9.2	6.2	4.6	6.2

Source: World Health Statistics Report (World Health Organization: Geneva, 1968), Vol. 21, No. 6, Table 2.

put forth the notion that a religion exerts a beneficial or preservative influence not because of the particular characteristics of the religious ideas it embodies but because it fosters a collective life of sufficient intensity through numerous and strong beliefs and practices common to all its members. Thus he observed that because the Protestant church does not foster the same degree of integration and social organization among its members as does Catholicism or Judaism, it therefore has less of a moderating influence on suicide.

Attempts to determine whether this interrelationship between religious affiliation and suicide exists to any degree in the United States are considerably hampered by the fact that religion is not recorded on the standard death certificate nor in the decennial census. Consequently, there is no base for conducting studies in this areas on a national scale. A few studies, cited by Dublin (1963), have been carried out in certain communities or areas of the nation such as an early study by Stearns in Massachusetts, where he found the suicide rate for Protestants to be higher than for Catholics and Jews, and studies conducted in St. Louis and New York, where the suicide rate for Jews was found to be lower than that for the total population.

Another manifestation of the possible influence of religion upon the incidence of suicide is provided by an examination of the suicide rates of those countries in which certain religious groups are predominant. In line with Durkheim's thesis and the findings of subsequent studies mentioned above. it is seen that some of the European countries in which the Catholic faith predominates had reported the lowest rates in 1960 (Table 7.15). For example, in Ireland (Irish Free State) the rate was only 3.0 per 100,000, in Greece 3.8 per 100,000, in Spain 5.5 per 100,000, in Italy 6.1 per 100,000, in Poland 8.0 per 100,000, and in Portugal 8.7 per 100,000. On the other hand, certain of the Protestant countries had high suicide rates, such as Finland, with a rate of 20.5 per 100,000, Denmark, with 20.3, Germany, with 18.8 and Sweden, with 17.4. There are exceptions, however, such as the low rates among predominantly Protestant countries as Northern Ireland (4.4 per 100,000), Norway (6.4), the Netherlands (6.6), and Scotland (7.7), and high rates among Catholic countries such as Hungary (24.9 per 100,000), Austria (23.1), Czechoslovakia (20.6), and France (15.9). In view of the exceptions it becomes quite clear, as Dublin (1963) points out that "the suicide rate of a nation is influenced by many factors besides the religion of its population, such as economic conditions, social traditions, degree of urbanization, and even the prevailing political climate." Hence, the data presented above can only serve to indicate the possible influence of religion.

SOCIOECONOMIC FACTORS AND SUICIDE

Attempts to assess the relationship between socioeconomic status and suicide are severely limited by the fact that data on certain socioeconomic characteristics, such as education and income, do not appear on the standard death certificate in the United States, or, if reported, as is the case with occupation, the differences in definition of occupational categories found on the death certificate and on the U.S. census record, owing to differences in reporting practices and in coding procedures, have cast some doubt upon the accuracy of mortality rates computed from the two sources. One approach to circumvent these problems has been used in a study conducted by the Population Research and Training Center of the University of Chicago with the cooperation of the National Center for Health Statistics and the Bureau of the Census in which death certificates for persons who died within the first four months after the 1960 census were matched to their 1960 census schedules. In this way, those social and economic characteristics of the decedents are obtainable from the census record. Thus, mortality rates for specified population groups based on the census data can be considered to have somewhat greater reliability since both numerator and denominator data are obtained from the same source. The procedures for carrying out this matching study were virtually identical with those described in Chapter 6 for the Louisiana-Maryland study.

Only data on educational level were available from the matching study for this monograph and, because of the very small number of suicides, findings could be cited only for suicides of males. According to Kitagawa and Hauser (1968), mortality from suicide of the least educated adult men (25 years of age and over) was almost twice that of the best educated. These results, the authors point out, though clearly significant, are subject to relatively high sampling variance in view of the small number of deaths. The information on usual occupation of the decendent appearing on the standard death certificate has not been used to any great extent to examine the incidence of suicide among various occupational groups. A study of mortality by occupation for 1950 conducted by the National Office of Vital Statistics showed that among males 20 to 64 years old with work experience, standard mortality ratios* with respect to suicide were highest for laborers and agricultural workers, whereas there was little difference in ratios among the other occupation groups, ranging from professionals to semiskilled workers (Guralnick, 1969).

These findings were not entirely consistent with those from reports of the Registrars General of England and Wales, in which mortality from suicide among males in various social classes, based primarily on occupation, was examined. The five social classes were defined as follows: Class I – persons in the professions and the highest ranks of business life; Class II – entrepreneurs, managers, retail traders, clerks, teachers, and farm owners; Class III – skilled workers; Class IV – unskilled laborers. Data for the period 1949-53 showed that among males 20-64 years of age suicide rates relative to the average rate for all civilian males were highest in Class I, next highest in Class V, and were followed by Classes II, IV, and III, in that order (the Registrar General's Decennial Supplement, 1958). Similar findings were encountered by Powell (1958) in his examination of suicides by occupational category for adult white males in Tulsa County, Oklahoma, during the period 1937-56. Both extremes of the occupational hierarchy, the professional-managerial and unskilled labor categories, generated the highest suicide rates, while the middle groups – sales-clerical, craftsmen, and operatives – had considerably lower rates. Schmid and Van Arsdol (1955), on the other hand, conducting a study in Seattle for the period 1948-52, found that, in general, members of the "white-collar" occupations and professions had lower rates of both completed and attempted suicides than persons employed in "blue-collar" occupations. As the authors point out, however, these findings are open to some question owing to the incompleteness of their data.

In the absence of good sources of socioeconomic data on suicides, another approach has been to examine the incidence of suicide in areas characterized by the general socioeconomic level of their

---

*This ratio is the actual number of deaths in a given class, divided by the expected number, where the latter figure is the sum of the number of deaths expected in each age group, if average mortality for the population in study in the same age group prevailed.

populations. Thus, Sainsbury (1955) in his ecological study of suicides in London found that boroughs of the city with high proportions of the "middle-class, moderately well-to-do" had suicide rates higher than average, whereas the "poorer" boroughs had rates below the average. Weiss (1954), delineating neighborhood districts of New Haven, Connecticut, into four class levels found that the average yearly suicide rate for those neighborhoods in the two combined "upper class" groupings was 12.3 per 100,000 population compared to a rate of 8.0 for neighborhoods in the two combined "lower class" groups.

In a study utilizing 1957 data concerning sociological and suicide information from Los Angeles County, Schneidman and Farberow (1960) divided the county into 100 relatively stable and homogeneous study areas. These areas were distributed among nine area types according to urbanization and social rank as follows: I – most advantaged suburbs; II – most advantaged residential communities; III – most advantaged apartment house areas; IV – most moderately advantaged suburbs; V – moderately advantaged natural communities; VI – moderately advantaged multiple dwelling areas; VII – least advantaged rural areas; VIII – least advantaged industrial communities; and IX – least advantaged rooming-house and apartment areas. Suicide rates for the nine area types ranged from 3 to 22 per 100,000 population, with the areas ranked from high to low according to their rates as follows: Type III – 22 per 100,000; Type VI – 21; Type IX – 19; Type II – 16; Type V – 14; Type VIII – 13; Type I – 12; Type IV – 8; and Type VII – 3.

The inconsistencies encountered in the findings of the studies cited can probably be attributed to such factors as inadequacies in the data available to the investigators, differences in methodology, differences in the types of populations or the area units studied, and differences in the time periods in which the various studies were carried out. Because of these inconsistencies no definite conclusions can be drawn concerning the relationship between socioeconomic status and the frequency of suicide.

MENTAL ILLNESS AND SUICIDE

The taking of one's own life is generally considered to be a deviant act in all but those few societies where it is regarded as a socially acceptable form of conduct. Thus, in the minds of many, suicide presumes the presence of mental illness. However, as Dublin (1963) points out, it is almost impossible to quantify the relationship between mental disease and suicide with any precision, owing to the facts that (1) the dividing line between "normality" and mental illness is never clear-cut; (2) the classification and nomenclature of mental disorders tend to vary not only over time but also from place to place; (3) there is no adequate means of assessing the *total* number of persons in a community who may be mentally ill, and thus it is difficult to judge what proportion of these are comprised of suicides of individuals who have exhibited such symptoms. All of these factors were mentioned earlier in the discussion of problems in psychiatric diagnosis.

Despite these difficulties, a number of studies in recent years have attempted to determine the proportion of persons committing suicide who were identified as having had some form of mental illness. As seen from Appendix Table 15, these percentages range from as low as 7 to as high as 94. Differences with respect to the place of study, source of data, size of the sample, and, most particularly, criteria for "mental illness" used by the investigator probably account, in part, for the wide variation observed in these percentages.

The relationship between mental illness and suicide has also been examined from the standpoint of the incidence of suicide among patients with mental disorders. The findings from selected areas of the United States and from studies conducted elsewhere, as shown in Appendix Table 16, indicate that suicide rates among mental patients or former mental patients are higher, and in some instances considerably higher, than those for the general population. The variation in suicide rates among the patient populations shown in the table can be attributed in part to differences in the types of populations represented; i.e., hospital versus case register populations. However, the diagnostic make-up of these populations might also contribute to the differences in rates, since it appears that certain categories of mental illness seem to generate a greater incidence of suicide, as seen in Table 7.21. The data in this table, taken from four sources and grouped into nearly similar diagnostic categories, indicate that, except for the New York State mental hospitals in 1961-62, the highest suicide rates appear to occur among patients with affective disorders (manic-depressive and involutional

Table 7.21 Average annual suicide rate for psychiatric populations, by diagnostic category: specified areas, various years

<table>
<tr><th>Diagnosis</th><th>New York 1957-59[a]</th><th>New York 1961-62[b]</th><th>California 1964-66[c]</th><th>Monroe City, New York 1960-62[d]</th></tr>
<tr><td>Total</td><td>34.0</td><td>35.6</td><td>50.1</td><td>160</td></tr>
<tr><td>Alcoholism</td><td>--</td><td>22.8</td><td>--</td><td>294</td></tr>
<tr><td>Cerebral arteriosclerosis</td><td>31.9</td><td rowspan="2">11.0</td><td rowspan="2">11.2</td><td rowspan="2">89[e]</td></tr>
<tr><td>Diseases of senium</td><td>--</td></tr>
<tr><td>Schizophrenia</td><td>30.1</td><td>43.2</td><td>42.5</td><td>146[f]</td></tr>
<tr><td>Manic-depressive phychosis</td><td>87.4</td><td>20.2</td><td>156.1</td><td rowspan="2">351</td></tr>
<tr><td>Involutional psychosis</td><td>80.4</td><td rowspan="2">88.8</td><td rowspan="2">108.4</td></tr>
<tr><td>Other psychosis</td><td rowspan="4">46.1</td><td>--</td></tr>
<tr><td>Psychoneurosis</td><td>209.6</td><td>109.5</td><td rowspan="2">151</td></tr>
<tr><td>Personality disorders</td><td>--</td><td rowspan="2">59.4</td></tr>
<tr><td>Other diagnoses</td><td>--</td><td>--</td></tr>
</table>

[a] Source: Dublin, Louis I., Suicide: A Sociological and Statis- Study, (New York: The Ronald Press, 1963), Table 18. Data refer to suicides among patients with mental diseases in New York State Mental Hospitals.

[b] Source: Annual Reports, New York State Department of Mental Hygiene. Data refer to patients resident in state mental hospitals.

[c] Source: Annual Reports, California Department of Mental Hygiene. Data refer to patients in state and county mental hospitals.

[d] Source: Gardner, Elmor A., Bahn, A.K. and Mack, M. "Suicides and Psychiatric Care in the Aging," Archives of General Psychiatry, Volume 10, June 1964, Table 3. Data refer to patients seen by psychiatric inpatient units, clinics, emergency services and all but 3 of 50 psychiatrists in private practice in Monroe County.

[e] Rate shown is for category "chronic brain syndrome"

[f] Includes paranoid reaction.

psychoses). Other diagnostic groups seen to have high rates are the psychoneurotics and, among the case register population, the alcoholics. The small number or lack of suicides among alcoholic patients in state mental hospitals can probably be attributed to the rapid turnover of this particular diagnostic group.

In another study of 134 suicides in St. Louis County, Missouri, over a one-year period 1956-57, Robins et al. (1959) found that 101 of these persons had one of five specific psychiatric illnesses (manic-depressive depression, which included psychotic depressive reaction and involutional psychosis, chronic alcoholism, schizophrenia, chronic brain syndrome, and drug addiction) and that of these approximately 60 percent suffered from manic-depressive reaction and 30 percent were chronic alcoholics. In another approach to the discussion of mental illness and suicide, Gibbs (1967), recognizing that the existence of concurrent mental illness is the dominant thesis in most research on the characteristics of persons committing suicide, feels that although this thesis has merits when applied to individual cases, it has little or no value in explaining variations in suicide rates. To support this view he maintains that to date no investigation has found a close relation between measures of the incidence of psychopathology and the suicide rate by sex, race, age, marital status, and societies or territorial divisions of societies (i.e., from community to community or from region to region), and, furthermore, that despite the fact that all measures of incidence of mental illness are subject to question, it is improbable that the incidence of mental illness has fluctuated as much as the suicide rate since 1900 or that there has even been a close correlation between the two trends. In a concluding observation he states that "even if it should be shown that the two trends have been closely related, one could argue that some social condition underlies both rates, which means that the rate of psychopathology and the rate of suicide are co-dependent variables rather than the former being the cause of the latter."

Brief reference has been made to some of the various approaches that have been pursued in the past to determine what sort of linkage may exist between the act of suicide and the mental status of the individual committing that act. In recent years, according to Yolles (1967) in his presentation at a 1965 symposium on suicide, investigations of suicide have taken a new direction which have led, after repeated testings, to the formulation of several new hypotheses concerning the act of suicide. These, he states, hypothesize that "(1) the tendency to suicide is a symptom of a hitherto unnamed psychic disease which only in the rarest of cases is a genuine mental illness; instead it is a neurosis which is a disturbance in mental balance often brought about by unresolved conflicts with the environment; (2) this disease generally begins in childhood and develops continually, however, it is avoidable and its fatal outcome can be prevented; and (3) suicidal patients are just as disinclined to be ill as, for instance, tuberculosis patients; they are not free in making their decisions to die."

8 / Prospects for the Future

The patterns of use of psychiatric facilities in 1966 as described in this volume were shaped by the events and actions that occurred in the twenty-year interval following the passage of the National Mental Health Act (P.L. 79-487) in 1946, referred to in Chapter 3. Thus, the data presented in this monograph serve as baselines against which to compare data reflecting further changes in mental health programs which are already occurring as a result of major federal legislation and expansion of private health insurance coverage.

In 1963 Congress enacted legislation which was destined to change the patterns of use of mental hospitals and other types of psychiatric services: the Mental Retardation and Community Health Centers Construction Act of 1963 (P.L. 88-164). This legislation, which authorized funds for constructing comprehensive mental health centers throughout the nation, has led to an intensified national effort to prevent and control mental disorders and to make psychiatric services more widely available to the public so as to change existing patterns of usage of psychiatric facilities and to promote mental health. Amendments were added subsequently to the basic law which authorized: (*a*) funds to assist in the initial cost of staffing these new centers (P.L. 89-105, 1965); (*b*) federal grants for the construction and staffing of community facilities and services for alcoholics and narcotic addicts and to permit states to use a portion of their allotment for centers to defray costs of state planning for community mental health services (P.L. 90-574, 1968; P L. 91-211, 1970); and (*c*) grants for services for children, including construction, staffing, training, and evaluation (P.L. 91-211, 1970). In addition these amendments extend the duration of all staffing grants to eight years: authorize a higher percentage of construction and staffing funds for programs in poverty areas; provide grants to developmental service programs in poverty areas; and permit additional staffing grants for consultation personnel in all four programs.

The Community Mental Health Centers Program has as its objective the establishment of a network of comprehensive community mental health center programs which will integrate and coordinate the elements of comprehensive services at the local level so as to maintain patients close to their own environment and to protect their links with family and community. The five essential elements of service to be provided by every center include: (1) inpatient services providing 24-hour care for treatment of acute disorders; (2) outpatient services; (3) partial hospitalization services such as day care, night care, and weekend care; (4) emergency services 24 hours per day which must be available within at least one of the first three services listed above; (5) consultation and education services to community agencies and professional personnel. To reach the goal of comprehensive services, five additional services will be needed: (6) diagnostic services; (7) rehabilitative services, including vocational and educational programs; (8) pre-care and after-care services in the community, including foster home placement, home visiting, and half-way houses, (9) training; and (10) research and evaluation.

As of July 1, 1970, 420 centers had been funded and 260 were already in operation. The intent of the legislation was that there would be an equivalent of one center for every 100,000 population by 1980.

Other major developments will continue to affect the patterns of use of psychiatric services. One of these is the expansion of private voluntary health insurance to cover mental health care, which has resulted in increasing numbers of persons having such coverage. This has been responsible, to a large extent, for the growth of psychiatric services in general hospitals and the increase in numbers of persons utilizing these services.

Another development is the federal legislation creating health insurance for the aged (P.L. 89-97, Sections XVIII and XIX, 1965). This amendment to the Social Security Act provides insurance benefits for the care of the aged mentally ill. The benefits under Section A of Title XVIII encouraged the use of general hospitals, extended care facilities, and services provided by home health agencies. The supplementary medical insurance benefits of Part B provide additional coverage for outpatient psychiatric services and for additional home health services. These benefits will undoubtedly increase the number of the aged mentally ill admitted to general hospitals and to nursing homes. Title XIX also provides grants to states for medical assistance for aged persons in mental institutions. To participate a state must meet certain standards and provide evidence that it is making satisfactory progress toward developing and implementing a comprehensive mental health program. This will require intensive welfare services so as to develop programs that will achieve these goals, particularily as they relate to the aged.

All of these developments are already beginning to have a profound effect upon the demand for mental health services and upon the number and characteristics of the persons who received them. Continued measurement of the kind of medical care data presented in this volume will undoubtedly reflect the impact of these new programs.

The regulations governing the implementation of the Community Mental Health Center legislation referred to above require such measurement and direct administrators who wish to qualify for funds for construction and staffing of centers to develop plans which take into account the need for mental health services within the boundaries of their states and localities. They further require that subareas within states be ranked in priority order according to need for mental health services. Development of these plans, therefore, requires knowledge of the demographic, social, and economic characteristics of the state, of patterns of utilization of psychiatric and related facilities, and, in particular, of factors that influence the occurrence and distribution of mental disorders and associated disabilities in the various subgroups of the population designated as the recipients of the mental health services.

It should be clear from the material presented in this volume that data on the characteristics of populations and on the patterns of utilization of psychiatric and related facilities required for these plans can be obtained, although doing so in a systematic way is a complex task. Sound techniques for estimating the need for mental health services in a community, on the other hand, do not exist. It cannot be emphasized enough that the expected changes in rates at which persons will come under psychiatric care in the future will not reflect changes in true incidence or prevalence of mental disorders in various segments of the population. The new programs mentioned above are designed to bring services to persons who are mentally ill but who hitherto have not been receiving services for a variety of reasons. Thus, the measurement of the actual level of mental disorder in a population and the number of individuals with such disorders who are in need of mental health services remains a problem yet to be solved.

Appendices

Appendix Tables

References

Index

Appendix A
Relationship of Admission Rate to Resident Patient Rate

Knowledge of two basic variables is essential to explain the differences between the composition of resident patient and annual first admission populations, namely, rates at which different categories of patients are admitted and the numerical size of these categories, and duration of stay of each category of patient, which is dependent on rates at which patients are returned to the community or die in the hospital. To illustrate this fact, consider how three hypothetical mental hospital populations developed.

Assume that there are two communities of the same size that have always been free of mental disorder. Suddenly, on January 1, 1940, 1,000 individuals became mentally ill for the first time in each community. To simplify the problem further, assume that these people are all afflicted with the same disorder and are hospitalized immediately on January 1. Thereafter, on January 1 of every year, 1,000 new cases of the same disorder always appear in each community and the sick individuals are hospitalized immediately. Let us also assume that the members of each annual cohort of admissions are returned to the community at some specified rate. Table A.1 indicates what would be the resident patient count on January 1 of each year under the following assumptions with respect to the way patients in each community are released from the hospital: (1) that 100 people annually are separated from each cohort of first admissions, and (2) that for each cohort of 1,000 new admissions, 10 percent of those in the hospital at the beginning of each year are separated during that year.

Although the annual number of first admissions in each year is the same, the populations resident in the hospital on January 1 of each year start to differ considerably as between communities after the first two years and eventually reach quite different levels. Thus, the resident patient count in example 1 increased to a total of 5,500 patients on January 1, 1949, and then stabilized at that level. In example 2, the resident patient count reached a total of 6,511 on January 1, 1949, and continued to increase. It can be shown that this population will stabilize eventually at 10,000. A third example is included in which in a community, identical in size with the other two, the annual number of new admissions to the mental hospital is assumed to be 2,000. In this population, however, 40 percent of each cohort still in the hospital at the beginning of a year are returned to the community during that year. In this population the resident patient count increased to 4,969 on January 1, 1949, and will stabilize at 5,000, a level less than in the other two examples.

Although the above illustrations dealt with admissions to hospitals in three hypothetical communities, they might also be used to illustrate how differences develop in a single hospital between the percentage distribution of diagnoses among first admissions as compared to that among resident patients. For example, assume that in a single hospital there are annually 1,000 admissions for disease type A, 1,000 of type B, and 2,000 of type C subjected to the rates of release in examples 1, 2, and 3 above, respectively. Table A.2 shows the percentage distribution (for each of the three disease categories A, B, and C) at time of admission and on January 1 of every year following the date the number of residents in each category stabilized. Thus, although the admission rate for one type of disorder is high, if the release rate is also high (i.e., average duration of stay is short), patients with this disorder will constitute a relatively small proportion of the resident population. On the other hand, a disorder with a relatively low admission rate may constitute a high proportion of resident patients because of a relatively long duration of stay.

These illustrations demonstrate that resident patient counts are a function of annual numbers of admissions and duration of stay of patients in each cohort of admissions. Explanations of differences in resident patient counts are not possible without knowledge of these two basic variables. Of course the preceding examples present a highly simplified representation of what actually goes on, since for each hospital we have assumed a constant annual number of admissions, a constant annual separation pattern for each cohort of admissions, and no readmissions. What makes a mental hospital population such a complex population unit to study is that its composition is a result of medical, social, environmental, economic, and administrative factors which have produced current and past rates of first admission, current and past rates at which patients are released to the community or die in the hospital, and current and past rates at which patients are readmitted to the hospital.

Table A.1 Illustration as to how three hypothetical mental hospital populations develop under various assumptions of admission and release of patients.

Example 1. Assumptions: 1,000 first admissions annually, all of whom are hospitalized on January 1 of specified year, and 100 patients annually are separated from each cohort of such first admissions

Cohort of year	Patients in hospital on Jan. 1 of specified year										
	1940	1941	1942	1943	1944	1945	1946	1947	1948	1949	1950
1940	1,000	900	800	700	600	500	400	300	200	100	0
1941		1,000	900	800	700	600	500	400	300	200	100
1942			1,000	900	800	700	600	500	400	300	200
1943				1,000	900	800	700	600	500	400	300
1944					1,000	900	800	700	600	500	400
1945						1,000	900	800	700	600	500
1946							1,000	900	800	700	600
1947								1,000	900	800	700
1948									1,000	900	800
1949										1,000	900
1950											1,000
Total	1,000	1,900	2,700	3,400	4,000	4,500	4,900	5,200	5,400	5,500	5,500

Example 2. Assumptions: 1,000 first admissions annually, all of whom are hospitalized on January 1 of specified year, and 10% of those in the hospital at the beginning of each year are separated during that year.

Cohort of year	Patients in hospital on Jan. 1 of specified year										
	1940	1941	1942	1943	1944	1945	1946	1947	1948	1949	1950
1940	1,000	900	810	729	656	590	531	478	430	387	348
1941		1,000	900	810	729	656	590	531	478	430	387
1942			1,000	900	810	729	656	590	531	478	430
1943				1,000	900	810	729	656	590	531	478
1944					1,000	900	810	729	656	590	531
1945						1,000	900	810	729	656	590
1946							1,000	900	810	729	656
1947								1,000	900	810	729
1948									1,000	900	810
1949										1,000	900
1950											1,000
Total	1,000	1,900	2,710	3,439	4,095	4,685	5,216	5,694	6,124	6,511	6,859

Example 3. Assumptions: 2,000 first admissions annually, all of whom are hospitalized on January 1 of specified year, and 40% of those in the hospital at the beginning of each year are separated during that year.

Cohort of year	Patients in hospital on Jan. 1 of specified year										
	1940	1941	1942	1943	1944	1945	1946	1947	1948	1949	1950
1940	2,000	1,200	720	432	259	155	93	56	34	20	12
1941		2,000	1,200	720	432	259	155	93	56	34	20
1942			2,000	1,200	720	432	259	155	93	56	34
1943				2,000	1,200	720	432	259	155	93	56
1944					2,000	1,200	720	432	259	155	93
1945						2,000	1,200	720	432	259	155
1946							2,000	1,200	720	432	259
1947								2,000	1,200	720	432
1948									2,000	1,200	720
1949										2,000	1,200
1950											2,000
Total	2,000	3,200	3,920	4,352	4,611	4,766	4,859	4,915	4,949	4,969	4,981

Table A.2 Comparison of distribution of numbers and percent of patients in three diagnostic groups in the annual first admissions and stabilized resident patient population of a hypothetical mental hospital according to certain assumptions of annual number of first admissions and length of stay

Type of mental disease	Number in: Annual first admissions	Number in: Stabilized population	Percent in: Annual first admissions	Percent in: Stabilized population	Average duration of stay of first admissions (in years)
Total	4,000	20,500	100.0	100.0	--
A	1,000	5,500	25.0	26.8	5.00
B	1,000	10,000	25.0	48.8	9.50
C	2,000	5,000	50.0	24.4	1.96

Assumptions as to annual first admissions and length of stay:

Disease Group A - One thousand new admissions annually, and 100 patients separated annually from each cohort of admission.

Disease Group B - One thousand new admissions annually, and 10 percent of each cohort in the hospital at the beginning of the year is separated during that year.

Disease Group C - Two thousand new admissions annually, and 40 percent of each cohort still in the hospital at the beginning of the year is separated during that year.

Appendix B
Relationship of First Admission Rate To a Mental Hospital to "True" Incidence Rate

If in population group, i,

N_i = number of persons in the midyear population of the year in question*

a_i = number of persons becoming mentally ill during the year (first attacks),

h_i = number of persons first hospitalized during the year among a_i,

h_i' = number of persons first hospitalized during the year among those who had become mentally ill in previous years and who had never been hospitalized,

then

$$I_i = \text{incidence rate for the year} = \frac{a_i}{N_i},$$

and

F_i = first admission rate for the year =

$$\frac{h_i + h_i'}{N_i} = \frac{a_i}{N_i} \cdot \frac{h_i + h_i'}{a_i},$$

*Use of the total midyear population as a denominator for the incidence and first admission rates yields only an approximation to their actual values. Theoretically, for the incidence rate, the population should be adjusted for the number of people who have had previous attacks of mental illness and, for the first admission rate, previous episodes of hospitalization.

that is,

$$F_i = I_i \left(\frac{h_i + h_i'}{a_i}\right).$$

Thus, the annual first admission rate is a function not only of the incidence of mental disorder but also of the ratio of first hospitalized patients to new patients. Indeed, the ratio of first admission rates in 2 population groups is equal to the ratio of the incidence rates only if:

$$\frac{h_1 + h_1'}{a_1} = \frac{h_2 + h_2'}{a_2};$$

that is, only when the ratio of the total number of persons first hospitalized during the year to the number becoming mentally ill during the year is constant between groups.

Studies which have used differences in first admission rates as an index of differences in incidence in population groups have made one of the following assumptions: (1) that the ratio of the number of persons becoming hospitalized in some specified interval of time to the number becoming mentally ill during that period is constant from group to group, in which case the ratio of first admission rates gives a true measure of relative morbidity risks; or (2) that the difference in incidence is so great that, regardless of the differences in the ratio of the number of persons hospitalized to the number becoming ill, the difference in first admission rates would still be in the same direction as the true difference in incidence.

Appendix C
The Classification of Mental Disorders

The diagnosis on the records of patients admitted to a psychiatric facility – be it a mental hospital, psychiatric service in a general hospital, or outpatient clinic – is the basic item from which annual, national statistics on care of patients with specific mental disorders are produced. Over the years several different classifications of mental disorders have provided the nomenclature which psychiatrists have used in recording these diagnoses. This appendix will provide a brief historical description of the development of these classifications in the United States, with particular emphasis on the two systems of psychiatric nomenclature on which the statistics in the volume are based.

HISTORICAL BACKGROUND

The federal government has collected and published statistical data on the mentally ill in the United States since the decennial census of 1840. In that census, the idiotic and insane were enumerated as a single class and no distinction was made between these two categories of persons. In the decennial census of 1850, the mentally ill were enumerated for the first time as a separate class, and the cases were not classified by type of illness. It was not until 1880 that an attempt was made to classify by type of mental disorder the number of mentally ill in the United States, both those in institutions and those not institutionalized. The following quote from the "Introductory Remarks on the Defective, Dependent and Delinquent Classes of the United States (June 1, 1880)" (Census Office, 1888) provides an interesting historical perspective on the problems surrounding the development of classification of mental disorders within our country. Indeed, many of the same problems are still with us:

> Much effort has been put forth to secure uniformity in the classification of the insane in every country of the world, but it seems impossible for those best qualified to form an opinion to agree upon any scheme which can be devised. Some classifications are based upon symptoms and some upon physical causes; others are a mixture of the two; and still others take into

> account the complications of insanity. For the purpose of the census, it seemed to me* advisable to disregard all minute subdivisions and to adopt a simple analysis on the broadest possible outlines. On consultation with the members of the New England Psychological Association and with other expert alienists (who concurred in this opinion), it was decided to make but seven distinctions as to the form of insanity, namely; Mania, which manifests itself in a state of nervous, intellectual and emotional exaltation and excitement; Melancholia, or a state of depression; Monomania, which it is difficult to define, but which is characterized by fixed delusions on particular subjects, which sometimes or often appear at a very early period in life; Paresis, or general paralysis of the insane; Dementia, which is the condition of imbecility into which mania and melancholia ultimately degenerate, where they do not terminate in death; Dipsomania, or alcoholic insanity and epilepsy.

The classification used in the census of 1880 was also used in the collection of statistics on the mentally ill in the census of 1890 but was not used thereafter. It was not until the special census of patients in hospitals for mental disease carried out in 1923 (Bureau of the Census, 1926) that extensive diagnostic statistics on the mentally ill in the United States were again published. The classification of mental disorders used in that census was developed collaboratively by the American Psychiatric Association (then the American Medico-Psychological Association) and the former National Committee for Mental Health. These efforts resulted in a classification of mental disorders and a plan for uniform statistics in hospitals for mental diseases, which were adopted by the American Psychiatric Association in May 1917 (American Medico-Psychological Association, 1920). This classifcation was used with only minor modifications until 1934, when it was revised to conform to the more extensive classification of mental diseases contained in the first edition of the Standard Nomenclature of Diseases (Jordan, 1933). This classification served as a basis for the collection of statistics on the diagnostic characteristics of patients admitted to mental hospitals

---

***This refers to Mr. Frederick Howard Wines, the Special Agent of the Census Office (then located in the Department of Interior) who was in charge of the census of the defective, dependent, and delinquent classes and prepared the introductory remarks.**

in the United States until 1952, when the American Psychiatric Association published the first edition of the Diagnostic and Statistical Manual, DSM-1 (American Psychiatric Association, 1952).

From 1934 to 1952 mental hospital psychiatrists used diagnostic terms that conformed to the nomenclature and definitions in the tenth edition of the *Statistical Manual for Use of Hospitals for Mental Diseases* (to be referred to hereafter as SMHMD) (American Psychiatric Association and National Committee for Mental Hygiene, 1942). Since the diagnostic classification in SMHMD was identical to that contained in the *Standard Nomenclature of Diseases* (1933), the diagnostic nomenclature of the psychobiologic section of the *Standard Nomenclature* became the official psychiatric nomenclature in the United States. However, this classification had been developed primarily for use in mental hospitals; consequently, it was found inadequate for diagnosing many of the types of disorders that were being seen by psychiatrists working in the induction stations, the armed forces, and the Veterans Administration during World War II. The *Standard Nomenclature* classification was also found to be inadequate by psychiatrists working in outpatient psychiatric clinics, in psychiatric services in general hospitals, which were developing at an accelerated pace following World War II, and in private practice. As a result, various groups modified the classification to meet their own needs. Thus, by 1948, three nomenclatures were in use in the United States – The *Standard,* armed forces, and Veterans Administration, and various teaching centers modified each of these for their own use.

The situation became more complicated when the sixth revision of the *Manual of the International Statistical Classification of Diseases, Injuries and Causes of Death* came into force in 1948. Its section on mental disorders was not completely compatible with the various classifications of mental disorders then in use in the United States. Accordingly, the Committee on Nomenclature and Statistics of the American Psychiatric Association was assigned the task of developing a revised classification of psychiatric disorders which would meet the needs of psychiatrists working not only in mental hospitals but also in general hospitals, outpatient facilities, and private practice. The committee started work on this assignment in 1948 and completed it with the publication of the *Diagnostic and Statistical Manual of Mental Disorders* in 1952 (A.P.A., 1952). This classification (to be referred to hereafter as DSM-1) was also adopted as the psychobiologic unit of the fourth edition of the *Standard Nomenclature of Diseases and Operations,* published in 1952 (Plunkett and Hayden, 1952). It thus provided the psychiatric nomenclature for use not only in psychiatric but also in general medical practice.

DIFFERENCES BETWEEN MAJOR CLASSIFICATIONS

The span of years covered in this monograph includes the period during which the diagnostic nomenclature used in psychiatric facilities (particularly mental hospitals) was changed. It is important, therefore, for the reader to be aware of the major differences between the diagnostic classifications in SMHMD (10th edition) and that in DSM-1, and of the difficulties of converting some of the diagnoses from the former classification to those in DSM-1. It is also important since all diagnostic data presented in this volume are arranged in categories from the DSM-1 classifications. The following paragraphs highlight the differences between the conceptual schemes of each system, their nomenclature, and the contents of major diagnostic categories.

The nomenclature in use *prior* to 1952 subdivided the mental disorders into the following major categories:

1. "Psychoses" associated with known organic etiologic factors
2. Disorders of psychogenic origin or without clearly defined tangible cause or structural change in the brain, subdivided into:
   (a) Psychoses
   (b) Psychoneuroses
   (c) Conditions "without mental disorder," a category which contained a limited number of mental disorders without psychoses:
      1. epilepsy
      2. alcoholism
      3. drug addiction
      4. mental deficiency
      5. disorders of personality due to epidemic encephalitis
      6. psychopathic personality
   (d) Primary behavior disorders
      1. simple adult maladjustment
      2. primary behavior disorders in children

The detailed inclusions in each of the above categories is given in Appendix D.

The limited and heterogeneous content of the category "without mental disorder" is a reflection of the stage of development of psychiatric services and practice in 1934, the date the classification in the SMHMD was first published. At that time the mental hospital was the primary resource for the care, treatment, and rehabilitation of the mentally ill. Relatively few outpatient psychiatric clinics existed in the United States, and only a small number of general hospitals had psychiatric units. The instruction for the use of this category is revealing of the state of psychiatric practice at that time: "This diagnosis is to be used in psychiatric clinics. Also in psychiatric and psychopathic hospitals, to account for patients submitted for observation and allowed to remain in hospitals for other legitimate reasons."

Classification DSM-1, 1952

The first revision of the nomenclature in the SMHMD was published in 1952 by the American Psychiatric Association. The revised classification was based on a conceptual scheme that differed considerably from that of the earlier classification. Many new diagnostic rubrics and terms, broader in scope than the old, were introduced to reflect a basic concept that some disorders or reactions formerly considered as separate clinical entities are really expressions of a single disease. These mental disorders are classified in the "fourth" edition of the *Standard Nomenclature of Diseases and Operations* under revised captions as follows:

A. Disorders caused by or associated with impairment of brain tissue function
   1. Acute brain disorders
   2. Chronic brain disorders
B. Mental deficiencies
C. Disorders of psychogenic origin or without clearly defined physical cause or structural change in the brain
   1. Psychotic disorders
   2. Psychophysiologic, autonomic, and visceral disorders
   3. Psychoneurotic disorders
   4. Personality disorders
   5. Transient situational personality disorders

The detailed inclusions in these categories are compared with those in SMHMD in Appendix D.

The following quotation from the introduction to the nomenclature of DSM-1 provides a more detailed statement of the purpose of the revision and a summary of changes in the old nomenclature and in the content of the major categories of disorders:

> This revision of psychiatric nomenclature attempts to provide a classification system consistent with the concepts of modern psychiatry and neurology. It recognizes the present day descriptive nature of all psychiatric diagnoses, and attempts to make possible the gathering of data for future classification of ideas concerning etiology, pathology, prognosis and treatment in mental disorders. It attempts to provide for inclusion of new ideas and advances yet to be made without radical revision of the system of nomenclature.
>
> This nomenclature limits itself to the classification of the disturbance of mental functioning. It does not include neurologic conditions or diagnoses of intracranial pathology, per se. Such conditions should be diagnosed separately, whether or not a mental disturbance is associated with them. When an intracranial lesion is accompanied by a mental disorder, it is the mental disorder which is diagnosed in this present classification. Provision is made for contributory etiological factors to be stated as a part of the diagnosis, or as an additional diagnosis, as necessary . . .
>
> This diagnostic scheme employs the term "disorder" generically to designate a group of related psychiatric syndromes. Insofar as is possible, each group is further divided into more specific psychiatric conditions termed "reactions." The code numbers are assigned in accordance with the overall plan of the Standard Nomenclature of Diseases and Operations, a system fully explained in that publication.
>
> All mental disorders are divided into two major groups:
>
> 1. Those in which there is disturbance of mental function resulting from, or precipitated by, a primary impairment of the function of the brain, generally due to diffuse impairment of brain tissue, and

2. Those which are the result of a more general difficulty in adaptation of the individual, and in which any associated brain function disturbance is secondary to the psychiatric disorder.

Perhaps the greatest change in this revision from previous listings lies in the handling of the disorders with known organic etiologic factors. In these disorders (Group 1) the psychiatric picture is characterized by impairment of intellectual functions, including memory, orientation and judgment, and by shallowness and lability of affect. This is a basic condition, and may be mild, moderate or severe. It may be, and more often than not is, the only mental disturbance present, or it may be associated with additional disturbances which in this nomenclature are descriptively classified as "psychotic," "neurotic" or "behavorial" reactions. These associated reactions are not necessarily related to severity to the degree of the organic brain syndrome, and are as much determined by inherent personality patterns, the social setting, and the stresses of interpersonal relations as by the precipitating organic impairment. For this reason, these associated reactions are to be looked upon as being released by the organic brain syndrome and superimposed upon it. The organic brain syndrome thereupon becomes the proper focus of diagnosis; associated reactions should be specified, when necessary, by adding to the diagnosis a qualifying phrase describing the manifestation: .x1 with psychotic reaction, .x2 with neurotic reaction, or, .x3 with behavorial reaction. It is anticipated that the majority of organic disorders will require no qualifying phrase.

When the organic brain syndrome is produced by prenatal or natal factors or in the formative years of infancy and childhood, the disturbance in intellectual development and learning ability may be prominent. Such disturbances, formerly diagnosed "Mental deficiency, secondary" are here listed under the chronic brain syndromes, where they seem more properly to belong. In these cases when it is desired to stress the disorder of intelligence as the primary clinical problem, the diagnosis may be qualified with the phrase, .x4 with mental deficiency, .x41 mild, .x42 moderate, or .x43 severe, and the current intelligence quotient will be included in the diagnosis. This categorization relegates the defect of intelligence to the sphere of symptomatology, rather than recognizing it as a primary mental disturbance . . .

It was necessary to retain a term for those cases presenting clinically primarily a disturbance of intellect, with no recognizable organic brain impairment prenatally, at birth or in childhood. Since no adequate substitution could be found, the title "Mental Deficiency" was retained for this group. Degree is indicated by the terms "mild," "moderate," or "severe." No I.Q. limit has been set for these qualifying terms, as it is believed that such arbitrary usage of a variable measure is not justifiable in clinical work.

The Schizophrenic reactions have been increased in number and type to allow more detailed diagnosis. The Manic depressive reactions have been reduced in number, and, with a Psychotic depressive reaction, have been grouped into the "Affective reactions."

The "psychosomatic" disorders have been given a separate category to allow more accurate accumulation of data concerning them. The generic term "Psychophysiologic, Autonomic and Visceral disorders" has been selected for this group because it seems to express best the interplay of psychic and somatic factors involved in these disturbances.

The Psychoneurotic Disorders have been classified on the basis of their psychopathology as it is generally understood today. The titles of Personality Disorders and Transient Situational Disorders have been elaborated and expanded.

As stated above, this revised nomenclature introduced another new feature – the qualifying phrases. Thus, one of the following phrases – .x1 with psychotic reaction, .x2 with neurotic reaction, .x3 with behavioral reaction – could be added to any of the primary diagnoses when needed to define or describe further the clinical picture. According to the manual, these phrases are applied:

> Only when superimposed picture symptoms are so marked that they definitely color the clinical picture. Mild or transient superimposed symptoms will not justify the use of a qualifying phrase. It is anticipated that a diagnosis of chronic brain syndrome will be sufficient in itself under ordinary conditions, and qualifying phrases will be needed only for further refinement of the diagnosis.

> A qualifying phrase will not be used where such use is redundant. In general, the phrase will be redundant when it repeats the major heading of any group of diagnoses; e.g., .x1 is redundant when used with a diagnosis listed under Psychotic Disorders; .x2 is redundant when used with Psychoneurotic Disorders; .x3 is redundant when used with Personality Disorders.
>
> A qualifying phrase is not needed with a diagnosis of acute brain syndrome, but a qualifying phrase may be used when superimposed manifestations warrant such use by their significant modification of the clinical picture.

During the first two years of the use of the new nomenclature, the National Institute of Mental Health carried out studies in a selected number of state mental hospital systems to determine the extent of usage of qualifying phrases with diagnoses in chronic brain syndrome categories. The phrase most frequently used was "with psychotic reaction." Since it was not possible to carry out studies to determine the consistency with which these phrases were being used across all hospitals in the United States, national data were collected on the categories of acute brain disorders and chronic brain disorders, specific for certain etiologic factors only. No attempt was made to gather data on these disorders further subdivided by each qualifying phrase except in the first two years following introduction of the new nomenclature. This was done to determine how frequently diagnoses of chronic brain syndromes were modified by a qualifying phrase. In a very high proportion – 80 to 90 percent – either no qualifying phrase was used or when used, the phrase was "with psychotic reaction."

It should also be noted that several diagnoses included in the classification of 1934 were not included in that of 1952. For example, the diagnosis "psychosis with psychopathic personality" was deleted from the 1952 classification. When a patient manifested both a psychotic disorder and a sociopathic personality disturbance, the sociopathic disturbance was not diagnosed if the latter was a manifestation of a more primary personality disturbance; e.g., schizophrenic reaction. In such instances, the schizophrenic reaction would be diagnosed. As stated in the manual: "Sociopathic reactions are very often symptomatic of severe underlying personality disorder, neurosis, or psychosis, or occur as a result of organic brain injury or disease. Before a definitive diagnosis in this group is employed, strict attention must be paid to the possibility of the presence of a more primary personality disturbance; such underlying disturbances will be diagnosed when recognized. Reaction will be differentiated as defined below."

CATEGORIES OF MENTAL DISORDERS USED IN THE MONOGRAPH

The categories of mental disorders for which time series are presented in this monograph are based on DSM-1. The conversion table given in Appendix D was used to convert the diagnostic terms from the 1934 classification into the most appropriate term in DSM-1. The following categories are used, and the code numbers are those published in DSM-1 (American Psychiatric Association, 1952, pp. 78-86) for use in tabulating diagnostic distributions of mental disorders:

All Mental Disorders
- Brain Syndromes 01.0 – 19.43 (except 02.1 and 13.00 - 13.03)
  - Diseases of the Senium 15.0 and 17.1
  - Cerebral Arteriosclerosis 15.0
  - Senile Brain Disease 17.1
  - Syphilitic 11.0 - 11.2
  - Other (except Alcoholics)
- Functional Psychoses 20-24
  - Schizophrenic Reaction 22
  - Affective and Involutional 20-21
  - Other 23-24
- Disorders associated with Alcoholism
  - Brain Syndromes 02.1 and 13.00 - 13.03
  - Addiction 52.3
  - Psychoneurosis 40
  - Personality Disorders (except Alcoholism) 50-54 (excluding 52.3)
  - All other

INCOMPATIBILITY OF DSM-1 AND SECTION V OF ICD (SIXTH REVISION)

The categories of mental disorders in the ICD (section V) were not used in the collection of diagnostic data from psychiatric facilities (W.H.O., 1948; 1957), since these statistical categories were quite unsatisfactory for classifying many of the diagnostic terms that were introduced in DSM-1. For example, with certain exceptions, ICD-6 did not provide rubrics for coding chronic brain syndromes (associated with various diseases or conditions) with neurotic or behavorial reactions or without qualifying phrases, nor did it provide for the transient situational personality disorders. The exceptions were post-encephalitic personality and character disorders among the chronic brain syndromes, alcoholic delirium among the acute brain syndromes, and gross stress reaction among the transient disorders.

The shortcomings of ICD-6 (and of ICD-7, the seventh edition in 1955, which did not revise the section on mental disorders), pointed up the unsuitability of its use in the United States for compiling statistics on the diagnostic characteristics of patients with mental disorders or for indexing medical records in psychiatric treatment facilities. Moreover, the section on mental disorders was not self-contained. For example, certain mental disorders occurred in other sections of the ICD. General paralysis was classified under syphilis and post-encephalitic psychosis under the late effects of acute infectious encephalitis. Also, many of the psychoses associated with organic factors were grouped in a catch-all category of "psychoses with other demonstrable etiology."

The United States was not the only country which found the section on mental disorders in ICD-6 unsatisfactory. In 1959 Professor E. Stengel, under the auspices of W.H.O., published a study revealing general dissatisfaction in all W.H.O. member countries (Stengel, 1959). This finding, combined with the growing recognition of mental disorders as a major international health concern, led W.H.O. to urge its member states to collaborate in developing a classification of these disorders that would overcome the ICD's shortcomings and gain general international acceptance. Such a classification was recognized as indispensable for international communication and data collection.

As a result of a very extensive collaborative effort, the eighth revision of the ICD (ICD-8) now includes a section on mental disorders which eliminated many of the objections to the section that were in the sixth and seventh editions (W.H.O., 1967). The American Psychiatric Association has now developed a psychiatric diagnostic nomenclature (DSM-2) which is compatible with ICD-8 and which is being used in psychiatric facilities throughout the United States. This will now make it possible to use ICD-8 as a basis for statistical tabulations of mental disorders in the United States.

Appendix D
Conversion of Terms in 1934 Classification of Mental Disorders to Those in the 1952 Revision

Appendix Table D.1 relates the various titles in the 1934 *Statistical Classification of Mental Disorders* to the appropriate titles in the 1952 revision of the classification. It was used by mental hospitals to convert historical statistical series of admissions, deaths, discharges, and resident patients by mental disorder into the 1952 classification so that some degree of continuity could be kept between these old series and those that were evolved on the basis of the new nomenclature. In making these conversions the term in the new classification that most closely approximates the old was selected. In most instances there is a one-to-one correspondence between a title in the old classification and a title in the new. However, in certain instances it was necessary to review the case histories in order to decide which of the new titles applied, as, for example, in deciding whether a given mental disorder should be reclassified as an acute or chronic brain syndrome.

In the left-hand column of the table is the code number of the classification of mental disorder with the appropriate title as given on pages 19 through 22 of the *Statistical Manual for the Use of Hospitals for Mental Disease, Tenth Edition, 1942.* These code numbers have been generally used in coding diagnoses for statistical tabulations, especially in those states that use machine tabulating equipment. In the right-hand column is the four-digit code number for tabulating the 1952 revised classification of mental disorders together with the name of the disorder as given on pages 78 through 86 of the *Diagnostic and Statistical Manual of Mental Disorders* published by the American Psychiatric Association in 1952. The code consists of four digits in which the first digit represents the broad class of mental disorder; the second, major categories within each of these broad classes; the third, subdivisions within each of these major categories; and the fourth, qualifying phrases where applicable. Where no subdivision exists within a major category, the third digit was coded as an "X." Where no qualifying phrase was applicable, the fourth digit was also coded as an "X" except in the *chronic brain disorders,* where diagnoses without qualifying phrases were coded "O" in the fourth digit. If a diagnosis was modified by a qualifying phrase the following numbers were used in the fourth digit: (1) with psychotic reaction; (2) with neurotic reaction; (3) with behavorial reaction. The qualifying phrase selected for the purpose of the conversion was the one which, when added to the new diagnostic term, approximated the term in the old nomenclature most closely. For example, the old term "psychosis with cerebral arterioclerosis" (old code 08) became "chronic brain syndrome associated with cerebral arteriosclerosis with psychotic reaction" and was coded 15.01, in which:

(a) the *first digit* "1" represents the broad category *chronic brain disorder*

(b) the *second digit* "5" represennts *chronic brain syndrome associated with circulatory disturbance*

(c) the *third digit* "0" represents the classification *cerebral arteriosclerosis* within the category *with circulatory disturbance*

(d) the *fourth digit* "1" represents the qualifying phrase *with psychotic reaction*

Appendix Table D.1. "Relationship between titles of 1934 Classification of Mental Disorders and those of the 1952 revision"

CLASSIFICATION OF MENTAL DISORDER (1934 REVISION)		CLASSIFICATION OF MENTAL DISORDER (1952 REVISION)	
CODE NO.[a/]	DISORDER	CODE NO.[b/]	DISORDER
01	Psychoses with syphilitic meningo-encephalitis (general paresis)	11.01	CBS[c/] with meningoencephalitic syphilis with psychotic reaction[e/]
02	Psychoses with other forms of syphilis of central nervous system:		
	021 Meningo-vascular type (cerebral syphilis)	11.11	CBS with meningovascular syphilis with psychotic reaction[e/]
	022 With intracranial gumma	11.21	CBS with other central nervous system syphilis with psychotic reaction[e/]
	023 Other types	11.21	CBS with other central nervous system syphilis with psychotic reaction[e/]
03	Psychoses with encephalitis	(01.0X	ABS[d/] with epidemic encephalitis
		(or	
		(12.01	CBS with epidemic encephalitis with psychotic reaction[e/]
04	Psychoses with other infectious diseases:		
	041 With tuberculous meningitis	(01.1X	ABS with intracranial infection except epidemic encephalitis
		(or	
		(12.01	CBS with intracranial infection with psychotic reaction[e/]
	042 With meningitis (unspecified)	(01.0X	ABS with intracranial infection except epidemic encephalitis
		(or	
		(12.01	CBS with intracranial infection with psychotic reaction[e/]
	043 With acute chorea (Sydenham's)	01.0X	ABS with intracranial infection except epidemic encephalitis
	044 With other infectious disease	01.0X	ABS with intracranial infection except epidemic encephalitis
	045 With post-infectious psychoses	01.2X	ABS with systemic infection not elsewhere classified
05	Psychoses due to alcohol:		
	051 Pathological intoxication	None	No such term. Diagnose underlying psychiatric disorder
	052 Delirium tremens	02.1X	ABS with alcohol intoxication
	053 Korsakoff's psychosis	13.01	CBS with alcohol intoxication with psychotic reaction
	054 Acute hallucinosis	02.1X	ABS with alcohol intoxication
	055 Other types	(02.1X	ABS with alcohol intoxication
		(or	
		(13.01	CBS with alcohol intoxication with psychotic reaction[e/]
06	Psychoses due to a drug or other exogenous poison:		
	061 Due to a metal	(02.2X	ABS with drug or poison intoxication (except alcohol)
		(or	
		(13.11	CBS with drug or poison intoxication (except alcohol) with psychotic reaction[e/]
	062 Due to a gas	(02.2X	ABS with drug or poison intoxication (except alcohol)
		(or	
		(13.11	CBS with drug or poison intoxication (except alcohol) with psychotic reaction[e/]
	063 Due to opium or a derivative	(02.2X	ABS with drug or poison intoxication (except alcohol)
		(or	
		(13.11	CBS with drug or poison intoxication (except alcohol) with psychotic reaction[e/]
	064 Due to another drug	(02.2X	ABS with drug or poison intoxication (except alcohol)
		(or	
		(13.11	CBS with drug or poison intoxication (except alcohol) with psychotic reaction[e/]

Appendix Table D.1. "Relationship between titles of 1934 Classification of Mental Disorders and those of the 1952 revision" (continued)

CLASSIFICATION OF MENTAL DISORDER (1934 REVISION)		CLASSIFICATION OF MENTAL DISORDER (1952 REVISION)	
CODE NO.[a]	DISORDER	CODE NO.[b]	DISORDER
07	Psychoses due to trauma:		
	071 Delirium due to trauma	03.XX	ABS with trauma
	072 Personality disorder due to trauma	14.-3	CBS with trauma (specify type) with behavioral reaction[f]
	073 Mental deterioration due to trauma	14.-0	CBS with trauma (specify type) without qualifying phrase[g]
	074 Other types	(03.XX	ABS with trauma
		(or	
		(14.-1	CBS with trauma (specify type) with psychotic reaction[e]
	Psychoses with cerebral arteriosclerosis	15.01	CBS with cerebral arteriosclerosis with psychotic reaction[e]
	Psychoses with other disturbances of circulation:		
	091 with cerebral embolism	15.11	CBS with other circulatory disturbances with psychotic reaction[e]
	092 with cardio-renal disease	(04.XX	ABS with circulatory disturbance
		(or	
		(15.11	CBS with other circulatory disturbance with psychotic reaction[e]
	093 Other types	(04.XX	ABS with circulatory disturbance
		(or	
		(15.11	CBS with other circulatory disturbance with psychotic reaction[e]
	Psychoses due to convulsive disorder (epilepsy):		
	101 Epileptic deterioration	16.00	CBS with convulsive disorder without qualifying phrase
	102 Epileptic clouded states	05.XX	ABS with convulsive disorder
	103 Other epileptic types	(05.XX	ABS with convulsive disorder
		(or	
		(16.01	CBS with convulsive disorder with psychotic reaction[e]
	Senile psychoses:		
	111 Simple deterioration	17.10	CBS with senile brain disease without qualifying phrase
	112 Presbyophrenic type	17.10	CBS with senile brain disease without qualifying phrase
	113 Delirious & confused types	17.11	CBS with senile brain disease with psychotic reaction
	114 Depressed & agitated types	17.11	CBS with senile brain disease with psychotic reaction
	115 Paranoid types	17.11	CBS with senile brain disease with psychotic reaction
12	Involutional psychoses:		
	121 Melancholia	20.XX	Involutional psychotic reaction
	122 Paranoid types	20.XX	Involutional psychotic reaction
	123 Other types	20.XX	Involutional psychotic reaction
13	Psychoses due to other metabolic, etc. diseases:		
	131 With grandular disorder	06.XX	ABS with metabolic disturbance
	132 Exhaustion delirium	06.XX	ABS with metabolic disturbance
	133 Alzheimer's disease (presenile sclerosis)	17.21	CBS with presenile brain disease with psychotic reaction[e]
	134 With pellagra	(06.XX	ABS with metabolic disturbance
		(or	
		(17.31	CBS with other metabolic disturbance with psychotic reaction[e]
	135 With other somatic disease	(06.XX	ABS with metabolic disturbance
		(or	
		(17.31	CBS with other metabolic disturbance with psychotic reaction[e]

Appendix Table D.1. "Relationship between titles of 1934 Classification of Mental Disorders and the 1952 revision" (continued)

CLASSIFICATION OF MENTAL DISORDER (1934 REVISION)		CLASSIFICATION OF MENTAL DISORDER (1952 REVISION)	
CODE NO.[a/]	DISORDER	CODE NO.[b/]	DISORDER
14	Psychoses due to new growth:		
	141 With intracranial neoplasm	(07.XX	ABS with intracranial neoplasm
		(or	
		(18.01	CBS with intracranial neoplasm with psychotic reaction[e/]
	142 With other neoplasms	No such diagnosis. Classify under disorders of psychogenic origin in accordance with clinical picture.	
15	Psychoses due to unknown or hereditary cause but associated with organic change:		
	151 With multiple sclerosis	19.01	CBS with multiple sclerosis with psychotic reaction[e/]
	152 With paralysis agitans	19.31	CBS with other diseases of unknown or uncertain cause with psychotic reaction[e/]
	153 With Huntington's chorea	19.11	CBS with Huntington's chorea with psychotic reaction[e/]
	154 With other disease of the brain or nervous system	19.31	CBS with other diseases of unknown or uncertain cause with psychotic reaction except Pick's disease with psychotic reaction which is coded 19.21.[e/]
16	Psychoneuroses:		
	161 Hysteria:		
	Anxiety hysteria	40.3X	Phobic reaction, except if 40.1 (Dissociative reaction) or 40.2 (Conversion reaction)
	Conversion hysteria:		
	Anesthetic type	40.2X	Conversion reaction
	Paralytic type	40.2X	Conversion reaction
	Hyperkinetic type	40.2X	Conversion reaction
	Paresthetic type	40.2X	Conversion reaction
	Autonomic type	40.2X	Conversion reaction (except those that are classified as 30-39 under Psychophysiologic autonomic & visceral disorders
	Amnesic type	40.1X	Dissociative reaction
	Mixed	None	Diagnose major reaction
	162 Psychasthenia or compulsive states:		
	Obsession	40.4X	Obsessive-compulsive reaction
	Compulsive tics & spasms	40.4X	Obsessive-compulsive reaction
	Phobia	40.3X	Phobic reaction
	163 Neurasthenia	38.XX	Psychophysiologic nervous system reaction
	164 Hypochondriasis	40.6X	Psychoneurotic reaction, other
	165 Reactive depression	40.5X	Depressive reaction
	166 Anxiety state	40.0X	Anxiety reaction
	167 Anorexia nervosa	35.XX	Psychophysiologic gastrointestinal reaction
	168 Mixed psychoneurosis	None	Diagnose major reaction
17	Manic-depressive psychoses:		
	171 Manic type	21.0X	Manic-depressive reaction, manic type
	172 Depressive type	21.1X	Manic-depressive reaction, depressive type
	173 Circular type	21.2X	Manic-depressive reaction, other
	174 Mixed type	21.2X	Manic-depressive reaction, other
	175 Perplexed type	21.2X	Manic-depressive reaction, other
	176 Stuporous type	21.2X	Manic-depressive reaction, other
	177 Other types	21.2X	Manic-depressive reaction, other

Appendix Table D.1. "Relationship between titles of 1934 Classification of Mental Disorders and the 1952 revision" (continued)

CLASSIFICATION OF MENTAL DISORDER (1934 REVISION)		CLASSIFICATION OF MENTAL DISORDERS (1952 REVISION)	
CODE NO.[a/]	DISORDER	CODE NO.[b/]	DISORDER
18	Dementia praecox (schizophrenia):		
	181 Simple type	22.0X	Schizophrenic reaction, simple type
	182 Hebephrenic type	22.1X	Schizophrenic reaction, Hebephrenic type
	183 Catatonic type	22.2X	Schizophrenic reaction, catatonic type
	184 Paranoid type	22.3X	Schizophrenic reaction, paranoid type
	185 Other types	(Rediagnose under one of the following (22.4X to 22.9X):	
		(22.4X	Schizophrenic reaction, acute undifferentiated type
		(22.5X	Schizophrenic reaction, chronic undifferentiated type
		(22.6X	Schizophrenic reaction, schizoaffective type
		(22.7X	Schizophrenic reaction, childhood type
		(22.8X	Schizophrenic reaction, residual type
		(22.9X	Schizophrenic reaction, other and unspecified
19	Paranoia and paranoid conditions:		
	191 Paranoia	23.1X	Paranoia
	192 Paranoid conditions	23.2X	Paranoid state
20	Psychoses with psychopathic personality	52.01	Antisocial reaction with psychotic reaction
21	Psychoses with mental deficiency	60.01	Mental deficiency (familial or hereditary) mild with psychotic reaction
		60.11	Mental deficiency (familial or hereditary) moderate with psychotic reaction
		60.21	Mental deficiency (familial or hereditary) severe, with psychotic reaction
		60.31	Mental deficiency (familial or hereditary) severity not specified, with psychotic reaction
		61.01	Mental deficiency (idiopathic) mild with psychotic reaction
		61.11	Mental deficiency (idiopathic) moderate with psychotic reaction
		61.21	Mental deficiency (idiopathic) severe with psychotic reaction
		61.31	Mental deficiency (idiopathic) severity not specified with psychotic reaction
22	Undiagnosed psychoses	24.XX	Psychotic reaction without clearly defined structural change other than above
23	Without mental disorder:		
	231 Epilepsy	91.XX	Epilepsy (idiopathic) without acute or chronic brain syndrome
	232 Alcoholism	52.3X	Alcoholism (addiction)
	233 Drug addiction	52.4X	Drug addiction
	234 Mental deficiency	(60.0X	Mental deficiency (familial or hereditary) mild
		(60.1X	Mental deficiency (familial or hereditary) moderate
		(60.2X	Mental deficiency (familial or hereditary) severe
		(60.3X	Mental deficiency (familial or hereditary) not specified
		(61.0X	Mental deficiency (idiopathic) mild
		(61.1X	Mental deficiency (idiopathic) moderate
		(61.2X	Mental deficiency (idiopathic) severe
		(61.3X	Mental deficiency (idiopathic) not specified
	235 Disorders of personality due to epidemic encephalitis	12.03	CBS with epidemic encephalitis with behavioral reaction
	236 Psychopathic personality	52.0X	Antisocial reaction
	2361 With pathologic sexuality	52.2X	Sexual deviation
	2362 With pathological emotionality	51.0X	Emotionally unstable personality
	2363 With asocial or amoral trends	52.1X	Dyssocial reaction
	2364 Mixed types	None	Diagnose major personality disorder
	237 Other nonpsychotic diseases or conditions	None	See text[h/] page 119--classify under "other" classification in each group of disorders

Appendix Table D.1. "Relationship between titles of 1934 Classification of Mental Disorders and those of the 1952 revision" (continued)

CLASSIFICATION OF MENTAL DISORDER (1934 REVISION)		CLASSIFICATION OF MENTAL DISORDER (1952 REVISION)	
CODE NO. a/	DISORDER	CODE NO. b/	DISORDER
24	Primary behavior disorders:		
	241 Simple adult maladjustment	54.1X	Adult situational reaction
	242 Primary behavior disorders in children:		
	2421 Habit disturbance	54.3X	Adjustment reaction of childhood
	2422 Conduct disturbance	54.3X	Adjustment reaction of childhood
	2423 Neurotic traits	54.3X	Adjustment reaction of childhood

a/ This is the code number for the statistical classification of mental disorders as found on pages 19 through 22 of the Statistical Manual for the Use of Hospitals for Mental Disease, Tenth Edition, 1942. This code is generally used by mental hospitals as the code number for their various diagnostic categories in preparation of statistical tables.

b/ This code number is the four-digit code number for tabulating the revised classification of mental disorders and is found on pages 78 through 86 of the Diagnostic and Statistical Manual of Mental Disorders published by the American Psychiatric Association in 1952.

c/ The abbreviation "CBS" stands for Chronic Brain Syndrome.

d/ The abbreviation "ABS" stands for Acute Brain Syndrome.

e/ In order to simplify conversion from recorded diagnoses, the qualifying phrase, "with psychotic reaction", has been added in each instance. If review of the clinical records is feasible, many of these diagnoses will be recorded as CBS without qualifying phrase and should be so coded. See pp. 12-13, "Diagnostic & Statistical Manual".

f/ 14.13 CBS with brain trauma (gross force) with behavioral reaction
14.23 CBS following brain operation with behavioral reaction
14.33 CBS following electrical brain trauma with behavioral reaction
14.43 CBS with irradiational brain trauma with behavioral reaction
14.53 CBS with other trauma with behavioral reaction

g/ 14.10 CBS with brain trauma (gross force) without qualifying phrase
14.20 CBS following brain operation without qualifying phrase
14.30 CBS following electrical brain trauma without qualifying phrase
14.40 CBS with irradiational brain trauma without qualifying phrase
14.50 CBS with other trauma without qualifying phrase

h/ Diagnostic and Statistical Manual--Mental Disorders. Published by the American Psychiatric Association, Mental Hospital Service, 1952.

Appendix E
Problems of Sample Size and Sampling Variation in the Study of Patterns of Use of Psychiatric Facilities in Louisiana and Maryland, 1960

The interpretation of the results in the Louisiana-Maryland study were complicated by at least two factors -- the number of cases available for study and the size of the sampling variation in the rates. Although there were over 13,000 psychiatric admissions in each of the two states during the study year, limiting the present analysis to first admissions and to those living in families reduced this number to about 7,000 in each state. Moreover, since the patient data were obtained by matching the patient records against the 1960 census 25 percent sample records, the number of cases in the sample was further reduced to approximately one-fourth of the above number. Although each sample case was then multiplied by 4, when the data were classified simultaneously by several variables, many of the resulting multidimensional cells contained only four cases or none at all.

All of the rates presented in this study contain in their numerators, in addition to the number of matched cases, estimates of the number of cases for which matching census schedules could not be found. Thus, the computation of the variance of the given rate takes into account the fact that the numerator consists of two parts – one based on a 25 percent sample (matched cases) and the other based on a 10 percent sample (nonmatched cases) – and the fact that the denominator for this particular set of data is based on a 5 percent sample. The standard errors of the rates relative to the rates themselves are generally high, particularly when the number of nonmatched cases in a specific category is high in relation to the number of matched cases in that category. Because of these large standard errors, very few of the differences tested were statistically significant. For this reason, the results have not been presented in terms of statistical significance. However, the magnitude of the differences between certain rates or the consistency in certain patterns in both states may indicate areas for further investigation concerning the relationship between patient characteristics and disability from mental illness.

Appendix Table 1. Average annual age-adjusted first admission rates per 100,000 population to state and county mental hospitals, by diagnosis: United States, each geographic region and each state, 1959-61

Geographic area	All mental disorders	Brain syndromes: Total	Brain syndromes: Dis. of senium	Brain syndromes: Syphilitic	Brain syndromes: Other	Functional psychoses: Total	Functional psychoses: Schizophrenic reactions	Functional psychoses: Affect. and involt.	Functional psychoses: Other	Disorders assoc. with alcohol.	Psychoneurosis	Personality disorders
United States	80.3	20.5	15.4	0.4	4.6	26.3	19.7	5.9	0.8	12.0	6.3	8.5
Northeast Region	91.5	28.1	23.4	0.4	4.3	35.1	25.3	8.2	1.6	9.8	6.2	7.9
New England	105.7	28.0	22.5	0.2	5.3	30.8	21.4	8.4	1.0	18.4	11.2	9.9
Maine	75.6	21.5	17.9	0.3	3.3	22.0	17.4	4.1	0.5	8.4	10.5	6.5
New Hampshire	126.8	25.9	16.3	0.1	9.5	36.8	18.8	14.8	3.2	14.2	14.3	12.0
Vermont	108.3	23.7	17.4	0.2	6.1	33.2	19.3	13.3	0.6	12.5	15.1	8.2
Rhode Island	113.4	34.5	29.4	0.2	4.9	28.6	20.6	6.1	1.9	23.5	8.2	11.3
Connecticut	109.5	29.7	24.5	0.1	5.1	33.1	24.1	8.6	0.5	21.9	11.4	10.5
Mid-Atlantic	89.4	28.1	23.6	0.4	4.1	35.8	25.9	8.2	1.7	8.5	5.5	7.6
New York	106.3	33.3	28.7	0.4	4.2	46.7	33.0	11.0	2.7	9.0	5.6	8.1
New Jersey	103.6	36.3	29.9	0.5	5.9	28.2	19.5	7.4	1.3	14.4	8.9	10.9
Pennsylvania	56.7	16.2	12.8	0.3	3.1	23.7	18.9	4.3	0.6	4.6	3.5	5.2
North Central Region	74.4	16.6	12.0	0.4	4.2	21.5	16.7	4.3	0.6	12.4	6.6	9.6
East North Central	77.5	18.5	13.7	0.4	4.4	22.7	18.0	4.1	0.6	11.6	6.7	9.8
Ohio	94.9	18.3	11.9	0.7	5.7	31.9	23.8	7.1	1.0	10.4	10.1	12.6
Indiana	58.4	15.7	11.8	0.5	3.4	17.9	14.4	3.3	0.2	10.5	4.1	7.4
Illinois	83.8	24.1	18.7	0.3	5.1	20.3	16.3	3.3	0.7	18.3	5.3	5.8
Michigan	42.2	9.0	6.1	0.2	2.7	16.6	14.0	2.2	0.3	3.1	4.1	8.0
Wisconsin	106.7	23.8	19.7	0.1	3.9	23.6	19.7	3.2	0.6	15.3	9.9	20.0
West North Central	67.7	12.9	8.8	0.3	3.8	18.8	13.5	4.8	0.4	14.2	6.5	8.9
Minnesota	78.1	15.2	11.5	0.1	3.6	16.6	11.3	5.1	0.3	26.9	5.0	4.6
Iowa	60.0	9.9	6.8	0.2	2.9	15.3	8.9	5.9	0.5	10.6	6.2	11.3
Missouri	47.5	11.1	6.7	0.6	3.8	15.0	12.3	2.5	0.2	5.0	4.3	4.9
North Dakota	176.5	25.2	19.6	0.1	5.5	61.3	50.5	10.4	0.4	56.0	12.2	10.8
South Dakota	79.0	15.1	11.2	0.1	3.9	18.5	11.6	4.8	2.1	16.5	7.9	9.7
Nebraska	76.7	16.3	11.2	0.1	5.1	16.7	12.2	4.3	0.2	16.7	8.5	14.3
Kansas	63.7	11.2	6.8	0.3	4.0	22.9	15.7	6.5	0.7	3.6	9.0	15.3

Southern Region	80.2	20.9	14.9	0.6	5.4	26.2	19.9	5.8	0.5	12.7	5.7	6.2
South Atlantic	84.6	24.6	18.0	0.7	6.0	27.5	20.5	6.4	0.5	12.1	6.8	6.1
Delaware	152.3	50.5	39.5	0.7	10.3	39.5	20.3	16.7	2.5	28.0	11.1	18.1
Maryland	94.4	25.6	18.4	0.8	6.4	26.6	21.5	4.7	0.4	21.9	6.3	9.5
Dist of Col.	154.3	48.7	38.3	1.0	9.4	58.0	50.2	7.4	0.4	14.8	9.9	11.2
Virginia	72.5	25.3	18.2	0.8	6.3	17.7	14.5	2.9	0.4	12.8	4.3	7.1
West Virginia	100.6	23.5	16.2	1.1	6.3	31.2	23.7	6.9	0.6	14.4	6.4	8.1
North Carolina	102.5	26.0	18.9	0.5	6.6	31.3	20.8	9.8	0.7	15.4	16.1	7.6
South Carolina	102.5	36.1	29.1	0.5	6.5	29.1	24.4	4.2	0.4	13.0	9.5	4.9
Georgia	83.2	27.9	21.0	0.7	6.2	33.0	23.4	9.4	0.2	6.4	2.4	1.5
Florida	46.4	12.9	8.7	0.4	3.8	20.0	14.5	4.8	0.7	3.4	2.1	3.2
East South Central	79.9	18.6	12.7	0.5	5.4	26.6	19.5	6.4	0.6	12.5	5.0	6.7
Kentucky	71.3	18.9	13.6	0.4	5.0	17.7	12.7	4.5	0.5	15.4	5.9	6.7
Tennessee	81.8	23.0	15.5	0.6	6.9	25.1	19.2	5.2	0.7	8.9	6.9	7.9
Alabama	65.6	17.0	12.1	0.6	4.4	30.0	23.5	6.2	0.3	4.5	1.6	6.9
Mississippi	113.3	13.2	7.7	0.5	5.0	37.2	23.9	12.2	1.1	27.4	5.5	4.6
West South Central	72.8	16.2	11.4	0.5	4.4	23.5	19.0	4.2	0.2	14.2	4.5	6.0
Arkansas	95.4	22.4	14.2	0.2	7.9	20.8	15.5	4.7	0.6	17.1	7.3	5.4
Louisiana	80.6	12.5	8.0	0.6	3.9	24.1	19.8	4.0	0.3	13.9	7.4	7.8
Texas	66.1	15.2	11.7	0.5	3.9	23.8	19.5	4.2	0.1	13.8	3.1	5.5
Western Region	75.4	14.9	10.2	0.2	4.5	23.2	17.5	5.3	0.4	13.0	6.8	12.0
Mountain	85.3	19.4	13.0	0.3	6.1	23.6	18.1	4.7	0.8	14.5	7.9	12.6
Montana	130.5	29.2	16.2	0.5	12.4	29.8	23.0	6.0	0.9	40.5	7.9	16.3
Idaho	86.4	15.1	9.4	0.3	5.4	24.8	17.9	6.6	0.2	12.3	10.7	19.7
Wyoming	72.5	22.5	15.5	0.6	6.5	10.3	7.5	2.5	0.2	16.4	3.1	16.1
Colorado	89.1	18.7	13.7	0.2	4.7	20.4	16.6	3.0	0.7	16.3	7.5	12.0
New Mexico	71.2	16.6	11.6	0.2	4.7	20.8	17.0	3.6	0.2	9.7	9.5	8.1
Arizona	83.5	22.2	14.8	0.5	6.9	31.3	23.2	6.2	1.9	5.4	10.4	9.7
Utah	54.1	10.3	7.4	0.1	2.8	16.7	13.1	2.9	0.6	5.4	3.6	15.1
Nevada	113.7	27.1	15.9	0.4	10.8	36.8	24.7	10.7	1.3	25.2	7.4	9.7
Pacific	72.5	13.6	9.4	0.2	3.9	23.1	17.3	5.5	0.3	12.5	6.5	11.8
Washington	68.1	15.8	11.4	0.2	4.2	25.4	18.7	6.1	0.6	2.6	7.9	9.2
Oregon	134.7	29.0	20.2	0.2	8.7	31.3	23.0	7.6	0.7	28.7	13.2	25.5
California	67.3	11.3	7.6	0.2	3.4	22.1	16.7	5.2	0.2	12.9	5.8	11.3
Hawaii	52.8	8.5	6.4	0.0	2.1	15.3	11.6	3.4	0.4	6.0	1.0	3.6
Alaska	60.5	20.4	12.6	0.2	7.6	28.2	21.2	6.3	0.7	3.5	2.0	2.6

Appendix Table 2. Average annual age-adjusted first admission rates per 100,000 population to state and county mental hospitals and percent change in rates over time: United States, each geographic region and each state, 1939-41, 1949-51, and 1959-61

Geographic area	1960	1950	1940	1940-1960	1950-1960	1940-1950
United States	80.3	71.9	67.2	19.5	11.7	7.0
Northeast Region	91.5	82.9	79.1	15.7	10.4	4.8
Northeast States	105.7	94.4	66.9	58.0	12.0	41.1
Maine	75.6	54.6	48.9	54.6	38.5	11.7
New Hampshire	126.8	135.7	92.2	37.5	-6.6	47.2
Vermont	108.3	97.5	60.8	78.1	11.1	60.4
Rhode Island	113.4	116.8	72.6	56.2	-2.9	164.3
Connecticut	109.5	92.5	68.4	60.1	18.4	35.2
Mid-Atlantic States	89.4	81.2	81.0	10.4	10.1	0.2
New York	106.3	100.9	101.0	5.2	5.4	-0.1
New Jersey	103.6	89.8	78.1	32.7	15.4	15.0
Pennsylvania	56.7	48.9	54.1	4.8	16.0	-9.6
North Central Region	74.4	67.5	61.7	20.6	10.2	9.4
East North Central States	77.5	74.1	63.8	21.5	4.6	16.1
Ohio	94.9	76.3	49.7	90.9	24.4	53.5
Indiana	58.4	39.0	48.3	20.9	49.7	-19.3
Illinois	83.8	92.2	88.6	-5.4	-9.1	4.1
Michigan	42.2	57.9	53.9	-21.7	-27.1	7.4
Wisconsin	106.7	91.5	65.6	62.7	16.6	39.5
West North Central States	67.7	53.7	57.5	17.7	26.1	-6.6
Minnesota	78.1	70.5	69.0	13.2	10.8	2.2
Iowa	60.0	54.2	55.2	8.7	10.7	-1.8
Missouri	47.5	38.4	58.4	-18.7	23.7	-34.2
North Dakota	176.5	70.9	63.4	178.4	148.9	11.8
South Dakota	79.0	59.2	41.8	89.0	33.4	41.6
Nebraska	76.7	94.5	53.3	43.9	-18.8	77.3
Kansas	63.7	26.0	48.8	30.5	145.0	-46.7

Southern Region	80.2	60.3	59.4	36.0	33.0	1.0
South Atlantic States	84.6	61.2	60.3	40.3	38.2	1.5
Delaware	152.3	121.1	91.4	66.6	25.8	32.5
Maryland	94.4	52.7	56.7	66.5	79.1	-7.1
Virginia	72.5	64.8	94.4	-23.2	11.9	-31.4
West Virginia	100.6	74.4	53.8	87.0	35.2	38.3
North Carolina	102.5	57.1	57.9	77.0	79.5	-1.4
South Carolina	102.5	85.4	69.5	47.5	20.0	22.9
Georgia	83.2	65.3	42.6	95.3	27.4	53.3
Florida	46.4	35.0	40.7	14.0	32.6	-14.0
East South Central States	79.9	62.4	66.5	20.2	28.0	-6.2
Kentucky	71.3	53.4	58.3	22.3	33.5	-8.4
Tennessee	81.8	57.4	54.0	51.5	42.5	6.3
Alabama	65.6	53.0	58.7	11.8	23.8	-9.7
Mississippi	113.3	96.2	105.0	7.9	17.8	-8.4
West South Central States	72.8	57.6	52.7	38.1	26.4	9.3
Arkansas	95.4	81.3	75.3	26.7	17.3	8.0
Louisiana	80.6	60.7	56.3	43.2	32.8	7.8
Texas	66.1	50.0	37.7	75.3	32.2	32.6
Western Region	75.4	87.0	75.1	0.4	-13.3	15.8
Mountain States	85.3	76.6	68.7	24.2	11.4	11.5
Montana	130.5	70.1	55.4	135.6	86.2	26.5
Idaho	86.4	70.6	62.3	38.7	22.4	13.3
Wyoming	72.5	48.3	57.1	27.0	50.1	-15.4
Colorado	89.1	105.0	94.1	-5.3	-15.2	11.7
New Mexico	71.2	36.3	49.5	43.8	96.1	-26.7
Arizona	83.5	96.3	67.4	23.9	-13.3	42.9
Utah	54.1	51.6	58.8	-8.0	4.8	-12.2
Nevada	113.7	80.6	65.5	73.6	41.1	23.1
Pacific States	72.6	90.3	77.4	-6.2	-19.6	16.7
Washington	68.1	75.4	70.8	-3.8	-9.7	6.5
Oregon	134.7	90.3	79.8	68.8	49.2	13.2
California	67.3	93.5	78.4	14.2	-28.0	19.3

Appendix Table 3. Net releases alive per 1,000 average resident patients from state and county mental hospitals, by age: 23 selected States, 1962

State	Age (in years)							Age adjusted[a]
	Total	Under 25	25-34	35-44	45-54	55-64	65+	
Arkansas	686.4	875.0	917.7	962.5	642.1	554.2	456.5	651.6
California	653.7	1,707.5	1,406.2	1,167.5	704.7	349.3	155.3	646.1
Connecticut	734.4	1,825.1	1,927.5	1,417.5	861.5	373.3	202.0	786.9
Delaware[b]	421.3	1,594.2	976.6	831.5	448.2	220.0	66.8	446.3
District of Columbia	246.8	699.2	648.0	404.6	258.7	139.2	65.6	253.9
Florida	327.1	796.6	591.7	521.5	357.9	177.0	86.4	305.3
Georgia	363.6	770.9	770.0	556.5	346.4	224.8	80.2	331.2
Illinois	396.7	1,109.3	984.7	802.1	475.0	242.2	91.2	436.4
Kansas	754.1	1,086.0	1,174.4	983.0	755.3	484.8	439.0	691.2
Kentucky	735.1	2,355.1	1,580.0	1,145.8	655.7	402.5	337.1	745.5
Louisiana	717.2	1,331.9	1,234.4	1,048.9	668.3	394.5	365.5	659.5
Minnesota	617.6	1,535.5	1,220.9	1,032.9	680.5	387.6	400.4	677.3
Missouri	260.1	688.4	541.6	358.6	232.0	157.8	127.5	253.9
Nebraska	550.7	1,291.8	1,410.7	1,058.7	669.8	326.8	192.5	609.3
New York[b]	218.1	698.1	607.0	386.1	205.9	110.7	49.0	225.7
North Carolina	744.8	1,603.9	1,402.9	1,100.7	739.7	473.6	265.4	697.2
Ohio[b]	579.2	1,562.0	1,503.0	942.4	492.6	240.0	242.9	574.0
Oregon	825.0	3,011.4	2,375.0	1,475.7	919.6	472.3	270.4	946.5
Pennsylvania	199.2	980.3	615.1	349.6	169.0	75.8	1.3	204.9
South Carolina	415.7	1,519.4	746.8	572.6	378.2	197.4	105.8	376.3
Tennessee	673.5	2,105.3	1,406.2	1,063.6	676.7	328.0	198.4	652.8
Texas	659.5	1,718.8	1,361.7	1,098.8	706.3	361.1	221.8	655.1
Virginia	354.1	627.5	709.0	628.2	353.8	201.6	96.3	330.6

[a]The standard population is the sum of all the States in the study.

[b]Data not reported for 1 hospital.

Appendix Table 4. Death ratios per 1,000 average resident patients in state and county mental hospitals, by age: 23 selected states, 1962

State	Age (in years)							
	Total	Under 25	25-34	35-44	45-54	55-64	65+	Age adjusted[a]
Arkansas	91.9	30.6	12.0	24.1	33.4	64.6	291.7	113.4
California	76.3	11.7	5.3	8.9	23.5	52.4	184.5	73.2
Connecticut	128.7	14.6	13.2	21.6	29.7	68.6	311.9	118.5
Delaware[b]	122.1	--	--	5.4	36.8	56.7	305.7	111.2
District of Columbia	66.2	12.2	6.1	13.4	18.6	40.5	162.1	63.7
Florida	84.1	8.4	11.8	13.3	30.8	59.7	236.5	92.7
Georgia	87.6	16.5	12.7	17.3	37.5	63.2	248.1	99.4
Illinois	103.2	8.1	10.7	16.2	29.4	57.5	241.7	93.8
Kansas	72.4	8.1	8.2	22.7	17.9	80.3	211.4	88.1
Kentucky	103.9	18.7	12.7	11.9	33.7	68.7	290.4	111.7
Louisiana	64.0	10.8	14.8	22.7	31.3	58.1	188.2	79.9
Minnesota	105.2	17.7	15.7	12.2	28.9	49.5	234.3	90.2
Missouri	68.4	10.6	10.7	10.8	25.4	47.7	192.0	75.5
Nebraska	99.0	3.9	13.4	23.0	18.7	62.6	222.5	88.1
New York[b]	99.8	4.7	8.0	13.9	26.2	58.9	241.0	92.5
North Carolina	104.3	21.6	18.1	18.3	35.3	82.5	340.8	131.5
Ohio[b]	84.1	2.3	8.4	17.6	31.1	59.8	223.8	89.0
Oregon	120.9	5.7	10.7	15.5	25.9	77.1	248.8	99.2
Pennsylvania	95.8	5.6	11.6	15.5	28.6	65.1	253.5	98.7
South Carolina	90.3	14.1	18.0	17.2	44.4	66.6	279.5	111.1
Tennessee	95.5	9.3	14.3	17.1	37.5	63.9	265.3	104.4
Texas	102.7	18.8	15.6	19.3	34.6	65.5	286.2	111.3
Virginia	95.3	20.1	6.9	15.7	35.4	63.3	266.1	103.7

[a]The standard population is the sum of all the states in the study.

[b]Data not reported for 1 hospital.

Appendix Table 5. Average annual age-adjusted resident patient rates in state and county mental hospitals per 100,000 population, by diagnosis: United States, each geographic region and each state, 1959-61

Geographic area	All mental disorders	Brain syndromes				Functional psychoses				Disorders assoc. with alcohol.	Psycho-neurosis	Person-ality disorders
		Total	Dis. of senium	Syphi-litic	Other	Total	Schizo-phrenic reactions	Affect. and involt.	Other			
United States	296.7	67.3	35.1	11.5	20.8	178.8	151.1	22.6	5.1	11.3	3.8	6.6
Northeast Region	399.5	83.6	50.6	11.8	21.1	261.0	219.9	31.8	9.3	16.1	4.6	7.1
New England	321.7	68.1	39.9	6.7	21.5	198.0	164.5	28.9	4.6	14.5	6.2	5.9
Maine	290.7	63.3	36.9	7.6	18.8	183.4	130.1	50.8	2.5	8.4	8.7	3.7
New Hampshire	386.9	86.2	51.5	9.3	25.4	210.3	173.6	29.8	6.9	6.6	4.0	7.3
Vermont	289.0	66.6	27.1	5.8	33.7	158.2	127.5	27.3	3.5	4.8	4.2	7.5
Rhode Island	357.7	79.4	47.3	6.1	25.9	205.0	170.2	27.7	7.1	24.8	7.4	8.3
Connecticut	311.5	61.9	37.6	6.0	18.3	204.7	179.4	21.3	4.0	16.6	5.8	5.3
Mid-Atlantic	411.4	86.0	52.3	12.6	21.1	270.7	228.4	32.3	10.0	16.4	4.4	7.3
New York	498.7	104.3	67.2	14.4	22.7	338.2	290.8	36.8	10.5	22.4	4.4	6.7
New Jersey	332.6	84.1	52.9	8.7	22.5	193.0	153.9	30.2	9.0	12.5	4.9	10.6
Pennsylvania	321.1	59.3	29.6	11.9	17.7	209.5	173.4	26.2	9.9	9.2	3.9	6.6
North Central Region	281.8	61.7	29.3	12.4	19.9	166.8	143.3	17.9	5.6	11.7	4.1	8.4
East North Central	306.7	69.2	34.0	14.4	20.8	181.1	154.9	19.0	7.2	13.5	4.1	8.5
Ohio	288.7	65.9	26.5	17.6	21.7	163.4	132.7	22.3	8.4	12.5	4.0	8.4
Indiana	249.5	60.8	29.4	16.8	14.6	153.3	132.8	18.3	2.2	6.9	3.4	8.9
Illinois	335.7	81.1	43.5	13.8	23.7	199.0	174.4	19.5	5.1	20.5	4.8	5.0
Michigan	290.6	57.4	24.1	13.9	19.5	190.7	168.6	15.1	6.9	8.1	3.8	13.8
Wisconsin	366.6	75.3	48.4	6.7	20.2	190.2	156.3	17.6	16.3	14.7	4.2	7.0
West North Central	226.8	46.2	20.1	8.0	18.1	134.3	116.3	15.8	2.2	7.7	4.2	8.0
Minnesota	288.8	60.9	37.3	5.0	18.5	176.0	148.3	23.4	4.4	14.6	5.1	8.3
Iowa	143.6	30.1	11.8	3.9	14.4	83.3	67.7	13.7	1.8	4.9	2.8	5.7
Missouri	245.1	48.3	13.8	14.4	20.1	138.2	124.4	12.4	1.4	4.5	2.9	7.1
North Dakota	284.9	54.5	28.4	4.2	22.0	187.7	172.5	14.6	0.6	13.0	4.5	3.4
South Dakota	232.3	51.3	27.8	4.3	19.2	144.2	116.2	24.0	4.0	10.8	5.6	6.0
Nebraska	264.8	58.0	25.5	8.7	23.9	149.0	131.1	16.4	1.6	12.4	5.6	14.0
Kansas	161.4	30.4	10.9	6.3	13.1	101.1	88.3	11.7	1.1	2.2	5.8	10.2

Southern Region	262.8	65.6	30.4	11.9	23.4	146.3	120.5	22.9	3.0	5.9	3.2	4.3
South Atlantic	296.1	79.2	39.4	13.3	26.5	162.0	131.0	27.2	3.7	7.8	3.9	4.8
Delaware	406.6	126.6	68.6	19.8	38.1	199.0	152.6	33.7	12.7	22.5	4.9	22.6
Maryland	304.2	81.0	44.1	12.9	23.9	166.1	144.9	17.9	3.3	15.6	4.0	6.0
Dist. of Col.	862.7	219.3	125.9	42.9	50.4	537.4	450.3	45.9	41.2	31.0	18.4	19.5
Virginia	315.3	84.0	40.9	13.6	29.4	167.6	119.4	45.2	3.0	9.4	3.7	5.6
West Virginia	301.7	79.5	30.8	19.1	29.6	131.1	100.3	28.6	2.2	9.7	3.2	6.5
North Carolina	244.2	66.9	30.5	10.2	26.1	141.9	116.2	23.2	2.4	3.2	4.0	3.6
South Carolina	335.2	94.6	55.0	11.9	27.7	194.1	166.9	23.3	3.9	3.9	5.7	1.2
Georgia	338.2	89.5	46.7	10.6	32.3	183.0	147.9	34.4	0.7	4.8	2.6	2.0
Florida	183.9	50.1	23.4	10.8	15.9	96.8	78.3	16.9	1.7	3.7	2.1	3.7
East South Central	242.4	55.5	26.2	9.9	19.5	140.1	115.5	22.2	2.4	3.1	3.2	2.7
Kentucky	223.4	50.8	20.8	10.9	19.1	115.9	100.1	14.7	1.0	5.0	2.4	2.6
Tennessee	236.7	60.2	32.3	9.0	18.9	140.7	116.5	21.7	2.5	3.4	3.0	3.7
Alabama	252.3	51.3	23.8	9.4	18.1	158.3	127.4	27.7	3.3	0.9	1.8	2.4
Mississippi	266.6	61.9	27.7	10.7	23.5	146.6	117.6	26.1	2.9	3.2	1.5	1.3
West South Central	226.9	52.6	20.2	11.2	21.2	126.7	107.6	16.8	2.2	4.9	2.8	4.8
Arkansas	275.3	61.7	23.8	9.7	28.2	131.2	106.3	20.5	4.3	3.7	3.7	3.1
Louisiana	290.7	61.1	26.8	15.3	19.0	153.3	137.3	14.1	1.9	8.7	3.8	6.3
Oklahoma	298.5	60.6	4.1	12.3	44.2	169.6	148.8	16.5	4.3	1.9	5.0	10.9
Texas	179.7	46.1	22.3	9.8	14.1	106.7	88.2	17.3	1.3	4.7	1.7	3.2
Western Region	230.1	55.5	30.7	8.1	16.7	136.4	118.4	16.2	1.8	12.9	3.2	7.4
Mountain	214.7	59.6	31.6	8.0	20.0	105.2	94.4	9.4	1.4	11.9	3.0	5.7
Montana	253.5	68.2	24.8	7.5	35.9	135.7	126.3	6.8	2.7	12.6	2.4	3.7
Idaho	151.8	36.6	16.1	4.2	16.3	85.8	77.0	8.2	0.6	4.4	3.4	7.7
Wyoming	204.8	66.0	38.2	12.9	14.9	111.0	92.5	17.1	1.4	12.3	2.2	8.3
Colorado	346.9	96.2	55.6	12.8	27.8	157.9	146.8	9.3	1.8	27.9	3.4	9.0
New Mexico	123.1	34.9	16.0	7.4	11.5	59.8	54.6	5.2	0.0	1.9	2.5	2.3
Arizona	145.5	46.4	22.2	6.2	18.0	68.5	60.0	7.5	1.0	3.0	3.6	3.1
Utah	135.9	24.3	12.1	2.6	9.6	81.2	65.3	14.4	1.6	4.4	2.0	6.8
Nevada	211.5	64.7	44.2	4.8	15.7	82.7	64.8	15.5	2.5	15.8	2.5	1.9
Pacific	234.8	54.2	30.4	8.1	15.7	145.8	125.8	18.1	1.9	13.1	3.3	8.0
Washington	227.4	50.2	26.5	6.6	17.1	141.6	118.9	18.5	4.2	4.6	4.6	9.4
Oregon	246.4	64.7	37.7	6.9	20.1	137.3	114.3	18.9	4.1	13.8	4.6	9.2
California	235.2	53.9	30.5	8.6	14.8	147.4	128.2	18.0	1.2	14.9	3.0	7.8
Hawaii	233.5	39.0	21.5	4.0	13.6	171.4	147.1	21.0	3.3	8.0	1.9	4.8
Alaska	221.0	59.1	17.6	11.7	29.8	110.1	102.5	5.4	2.5	10.6	2.0	1.1

Appendix Table 6 Numbers and rates per 100,000 civilian population of patient care episodes[a] in psychiatric facilities, by type of facility, age, and sex: United States, 1966

Age (in years)	All facilities	Number: Public and private mental hospitals: Total	State and county hospitals	VA hospitals	Private hospitals	General hospitals with psychiatric services	Outpatient psychiatric clinics
Both sexes							
Total	2,764,089	1,029,168	802,216	122,979	103,973	548,921	1,186,000
Under 15	368,382	15,822	13,840	65	1,917	16,475	336,085
15-24	443,944	96,377	76,866	2,480	17,031	84,314	263,253
25-34	444,719	140,487	104,511	17,452	18,524	98,898	205,334
35-44	517,165	205,684	134,363	48,484	22,837	117,681	193,800
45-54	403,171	188,478	145,299	25,627	17,552	100,678	114,015
55-64	275,594	160,113	138,486	8,693	12,934	66,431	49,050
65+	311,114	222,207	188,851	20,178	13,178	64,444	24,463
Males							
Total	1,446,091	574,855	412,900	122,979	38,976	220,117	651,119
Under 15	250,261	10,886	9,634	65	1,187	8,584	230,791
15-24	228,734	58,079	47,485	2,480	8,114	33,678	136,977
25-34	208,168	83,957	60,340	17,452	6,165	35,439	88,772
35-44	267,761	126,415	70,015	48,484	7,916	45,344	96,002
45-54	210,584	106,588	74,514	25,627	6,447	41,822	62,174
55-64	139,370	85,071	71,389	8,693	4,989	29,276	25,023
65+	141,213	103,859	79,523	20,178	4,158	25,974	11,380
Females							
Total	1,317,998	454,313	389,316	b	64,997	328,804	534,881
Under 15	118,121	4,936	4,206		730	7,891	105,294
15-24	215,210	38,298	29,381		8,917	50,636	126,276
25-34	236,551	56,530	44,171		12,359	63,459	116,562
35-44	249,404	79,269	64,348		14,921	72,337	97,798
45-54	192,587	81,890	70,785		11,105	58,856	51,841
55-64	136,224	75,042	67,097		7,945	37,155	24,027
65+	169,901	118,348	109,328		9,020	38,470	13,083

	Rate per 100,000 civilian population						
Both sexes							
Total	1,427.0	531.3	414.2	63.5	53.6	283.4	612.3
Under 15	613.3	26.3	23.0	0.1	3.2	27.4	559.6
15-24	1,473.0	319.7	255.0	8.2	56.5	279.8	873.5
25-34	2,043.8	645.6	480.3	80.2	85.1	454.5	943.7
35-44	2,172.4	864.0	564.4	203.7	95.9	494.3	814.1
45-54	1,814.0	848.0	653.7	115.3	79.0	453.0	513.0
55-64	1,597.1	927.9	802.5	50.4	75.0	385.0	284.2
65+	1,685.6	1,203.9	1,023.2	109.3	71.4	349.2	132.5
Males							
Total	1,541.6	612.7	440.2	131.1	41.4	234.7	694.2
Under 15	818.5	35.6	31.5	0.2	3.9	28.1	754.8
15-24	1,592.0	404.3	330.5	17.3	56.5	234.4	953.3
25-34	2,001.8	807.3	580.2	167.8	59.3	340.8	853.7
35-44	2,338.1	1,103.9	611.4	423.4	69.1	395.9	838.3
45-54	1,958.6	991.3	693.0	238.3	60.0	389.0	578.3
55-64	1,690.9	1,032.1	866.1	105.5	60.5	355.2	303.6
65+	1,764.2	1,297.5	993.5	252.1	51.9	324.5	142.2
Females							
Total	1,319.3	454.8	389.7	b	65.1	329.1	535.4
Under 15	400.7	16.8	14.3		2.5	26.8	357.1
15-24	1,364.6	242.8	186.3		56.5	321.1	800.7
25-34	2,082.6	497.7	388.9		108.8	558.7	1,026.2
35-44	2,018.8	641.7	520.9		120.8	585.5	791.6
45-54	1,678.5	713.7	616.9		96.8	513.0	451.8
55-64	1,511.4	832.6	744.4		88.2	412.2	266.6
65+	1,625.4	1,132.2	1,045.9		86.3	368.0	125.2

[a] Patient care episodes--the sum of residents at the beginning plus admissions during the year. For clinic residents refer to patients carried over at beginning of year.

[b] Female patients excluded because number is negligible.

Appendix Table 7 Numbers and rates per 100,000 civilian population of total admissions to psychiatric facilities, by type of facility, age, and sex: United States, 1966

Age (in years)	All facilities	Number: Public and private mental hospitals: Total	State and county hospitals	VA hospitals	Private hospitals	General hospitals with psychiatric services	Outpatient psychiatric clinics
Both sexes							
Total	1,637,432	481,954	327,014	65,025	89,915	526,186	629,292
Under 15	210,203	8,982	7,706	65	1,211	15,793	185,428
15-24	288,478	64,987	48,953	2,016	14,018	80,822	142,669
25-34	291,977	89,237	61,874	10,729	16,634	94,802	107,938
35-44	330,190	118,812	67,864	30,171	20,777	112,807	98,571
45-54	239,770	86,598	55,976	15,021	15,601	96,508	56,664
55-64	139,152	50,169	36,120	2,666	11,383	63,679	25,304
65+	137,662	63,169	48,521	4,357	10,291	61,775	12,718
Males							
Total	829,078	277,379	178,942	65,025	33,412	211,000	340,699
Under 15	141,606	5,956	5,189	65	702	8,229	127,421
15-24	144,891	38,336	29,704	2,016	6,616	32,283	74,272
25-34	130,532	51,248	35,073	10,729	5,446	33,971	45,313
35-44	163,515	73,713	36,325	30,171	7,217	43,466	46,336
45-54	119,845	50,796	30,062	15,021	5,713	40,090	28,959
55-64	67,396	26,727	19,684	2,666	4,377	28,063	12,606
65+	61,293	30,603	22,905	4,357	3,341	24,898	5,792
Females							
Total	808,354	204,575	148,072	a	56,503	315,186	288,593
Under 15	68,597	3,026	2,517		509	7,564	58,007
15-24	143,587	26,651	19,249		7,402	48,539	68,397
25-34	161,445	37,989	26,801		11,188	60,831	62,625
35-44	166,675	45,099	31,539		13,560	69,341	52,235
45-54	119,925	35,802	25,914		9,888	56,418	27,705
55-64	71,756	23,442	16,436		7,006	35,616	12,698
65+	76,369	32,566	25,616		6,950	36,877	6,926

	Rate per 100,000 civilian population						
Both sexes							
Total	845.3	248.8	168.8	33.6	46.4	271.6	324.9
Under 15	349.9	14.9	12.8	0.1	2.0	26.3	308.7
15-24	957.2	215.6	162.4	6.7	46.5	268.2	473.4
25-34	1,342.0	410.2	284.4	49.3	76.5	435.7	496.1
35-44	1,387.1	499.1	285.1	126.7	87.3	473.9	414.1
45-54	1,078.7	389.6	251.8	67.6	70.2	434.2	254.9
55-64	806.3	290.7	209.3	15.4	66.0	369.0	146.6
65+	745.9	342.3	262.9	23.6	55.8	334.7	68.9
Males							
Total	883.9	295.7	190.8	69.3	35.6	225.0	363.2
Under 15	463.1	19.5	17.0	0.2	2.3	26.9	416.7
15-24	1,008.3	266.7	206.7	14.0	46.0	224.7	516.9
25-34	1,255.3	492.9	337.3	103.2	52.4	326.7	435.7
35-44	1,427.8	643.7	317.2	263.5	63.0	379.5	404.6
45-54	1,114.6	172.4	279.6	139.7	53.1	372.9	269.3
55-64	817.5	324.2	238.8	32.3	53.1	340.4	152.9
65+	765.8	382.3	286.2	54.4	41.7	311.1	72.4
Females							
Total	809.2	204.8	148.2	a	56.6	315.5	288.9
Under 15	232.6	10.2	8.5		1.7	25.7	196.7
15-24	910.5	169.0	122.1		46.9	307.8	433.7
25-34	1,421.2	334.4	235.9		98.5	535.5	551.3
35-44	1,349.2	365.1	255.3		109.8	561.3	422.8
45-54	1,045.2	312.0	225.8		86.2	491.7	241.5
55-64	769.2	260.1	182.4		77.7	395.2	140.9
65+	730.7	311.6	245.1		66.5	352.8	66.3

[a] Female patients were excluded because numbers were negligible.

Appendix Table 8 Numbers and rates per 100,000 civilian population of patients resident in psychiatric facilities, by type of facility, and on rolls of outpatient psychiatric clinics at beginning of year, by age and sex: United States, 1966.

	Number						
		Public and private mental hospitals					
Age (in years)	All facilities	Total	State and county hospitals	VA hospitals	Private hospitals	General hospitals with psychiatric services	Outpatient psychiatric clinics
Both sexes							
Total	1,126,657	547,214	475,202	57,954	14,058	22,735	556,708
Under 15	158,179	6,840	6,134	--	706	682	150,657
15-24	155,466	31,390	27,913	464	3,013	3,492	120,584
25-34	152,742	51,250	42,637	6,723	1,890	4,096	97,396
35-44	186,975	86,872	66,499	18,313	2,060	4,874	95,229
45-54	163,401	101,880	89,323	10,606	1,951	4,170	57,351
55-64	136,442	109,944	102,366	6,027	1,551	2,752	23,746
65+	173,452	159,038	140,330	15,821	2,887	2,669	11,745
Males							
Total	617,013	297,476	233,958	57,954	5,564	9,117	310,420
Under 15	108,655	4,930	4,445	--	485	355	103,370
15-24	83,843	19,743	17,781	464	1,498	1,395	62,705
25-34	77,636	32,709	25,267	6,723	719	1,468	43,459
35-44	104,246	52,702	33,690	18,313	699	1,878	49,666
45-54	90,739	55,792	44,452	10,606	734	1,732	33,215
55-64	71,974	58,344	51,705	6,027	612	1,213	12,417
65+	79,920	73,256	56,618	15,821	817	1,076	5,588
Females							
Total	509,644	249,738	241,244	a	8,494	13,618	246,288
Under 15	49,524	1,910	1,689		221	327	47,287
15-24	71,623	11,647	10,132		1,515	2,097	57,879
25-34	75,106	18,541	17,370		1,171	2,628	53,937
35-44	82,729	34,170	32,809		1,361	2,996	45,563
45-54	72,662	46,088	44,871		1,217	2,438	24,136
55-64	64,468	51,600	50,661		939	1,539	11,329
65+	93,532	85,782	83,712		2,070	1,593	6,157

	Rate per 100,000 civilian population						
Both sexes							
Total	581.6	282.5	245.3	29.9	7.3	11.7	287.4
Under 15	263.3	11.4	10.2	--	1.2	1.1	250.8
15-24	515.8	104.1	92.6	1.5	10.0	11.6	400.1
25-34	702.0	235.6	196.0	30.9	8.7	18.8	447.6
35-44	785.4	364.9	279.3	76.9	8.7	20.5	400.0
45-54	735.2	458.4	401.9	47.7	8.8	18.8	258.0
55-64	790.6	637.1	593.2	34.9	9.0	15.9	137.6
65+	939.7	861.6	760.3	85.7	15.6	14.5	63.6
Males							
Total	657.8	317.1	249.4	61.8	5.9	9.7	331.0
Under 15	355.4	16.1	14.5	--	1.6	1.2	338.1
15-24	583.5	137.4	123.8	3.2	10.4	9.7	436.4
25-34	746.6	314.6	243.0	64.7	6.9	14.1	417.9
35-44	910.3	460.2	294.2	159.9	6.1	16.4	433.7
45-54	843.8	518.8	413.4	98.6	6.8	16.1	308.9
55-64	873.2	707.9	627.3	73.1	7.5	14.7	150.6
65+	998.5	915.3	707.4	197.7	10.2	13.4	69.8
Females							
Total	480.1	250.0	241.5	a	8.5	13.6	216.5
Under 15	167.9	6.4	5.7		0.7	1.1	160.4
15-24	454.1	73.8	64.2		9.6	13.3	367.0
25-34	661.1	163.2	152.9		10.3	23.1	474.8
35-44	669.7	276.6	265.6		11.0	24.3	368.8
45-54	632.2	401.6	391.0		10.6	21.2	210.4
55-64	715.3	572.5	562.1		10.4	17.1	125.7
65+	894.7	820.6	800.8		19.8	15.2	58.9

[a]Female patients were excluded because numbers were negligible.

Appendix Table 9. Total numbers and percent distribution by diagnoses of first admissions and resident patients in psychiatric facilities, by type of facility: United States, 1966

Diagnostic category	Public mental hospitals, state and county		Private mental hospitals		General hospitals with psychiatric facilities	Outpatient psychiatric clinics
	First admissions	Resident patients	First admissions	Resident patients	Discharges	Terminations
Total patients	150,702	452,329	51,104	14,808	446,931	593,000
Percent Distribution						
All diagnoses	100.0	100.0	100.0	100.0	100.0	100.0
Brain syndromes[a]	21.8	22.9	7.0	16.8	10.5	3.3
Disorders of senium	16.5	12.7	3.6	8.2	4.2	0.7
Other brain syndromes	5.3	10.2	3.4	8.6	6.3	2.5
Schizophrenic reactions	18.6	48.3	18.9	26.3	14.9	16.1
Depressive disorders	9.7	5.1	33.3	19.7	27.4	13.2
Affective reactions	2.5	4.1	9.1	7.6	6.2	2.1
Psychoneurotic depressive reactions	7.2	1.0	24.2	12.1	21.2	11.1
Alcoholic disorders[b]	17.8	4.8	7.7	5.3	11.8	3.2
Personality disorders[c]	11.7	2.2	7.7	8.8	7.0	22.6
Psychoneurotic disorders[d]	3.7	0.8	10.4	5.1	15.2	11.7
Transient situational personality disorders	3.8	0.8	3.3	2.7	3.4	18.2
Mental deficiency	2.5	7.9	0.3	2.2	0.8	1.5
All other disorders	4.6	5.0	8.9	7.3	7.4	3.3
Undiagnosed	5.0	1.8	2.1	6.9	1.2	5.9
Without mental disorder	1.4	0.3	0.5	0.3	0.4	1.1

[a] Brain syndromes: excludes brain syndromes associated with alcoholism.

[b] Alcoholic disorders: includes brain syndromes associated with alcohol and the category alcohol (addiction) from the personality disorders.

[c] Personality disorders: includes all personality disorders except alcohol (addiction).

[d] Psychoneurotic disorders: includes all psychoneurotic reactions except psychoneurotic depressive reaction.

Appendix Table 10. Age-adjusted suicide rates per 100,000 population by sex, color, and marital status: United States and each geographic region, 1959-61

Area, color, and sex	Total	Single	Married	Widowed	Divorced
United States					
White male	23.1	35.2	18.7	90.6	75.7
White female	6.9	8.2	5.8	12.0	20.6
Nonwhite male	12.2	17.0	9.9	39.5	21.3
Nonwhite female	3.0	2.5	2.4	6.0	4.3
New England					
White male	19.0	29.1	15.0	88.3	63.9
White female	5.2	5.8	4.4	13.3	24.8
Nonwhite male	13.8	25.0	10.2	6.8	0.0
Nonwhite female	3.8	0.0	2.6	12.2	4.9
Middle Atlantic					
White male	18.0	28.4	14.5	64.5	67.3
White female	6.1	7.5	5.3	7.6	15.2
Nonwhite male	12.4	17.7	8.3	40.3	28.9
Nonwhite female	3.6	3.7	3.3	6.9	2.2
East North Central					
White male	22.0	33.3	17.8	66.8	67.3
White female	6.3	7.4	5.3	11.7	17.4
Nonwhite male	10.8	9.3	9.5	36.1	13.7
Nonwhite female	3.0	2.8	2.3	3.7	2.7
West North Central					
White male	22.9	39.1	17.7	106.5	95.4
White female	5.6	6.7	4.7	10.1	16.8
Nonwhite male	13.5	19.7	12.2	1.6	20.3
Nonwhite female	4.5	4.5	2.9	19.2	13.9
South Atlantic					
White male	28.0	40.1	23.7	135.2	77.3
White female	7.4	9.4	6.4	14.3	22.3
Nonwhite male	10.9	12.7	10.1	37.4	17.9
Nonwhite female	2.2	2.0	1.8	6.7	4.1
East South Central					
White male	24.3	39.7	19.8	73.8	84.9
White female	5.0	6.9	4.2	10.0	12.0
Nonwhite male	9.5	12.5	8.1	50.6	24.3
Nonwhite female	1.9	1.3	1.6	1.1	3.0
West South Central					
White male	21.1	32.3	17.4	61.5	76.4
White female	5.4	6.9	4.8	11.5	16.8
Nonwhite male	10.4	15.7	8.2	27.0	22.0
Nonwhite female	1.9	0.3	1.7	3.3	2.0
Mountain					
White male	30.7	55.4	23.4	122.8	104.4
White female	8.0	13.0	6.9	10.9	26.7
Nonwhite male	30.3	39.3	24.5	0.0	67.3
Nonwhite female	9.1	15.0	6.2	1.4	17.3
Pacific					
White male	29.4	43.4	23.9	132.2	77.4
White female	11.8	15.7	9.6	19.8	30.3
Nonwhite male	19.4	31.5	12.7	80.6	25.7
Nonwhite female	6.9	3.1	4.4	20.6	7.9

Appendix Table 11. Suicide rates per 100,000 population by age, color, and sex: United States and each geographic region, 1959-61

Region, color, and sex	All ages										
	Age-adjusted	Crude	5-14	15-24	25-34	35-44	45-54	55-64	65-74	75-84	85+
Total U.S.	10.5	10.5	0.2	5.1	10.0	14.0	20.3	23.7	23.2	27.5	25.6
White male	17.3	17.5	0.4	8.2	14.6	21.9	33.1	40.7	42.2	55.6	62.4
female	5.2	5.2	0.1	2.3	5.8	8.0	10.4	10.6	9.2	8.2	4.9
Nonwhite male	9.1	7.5	0.1	6.5	14.4	12.1	13.6	15.8	13.6	17.6	12.8
female	2.3	1.9	0.1	1.9	3.6	3.5	2.9	3.6	2.9	3.0	4.1
New England	8.8	9.2	0.3	4.7	9.4	11.2	15.8	18.7	20.3	22.5	21.3
White male	14.3	14.7	0.6	8.0	13.7	17.6	24.5	30.3	36.7	45.2	54.8
female	3.9	4.2	0.0	1.5	5.0	5.3	7.8	8.5	7.6	7.1	2.9
Nonwhite male	10.1	8.8	0.0	1.7	22.4	7.4	18.3	25.6	7.1	18.7	83.5
female	2.9	2.5	0.0	1.7	1.5	7.4	0.0	12.8	0.0	16.0	0.0
Middle Atlantic	8.6	9.4	0.2	4.3	8.0	10.2	15.4	20.5	23.2	25.4	26.6
White male	13.5	14.7	0.3	6.8	11.0	14.7	23.9	32.6	39.2	48.6	62.9
female	4.6	5.1	0.0	1.9	4.9	6.3	8.6	10.8	10.8	9.5	6.6
Nonwhite male	9.3	8.4	0.2	7.1	16.1	13.0	11.9	14.1	17.1	10.9	12.6
female	2.7	2.6	0.2	2.5	4.2	4.5	3.0	4.0	3.0	1.7	15.8
East North Central	10.1	10.2	0.2	4.7	8.9	12.6	19.5	23.1	24.9	31.2	28.4
White male	16.5	16.8	0.4	8.1	13.1	18.9	31.0	38.2	44.5	63.1	68.4
female	4.8	4.8	0.1	1.8	4.8	7.3	9.9	10.5	9.3	8.4	4.9
Nonwhite male	8.1	7.0	0.2	4.9	14.2	12.5	10.7	13.8	11.4	10.1	0.0
female	2.2	2.0	0.0	1.6	4.0	3.5	4.5	2.7	1.2	0.0	0.0
West North Central	10.4	10.9	0.1	4.8	8.9	13.1	21.3	25.6	24.2	26.7	27.0
White male	17.3	18.1	0.4	7.7	12.8	20.9	34.9	44.4	42.8	51.8	60.3
female	4.3	4.4	0.1	1.7	5.1	5.8	8.8	9.2	8.1	7.6	5.3
Nonwhite male	10.0	8.4	0.0	10.0	14.4	13.2	17.7	8.3	24.7	5.2	0.0
female	3.5	2.9	0.0	3.7	3.7	7.6	5.2	4.0	4.0	0.0	0.0

South Atlantic	11.4	10.7	0.1	5.0	11.3	17.1	22.7	26.2	20.0	23.5	17.1
White male	20.9	20.3	0.3	8.1	18.2	31.0	42.6	50.9	41.0	52.9	48.9
female	5.6	5.5	0.1	2.7	6.9	8.9	11.0	11.7	7.4	6.5	3.0
Nonwhite male	8.1	6.4	0.1	5.7	12.0	11.8	13.3	15.1	10.8	11.0	0.0
female	1.6	1.4	0.1	1.6	2.7	2.0	2.0	3.2	1.8	2.1	0.0
East South Central	9.4	8.9	0.2	3.7	9.8	13.1	19.6	20.6	18.3	23.2	15.2
White male	18.2	17.5	0.4	6.3	16.7	24.2	38.7	42.6	39.7	53.8	37.9
female	3.8	3.7	0.1	1.7	4.7	6.4	7.4	6.8	6.0	5.6	3.6
Nonwhite male	7.0	5.5	0.0	4.4	10.7	6.4	13.3	14.3	12.1	13.5	16.3
female	1.4	1.1	0.0	0.8	3.5	2.2	1.7	1.6	1.3	1.1	0.0
West South Central	8.9	8.5	0.2	4.8	8.5	12.7	17.1	20.1	18.4	18.2	18.9
White male	15.8	15.2	0.4	7.2	12.8	21.3	30.7	37.5	38.5	41.7	53.6
female	4.1	3.8	0.1	2.8	5.1	6.7	7.2	7.7	5.4	3.9	1.6
Nonwhite male	7.7	6.1	0.1	4.9	11.6	10.4	12.8	16.1	10.2	9.4	0.0
female	1.4	1.2	0.1	1.9	1.3	1.6	2.7	2.1	2.1	1.1	0.0
Mountain	14.6	13.3	0.2	8.2	15.3	20.7	28.7	30.6	27.0	29.6	28.7
White male	23.0	21.2	0.6	12.2	20.7	32.0	44.5	51.8	47.7	58.8	64.5
female	6.0	5.4	0.0	3.0	7.8	9.4	13.4	10.4	8.0	4.4	4.2
Nonwhite male	22.8	18.2	0.0	30.1	53.6	29.3	20.3	14.3	11.4	27.6	0.0
female	6.9	5.3	0.0	7.4	13.9	11.4	5.6	12.6	0.0	0.0	0.0
Pacific	14.9	14.9	0.4	7.3	13.9	20.5	29.7	32.4	30.2	41.2	40.0
White male	22.2	22.1	0.8	11.0	19.0	28.2	42.2	51.3	49.3	75.6	88.3
female	8.9	8.9	0.2	3.6	9.5	14.7	19.9	16.2	14.5	13.5	8.0
Nonwhite male	14.4	12.3	0.2	10.7	16.2	15.5	19.6	26.6	28.3	86.4	103.8
female	5.2	4.2	0.2	2.9	5.4	6.5	4.6	9.9	19.0	27.0	48.5

Appendix Table 12a. **Suicide rates per 100,000 population of total persons according to whether born within or outside state of residence, or foreign-born: United States, each geographic region and state, 1959-61**

Geographic area	Total		Born in state	Born outside state			Foreign-born
	Crude	Age adjusted		Total	Contiguous states	Non-contiguous states	
New England							
Connecticut	9.4	9.1	6.5	10.5	11.6	9.8	22.1
Maine	12.3	11.9	11.1	12.3	17.6	11.7	25.9
Massachusetts	8.3	7.9	6.8	10.0	11.4	8.1	14.7
New Hampshire	11.8	11.1	8.6	14.0	17.0	9.5	24.6
Rhode Island	6.4	6.1	5.1	7.7	7.3	8.0	11.2
Vermont	15.2	14.0	13.5	15.2	18.6	10.4	31.4
Middle Atlantic							
New Jersey	8.3	7.7	6.0	8.9	9.9	7.6	18.6
New York	9.5	8.6	7.3	9.9	12.6	8.9	18.3
Pennsylvania	9.8	9.2	9.0	9.2	12.4	7.2	23.6
South Atlantic							
Delaware	11.6	11.9	9.6	12.5	14.6	10.6	31.9
Florida	13.0	12.8	5.8	16.1	14.3	16.6	25.4
Georgia	9.4	10.4	9.2	9.8	11.0	8.5	13.2
Maryland	10.4	10.8	9.0	11.1	12.2	10.1	24.1
North Carolina	9.5	10.6	9.4	10.3	12.1	8.6	6.1
South Carolina	7.1	8.3	6.4	10.1	20.9	7.5	20.9
Virginia	12.6	13.6	12.9	11.6	15.5	9.4	20.8
West Virginia	11.6	11.9	11.3	11.1	14.0	6.0	34.9
East North Central							
Illinois	9.4	8.8	7.9	9.2	11.7	8.2	22.3
Indiana	11.0	11.0	10.3	11.4	14.0	8.9	26.1
Michigan	10.0	10.4	7.7	12.4	19.0	11.0	23.7
Ohio	10.5	10.3	9.7	10.3	11.4	9.2	23.3
Wisconsin	11.0	10.8	10.2	10.6	10.9	10.5	25.8

East South Central							
Alabama	8.6	9.4	8.1	10.9	13.5	8.4	15.6
Kentucky	10.2	10.6	10.0	10.3	12.4	8.3	25.7
Mississippi	6.5	7.3	6.1	9.1	9.9	8.3	0.0
Tennessee	9.4	9.6	9.1	9.9	11.5	7.2	16.8
West North Central							
Iowa	11.7	11.0	11.1	13.0	15.7	9.1	21.3
Kansas	11.3	10.9	9.8	13.0	14.1	12.1	31.1
Minnesota	9.4	9.4	7.7	11.3	13.7	8.5	29.0
Missouri	12.0	11.1	11.2	12.9	16.7	8.9	23.1
Nebraska	11.0	10.2	10.1	12.9	16.8	9.0	14.9
North Dakota	8.4	9.1	7.0	11.6	9.3	14.1	16.7
South Dakota	8.9	9.2	7.8	11.3	7.8	10.6	16.1
West South Central							
Arkansas	7.6	7.5	6.3	11.0	10.7	11.4	31.3
Louisiana	7.6	8.4	6.6	10.8	10.5	11.2	22.9
Oklahoma	9.2	9.1	6.7	12.7	13.6	11.4	25.0
Texas	8.8	9.4	7.5	11.9	11.6	12.1	11.9
Mountain							
Arizona	12.2	13.6	5.8	14.7	14.7	14.7	18.0
Colorado	14.4	15.2	9.7	17.6	19.1	17.0	26.2
Idaho	12.8	13.5	8.2	16.4	12.5	18.4	42.9
Montana	14.9	15.3	9.3	19.8	14.8	22.0	32.6
Nevada	26.2	26.8	12.0	28.7	15.6	34.7	58.4
New Mexico	10.3	12.5	6.8	13.9	11.5	15.9	9.3
Utah	9.6	11.4	7.8	14.1	15.4	13.3	12.4
Wyoming	16.3	17.3	8.9	19.9	19.3	20.3	51.7
Pacific							
Alaska	14.9	19.7	9.1	15.3	-	-	48.6
California	15.6	15.6	8.0	19.4	17.4	19.5	26.6
Hawaii	8.1	9.7	4.9	9.3	-	-	24.7
Oregon	12.6	12.2	8.0	15.5	10.5	17.1	28.0
Washington	13.8	13.6	8.2	17.0	13.7	17.5	29.3

Appendix Table 12b. Suicide rates per 100,000 population of white persons according to whether born within or outside state of residence, or foreign-born: United States, each geographic region and state, 1959-61

Geographic area	Total		Born in state	Born outside state			Foreign-born
	Crude	Age Adjusted		Total	Contiguous states	Non-contiguous states	
New England							
Connecticut	9.7	9.2	6.6	10.8	11.7	10.1	22.5
Maine	12.2	11.8	11.0	12.6	17.6	12.0	25.8
Massachusetts	8.3	7.9	6.9	9.6	11.5	8.3	14.8
New Hampshire	11.8	11.1	8.6	14.1	17.1	9.7	24.8
Rhode Island	6.3	5.9	5.1	7.7	7.3	7.9	10.6
Vermont	15.2	14.0	13.4	15.3	18.6	10.5	31.6
Middle Atlantic							
New Jersey	8.7	7.9	6.2	9.5	9.9	8.7	18.7
New York	9.8	8.7	7.6	10.4	12.6	9.2	18.7
Pennsylvania	10.2	9.5	9.3	10.1	13.1	7.5	23.8
South Atlantic							
Delaware	12.2	12.4	10.2	13.3	14.7	11.9	30.3
Florida	15.1	14.4	7.5	17.5	18.3	17.4	26.5
Georgia	11.9	12.5	12.1	10.9	12.5	9.2	14.0
Maryland	11.6	11.7	10.2	12.0	13.2	10.9	23.7
North Carolina	11.4	12.1	11.5	11.1	12.9	9.8	6.7
South Carolina	9.7	10.5	9.2	11.0	15.1	8.1	16.1
Virginia	14.6	15.3	15.7	12.3	16.5	9.9	19.4
West Virginia	12.0	12.2	11.5	12.0	15.0	6.4	35.5
East North Central							
Illinois	10.0	9.2	8.3	10.7	12.1	9.9	22.5
Indiana	11.4	11.3	10.6	12.0	14.3	9.4	26.4
Michigan	10.6	10.9	8.0	14.2	19.2	12.7	23.8
Ohio	11.0	10.7	10.0	11.2	11.7	10.6	23.4
Wisconsin	11.2	10.8	10.3	11.2	11.1	11.3	26.2

East South Central							
Alabama	11.1	11.5	11.0	11.8	14.6	9.2	14.2
Kentucky	10.5	10.8	10.2	10.5	12.5	8.4	25.4
Mississippi	9.4	9.5	9.3	10.0	11.4	8.6	0.0
Tennessee	10.5	10.6	10.3	11.0	13.2	7.7	18.1
West North Central							
Iowa	11.7	11.1	11.1	13.4	15.9	9.6	21.7
Kansas	11.6	11.1	10.1	13.6	14.2	13.0	33.2
Minnesota	9.5	9.5	7.8	11.5	13.8	8.6	29.4
Missouri	12.7	11.5	11.7	14.1	16.7	10.6	23.8
Nebraska	11.2	10.3	10.2	13.3	16.8	9.5	15.1
North Dakota	8.4	8.9	7.0	11.6	8.9	14.4	16.9
South Dakota	8.8	8.9	7.5	11.5	11.9	10.9	16.4
West South Central							
Arkansas	8.8	8.3	7.4	12.0	12.2	11.7	28.5
Louisiana	9.8	10.4	8.9	12.3	12.0	12.5	22.1
Oklahoma	9.7	9.4	7.0	13.2	14.0	12.1	25.1
Texas	9.4	9.9	8.2	12.5	12.1	12.7	11.4
Mountain							
Arizona	12.3	13.3	4.1	15.1	14.6	15.2	18.2
Colorado	14.6	15.4	9.8	18.2	19.4	17.5	27.0
Idaho	12.8	13.4	8.0	16.6	12.7	18.6	42.9
Montana	15.2	15.4	9.4	20.2	14.6	22.2	33.4
Nevada	26.8	26.9	10.0	30.0	15.0	37.1	59.4
New Mexico	10.2	12.2	6.0	14.0	11.5	16.1	9.7
Utah	9.3	11.2	7.6	14.1	14.6	13.8	12.0
Wyoming	16.2	17.1	8.5	19.8	18.5	20.7	53.3
Pacific							
Alaska	16.4	21.7	8.0	16.4	-	16.4	46.8
California	16.2	16.0	8.3	20.5	17.3	20.7	26.5
Hawaii	8.7	10.5	5.4	9.8	-	9.8	21.9
Oregon	12.7	12.2	8.0	15.7	10.6	17.4	27.4
Washington	13.8	13.5	8.1	17.3	13.7	17.8	29.1

Appendix Table 12c. Suicide rates per 100,000 population of nonwhite persons according to whether born within or outside state of residence, or foreign-born: United States, each geographic region and state, 1959-61

Geographic area	Total		Born in state	Born outside state			Foreign-born
	Crude	Age adjusted		Total	Contiguous states	Non-contiguous states	
New England							
Connecticut	4.8	5.4	2.3	6.9	0.0	7.4	0.0
Maine	22.3	37.2	45.2	0.0	0.0	0.0	37.9
Massachusetts	4.8	5.2	1.8	5.9	8.0	5.8	11.2
New Hampshire	0.0	0.0	0.0	0.0	0.0	0.0	0.0
Rhode Island	9.6	12.4	6.1	8.0	0.0	8.9	51.0
Vermont	42.2	64.4	150.2	0.0	0.0	0.0	0.0
Middle Atlantic							
New Jersey	4.2	4.6	2.7	5.5	8.9	5.1	7.3
New York	6.1	6.6	2.7	8.3	10.7	8.2	9.9
Pennsylvania	4.7	5.2	3.1	6.4	4.1	6.7	9.0
South Atlantic							
Delaware	7.5	8.8	6.6	7.6	13.8	5.2	97.2
Florida	3.3	4.0	2.0	5.2	6.2	3.6	7.8
Georgia	3.2	4.0	3.3	2.2	2.4	1.9	0.0
Maryland	4.5	5.3	3.4	5.9	4.3	6.7	31.7
North Carolina	4.0	5.2	3.7	6.6	9.7	1.3	0.0
South Carolina	2.4	3.3	2.2	3.0	2.3	3.2	83.6
Virginia	5.2	6.2	4.5	7.4	10.1	4.8	37.2
West Virginia	4.4	5.1	5.1	3.2	2.3	3.9	0.0
East North Central							
Illinois	4.1	4.6	2.6	4.8	5.1	4.7	15.3
Indiana	5.1	6.1	2.4	7.2	9.2	6.6	14.9
Michigan	4.4	5.1	2.0	5.9	11.8	5.8	16.5
Ohio	4.7	5.2	3.6	5.6	5.7	5.6	11.8
Wisconsin	3.6	4.9	4.1	4.4	0.0	4.7	0.0

East South Central							
Alabama	2.8	3.5	2.8	4.4	6.9	1.3	38.6
Kentucky	6.7	7.7	6.0	8.8	11.0	7.6	30.2
Mississippi	2.6	3.4	2.5	4.8	4.4	5.7	0.0
Tennessee	3.5	4.1	3.0	5.2	5.7	3.2	0.0
West North Central							
Iowa	5.8	6.4	11.8	0.0	0.0	0.0	0.0
Kansas	4.0	4.5	2.2	5.8	12.1	2.8	0.0
Minnesota	4.7	6.0	5.7	4.0	0.0	4.4	0.0
Missouri	5.6	6.5	4.4	7.0	17.6	4.2	0.0
Nebraska	4.6	5.7	2.1	6.5	16.9	4.0	0.0
North Dakota	10.3	15.8	9.4	16.0	41.9	0.0	0.0
South Dakota	10.9	15.7	13.0	0.0	0.0	0.0	0.0
West South Central							
Arkansas	3.3	3.9	2.8	5.6	5.2	7.4	75.8
Louisiana	2.7	3.6	2.5	4.0	5.0	2.5	35.3
Oklahoma	4.5	5.7	4.1	5.2	7.2	3.3	24.2
Texas	4.2	4.9	3.7	5.7	8.3	2.7	35.6
Mountain							
Arizona	11.3	14.8	12.9	7.1	16.3	6.0	13.4
Colorado	7.5	8.4	7.4	7.2	4.7	7.9	10.8
Idaho	17.0	19.4	24.6	0.0	0.0	0.0	43.7
Montana	6.9	9.4	6.7	9.5	31.7	0.0	0.0
Nevada	18.3	21.1	28.3	10.6	33.9	6.3	42.2
New Mexico	12.0	16.3	12.8	9.8	10.3	9.2	0.0
Utah	21.8	25.3	28.1	14.8	45.2	0.0	20.7
Wyoming	18.7	23.9	15.8	25.1	141.2	0.0	0.0
Pacific							
Alaska	9.7	13.5	9.9	0.0	-	0.0	60.1
California	8.2	9.8	4.3	7.1	19.8	6.9	28.1
Hawaii	7.8	9.2	4.8	6.1	-	6.1	25.0
Oregon	8.2	10.0	6.7	3.6	0.0	4.3	40.3
Washington	12.1	14.9	9.6	8.8	16.3	8.4	31.2

Appendix Table 13. Suicide rates per 100,000 population according to region of birth and region of residence at time of death: United States and each geographic region, 1959-61

Region of birth	Region of residence								
	New England	Middle Atlantic	East North Central	West North Central	South Atlantic	East South Central	West South Central	Mountain	Pacific
New England	7.9	11.4	11.8	8.8	13.3	8.3	16.2	13.7	18.4
Middle Atlantic	13.1	8.0	13.7	12.7	14.6	11.5	13.4	22.2	21.4
East North Central	13.4	13.2	9.3	15.3	15.3	7.7	15.6	21.2	21.6
West North Central	13.9	14.1	13.4	10.4	19.1	11.0	14.9	19.4	22.6
South Atlantic	9.5	9.8	10.5	8.6	9.9	12.5	12.8	18.2	20.0
East South Central	10.1	10.7	9.5	13.9	13.7	8.7	15.0	19.2	19.9
West South Central	5.0	9.5	8.5	11.7	13.6	12.2	7.5	15.7	14.8
Mountain	21.9	13.0	13.6	12.0	13.9	9.7	11.6	9.2	21.8
Pacific	6.9	11.1	6.8	5.1	8.2	7.5	8.0	12.0	8.5

Appendix Table 14. Age-adjusted suicide rates[a] by sex: United States, 1900-65

Year	Total	Male	Female
1965	11.4	16.9	6.3
1964	11.0	16.6	5.8
1963	11.3	17.0	6.0
1962	11.0	16.9	5.6
1961	10.5	16.4	5.0
1960	10.6	16.6	5.0
1959	10.5	16.6	4.7
1958	10.5	16.8	4.7
1957	9.6	15.3	4.2
1956	9.7	15.5	4.4
1955	9.9	15.7	4.5
1954	9.9	16.0	4.1
1953	9.8	15.7	4.2
1952	9.7	15.3	4.3
1951	10.0	15.7	4.5
1950	11.0	17.3	4.9
1949	11.0	17.3	4.9
1948	10.8	16.7	5.1
1947	11.1	17.1	5.4
1946	11.1	16.8	5.6
1945	10.7	16.3	5.6
1944	9.6	14.2	5.3
1943	10.0	14.7	5.3
1942	11.8	18.0	5.8
1941	12.7	19.2	6.3
1940	14.3	21.9	6.8
1939	14.3	21.8	6.6
1938	15.5	23.9	7.0
1937	15.3	23.3	7.2
1936	14.8	22.4	7.0
1935	14.9	22.7	7.0
1934	15.7	24.1	7.1
1933	17.0	26.5	7.1
1932	18.6	29.3	7.5
1931	18.2	28.3	7.6
1930	17.0	26.2	7.4
1929	15.3	23.1	7.1
1928	15.0	22.9	6.8
1927	14.6	22.1	6.7
1926	14.0	20.9	6.8
1925	13.4	20.1	6.3
1924	13.4	20.2	6.2
1923	12.9	19.1	6.4
1922	13.3	19.8	6.3
1921	13.9	21.1	6.3
1920	11.5	16.3	6.3
1919	12.8	18.4	7.0
1918	13.6	20.0	6.9
1917	14.6	21.4	7.3
1916	15.4	23.2	7.1
1915	17.9	26.8	8.3
1914	17.8	26.6	8.3
1913	17.0	25.6	7.7
1912	17.3	26.0	7.9
1911	17.7	26.5	8.1
1910	16.9	25.5	7.7
1909	17.6	26.8	7.9
1908	18.6	28.3	8.3
1907	16.1	24.4	7.4
1906	14.3	22.0	6.2
1905	14.9	22.6	7.1
1904	13.4	20.7	6.3
1903	12.5	19.2	5.7
1902	11.5	17.5	5.6
1901	11.6	17.6	5.7
1900	11.3	17.7	5.0

Sources: U.S. Dept. of Health Education and Welfare, Public Health Service, "Suicide - Death Rates by Age, Race and Sex, U.S. 1900-1953," Vital Statistics - Special Reports, Vol. 43, No. 30, August 22, 1956; "Mortality Trends in the United States, 1954-1963," Vital and Health Statistics, Series 20, No. 2; and Vital Statistics of the U.S., Part II. Mortality, 1964 & 1965.

[a]Age-adjusted by authors from source data, using the total U.S. population of 1940 as standard.

Appendix Table 15. Listing of studies of mental disorders among persons who commit suicide

Reference and place of study	Source of data	Size of sample	Percent with mental disorders	Comments
Asuni, 1962 (Western Nigeria	Coroner's Records, 1957-60	221	24	All psychoses
Gorceix & Zimbacca, 1965 (Seine, France)	Medico-legally verified cases, 1962 (of 869 recorded)	148	30	Had been in mental hosp.or treated by psychiatrist
			20	Apparently mentally ill (additional cases)
Krupinski, et al, 1965 (Victoria, Australia)	Coroner's Records, 1963 -male	302	21	Previously under care of mental health department
	female	147	22	
McCarthy & Walsh, 1966 (Dublin, Ireland)	Coroner's Records, 1954-63 (31 incomplete records excluded)	284	62	Mental or personality factor appeared most important cause.
Dublin, 1963 (USA)	Industrial policy-holder	22,000	20	
Prokupek, 1967 (Czechoslavakia)	National Statistics, 1963-66	2,335	30	Psychoses
			20	Neuroses
			7	Psychopathic personalities
Ringel, 1961 (Vienna, Austria)	Admissions to suicide prevention center		1/3	
Robins, et al, 1959 (St.Louis,Mo.)	Consecutive suicide verdicts 1956-57	134	94	68% with manic-depressive psychosis or alcoholism. Survivors interviewed.
Sainsbury, 1955 (London, Eng.)	Coroners' and medical records, 5 boroughs, 1936-38	390	37	Principal factor
			47	Contributory factor
Seager & Flood, 1965 (Bristol,Eng.)	Coroner's Records, 1957-61	325	66	Some form of mental disorder
Yap, 1958 (Hong Kong)	Criminal Investigation Dept. Records,1953-54	218	8	"Insanity" alone
			20	Including reactive depression
Stengel & Cook,1958 (London,Eng.)	Coroners' Records, 1953	117	33	Psychoses

Source: World Health Organization, "Prevention of Suicide," Public Health Papers No.35, Geneva, 1968, Annex 2, Table 9.

Appendix Table 16 Listing of sources regarding incidence of suicide among patients with mental disorders

Source of data and place	Period covered	Type of patient population	Size of patient population (average annual)	Average annual suicide rate per 100,000 patient population
Australia, Victoria (Krupinski, et al, 1965)	1963	Under care of mental health department males	11,591	550
		females	12,245	260
Australia, Perth (James & Levin, 1964)	1955-61	Discharged patients	3,225	119
England & Wales (Registrar General, 1960)	1954-56	Mental hospital patients	Not stated	38
Finland, Helsinki (Achte, et al, 1966)	1956-63	Patients in mental hospitals in Helsinki	5,535-6,640per yr.	99
State of California (Dublin, 1963)	1950-56 (incl.)	Patients in mental hospitals	Not stated	63
State of California (Pokorny, 1964)	1949-63	Patients and ex-patients, VA hospitals	11,585	165
State of Massachusettes (Temoche, et al, 1964)	1969-52	Patients in hospital	37,479	18
		Former patients	69,725	48
New York State (Malzberg, in Dublin, 1963)	Apr., 1957-Mar., 1959	Patients in State mental hospitals	90,000 per yr. (av.)	34
Monroe County, N.Y. (Gardner, et al, 1964)	1960-62	Patients on psychiatric case register	Not stated	160
New York State (Annual Reports - Dept. of Mental Hygiene)	1961-62	Patients resident in State and county mental hospitals	88,603	36
State of California (Annual Reports - Dept. of Mental Hygiene)	1964-66	Patients resident in State and county mental hospitals	30,206	50
State of Maryland (Annual Report - Dept. of Mental Hygiene)	1965-67	Patients resident in State and county mental hospitals	8,346	68

Sources: Items 1-9: World Health Organization, "Prevention of Suicide," Public Health Paper 35, Geneva, 1968, Annex 2, Table 7.
Items 10 - 12: Based on data obtained from annual reports of Departments of mental hygiene for States indicated.

References

1. American Medico-Psychological Association. *Statistical Manual for the Use of Institutions for Mental Diseases.* Utica, N.Y.: State Hospitals Press, 1920.

2. American Psychiatric Association and National Committee for Mental Hygiene: Committee on Statistics. *Statistical Manual for Use of Hospitals for Mental Diseases.* Tenth Edition. Utica. N.Y.: State Hospitals Press, 1942.

3. American Psychiatric Association. Committee on Nomenclature and Statistics. *Diagnostic and Statistical Manual of Mental Disorders, DSM-I.* Washington, D.C., 1952.

4. American Psychiatric Association. Committee on Nomenclature and Statistics. *Diagnostic and Statistical Manual of Mental Disorders, DSM-II.* Washington, D.C., 1968.

5. American Psychopathological Association. *Trends in Mental Disease.* New York: King's Crown Press, Columbia University Press, 1945.

6. American Public Health Association. Program Area Committee on Mental Health. *Mental Disorders: A Guide to Control Methods.* New York: American Public Health Association, 1962.

7. Ash, P. "The reliability of psychiatric diagnoses." *Journal of Abnormal Social Psychology,* 44:272 (1949).

8. Babigian, H. M., Gardner, E. S., Miles, H. C., and Romano, J. "Diagnostic consistency and change in a follow-up study of 1215 patients," *American Journal of Psychiatry,* 121:895-901 (1965).

9. Babigian, H. M., and Odoroff, C. L. "The mortality experience of a population with psychiatric illness," *American Journal of Psychiatry,* 126:4 (1969).

10. Bahn, A. K., and Norman, V. B. "First national report on patients of mental health clinics," *Public Health Reports,* 74:943-956 (1959).

11. Bahn, A. K. "Methodological study of population of outpatient psychiatric clinics, Maryland, 1958-59," *Public Health Monograph* No. 65: Public Health Service Publication. Washington, D.C.: U.S. Government Printing Office (1961).

12. Bahn, A. K., et al. "Admissions and prevalence rates for psychiatric facilities in four register areas," *American Journal of Public Health,* 56:2033 (1966).

13. Baldwin, J. A., et al. "A psychiatric case register in north-east Scotland," *British Journal of Preventive and Social Medicine,* 19:38 (1965).

14. Beck, A. T. "Reliability of psychiatric diagnoses. 1. A critique of systematic studies," *American Journal of Psychiatry,* 121:895-901 (1962).

15. Belknap, I. *Human Problems of a State Mental Hospital.* New York: McGraw-Hill, 1956.

16. Bodian, Carol, Gardner, Elmer A., Willis, Ernest M., and Bahn, Anita K. "Socioeconomic indicators from census tract data related to rates of mental illness," *Papers Presented at the Census Tract Conference.* Washington, D.C.: U.S. Bureau of the Census (1963).

17. Brown, G. W., Bone, M., Dalison, B., and Wing, J. K. *Schizophrenia and Social Care.* London: Oxford University Press, 1966.

18. Cavan, R. S. *Suicide.* Chicago: University of Chicago Press, 1928.

19. Cole, J. C., and Gerard, R. W., eds. *Psychopharmacology Problems in Evaluation.* Washington, D.C.: National Academy of Sciences, National Research Council, Publication 583, 1959.

20. Conwell, M., Rosen, B. M., Hench, C. L., and Bahn, A. K. "The first national survey of psychiatric day-night services," in *Day Care of Psychiatric Patients.* (Epps, R. L., ed.), Springfield, Ill.: Charles C Thomas, 1964.

21. Cooper, J. E. "Diagnostic change in a longitudinal study of psychiatric patients," *British Journal of Psychiatry,* 113:129-142 (1967).

22. Cooper, J. E., Kendell, R. E., Gurland, B., Sartorius, N., and Farkas, J. "Cross national study of diagnosis of the mental disorders – results," *American Journal of Psychiatry,* 125:21-29 (1969).

23. Dayton, N. A. *New Facts on Mental Disorders.* Baltimore: Charles C Thomas, 1940.

24. Dublin, L. I. *Suicide: A Sociological and Statistical Study.* New York: the Ronald Press, 1963.

25. Dunham, H. W., and Weinberg, S. K. *The Culture of the State Mental Hospital.* Detroit: Wayne State University Press, 1960.

26. Dunham, H. W. "Social class and schizophrenia," *American Journal of Orthopsychiatry,* 34:634-642 (1964).

27. Durkheim, E. *Le Suicide.* Paris: Librairie Felis Alean, 1912.

28. Durkheim, E. *Suicide: A Study in Sociology.* Glencoe, Ill.: the Free Press, 1951.

29. Duvall, H. J., Locke, B. Z., and Kramer, M. "Psychoneuroses among first admissions to psychiatric facilities in Ohio, 1958-1961," *Community Mental Health Journal,* 2:237-243 (1966).

30. Faris, R. E. L., and Dunham, H. W. *Mental Disorders in Urban Areas.* Chicago: University of Chicago Press, 1939.

31. Federal Security Agency, Public Health Service and National Institutes of Health. *Proceedings of the First Research Conference on Psychosurgery.* Washington, D.C.: U.S. Government Printing Office, 1952.

32. Federal Security Agency, Public Health Service and National Institutes of Health. *Proceedings of the Second Research Conference on Psychosurgery.* Washington, D C.: U.S. Government Printing Office, 1952.

33. Federal Security Agency, Public Health Service and National Institutes of Health. *Proceedings of the Third Research Conference on Psychosurgery.* Washington, D.C.: U.S. Government Printing Office, 1954.

34. Ferber, A., et al. "Current family structure: psychiatric emergencies and patient fate," paper presented at the 122nd meeting of the American Psychiatric Association, Atlantic City, N.J., May 13, 1966.

35. Foulds, G. A. "Reliability of psychiatric and validity of psychological diagnoses," *Journal of Mental Science,* 101:851 (1955).

36. Fowler, I. A., Greenberg, E. M., McCaffery, I., and Rogot, E. "The relationship of city-sized geographic location and proximity to mental hospitals with hospitalized incidence of psychosis of the aged," in Technical Report of the

Mental Health Research Unit, New York State Department of Mental Hygiene. Syracuse: Syracuse University Press, 1956.

37. Freud, S. "Mourning and melancholia," *Collected Papers,* vol. IV, 152-170, London: Hogarth Press, 1949.

38. Frost, W. H. "Epidemiology in Nelson loose leaf system," *Public Health Preventive Medicine,* vol. 2. New York: Thomas Nelson and Sons, 1927. (Reprinted in papers of Wade Hampton Frost, M.D., *A Contribution to Epidemiologic Method* (K. F. Maxcy, ed.). New York: Commonwealth Fund).

39. Galioni, E. F., et al. "Intensive treatment of backward patients: a controlled pilot study," *American Journal of Psychiatry,* 109:576 (1953).

40. Gardner, E. A., et al. "All psychiatric experience in a community – a cumulative survey: report of the first year's experience," *Archives of General Psychiatry,* 9:369 (1963).

41. Gardner, E. A., et al. "Suicide and psychiatric care in the aging," *Archives of General Psychiatry,* 10:547 (1964).

42. General Register Office. *Studies on Medical and Population Subjects No. 22: A Glossary of Mental Disorders based on the International Statistical Classification of Diseases, Injuries and Causes of Death.* London: Her Majesty's Stationery Office, 1968.

43. Giesler, R., Hurley, P. L., and Person, P. H. *Survey of General Hospitals Admitting Psychiatric Patients.* Chevy Chase, Md.: National Clearinghouse for Mental Health Information, 1966.

44. Gibbs, J. P. "Sociological views of suicide," *Symposium on Suicide.* (Yochelson, L., ed.). Washington, D.C.: George Washington University, 1967.

45. Greenblatt, M., et al. *From Custodial to Therapeutic Patient Care in Mental Hospitals.* New York: Russell Sage Foundation, 1955.

46. Gregory, I. "Analysis of family data on 1,000 patients admitted to a Canadian mental hospital," *Acta Genetica et Statistica Medica,* 91:54096 (1959).

47. Grinker. R. R. "The psychodynamics of suicide and attempted suicide," *Symposium on Suicide* (Yochelson, L., ed.). Washington, D.C.: George Washington University, 1967.

48. Group for the Advancement of Psychiatry, Committee on Preventive Psychiatry. *Problems of Estimating Changes in Frequency of Mental Disorders.* New York: Publications Office of G.A.P., 1961.

49. Guralnick, Lillian. *The Study of Mortality by Occupation in the United States.* Washington, D.C.: U.S. Department of Health, Education, and Welfare, 1969.

50. Gurland, B. J., et al. "Cross national study of diagnosis of the mental disorders: some comparisons of diagnostic criteria from the first investigation," *American Journal of Psychiatry,* 125 (April Supp.): 30-38 (1969).

51. Gurland, B. J., Fleiss, J. L., Cooper, J. E., Sharpe, L., Kendell, R. E., and Roberts, P. "Cross national study of diagnoses of mental disorders: hospital diagnoses and hospital patients in New York and London," *Comprehensive Psychiatry,* vol. II, 18-25 (1970).

52. Hendin, H. *Suicide and Scandinavia.* New York: Grune and Stratton, 1965.

53. Henry, A. F., and Short, J. F., Jr. "The sociology of suicide," in *Clues to Suicide.* (Shneidman, E. S., and Faberow, N. L., eds.). New York: McGraw-Hill, 1957.

54. Hollingshead, A. B., and Redlich, F. C. *Social Class and Mental Illness.* New York: John Wiley, 1958.

55. Hunt, W. A., Wittson, C. L., and Hunt, E. B. "A theoretical and practical analysis of the diagnostic process," in *Current Problems in Psychiatric Diagnosis* (Hock, P. H., and Zubin, J., eds.). New York: Grune and Stratton, 1953.

56. Jaco, E. G. "Mental health of the Spanish-American in Texas," in *Culture and Mental Health* (Opler, M. K., ed.). New York: Macmillan, 1959.

57. Jaco, E. G. *The Social Epidemiology of Mental Disorders.* New York: Russell Sage, 1960.

58. Joint Commission on Mental Illness and Health. *Action for Mental Health.* New York: Basic Books, 1961.

59. Jordan, E. P., ed. *Standard Nomenclature of Diseases and Standard Nomenclature of Operations.* Chicago: American Medical Association, 1933.

60. Juel-Nielsen, N., et al. "Frequency of depressive states within geographically delimited groups: 3," *Acta Psychiatrica Scandinavica,* 37:69 (1961).

61. Kendell, R. E., Gourlay, J., and Cooper, J. E. "Differences in American and British usage of key diagnostic terms," in *Video Studies I,* presented at annual meeting of the American Psychiatric Association in Miami Beach, 1969.

62. Kitagawa, Evelyn M., and Hauser, Philip M. "Education differentials in mortality by cause of death, United States, 1960," *Demography,* 5(1):318-353 (1968).

63. Kramer, M., Goldstein, H., Israel, R. H., and Johnson, N. A. *An Historical Study of the Disposition of First Admissions to a State Mental Hospital. Experience of the Warren State Hospital During the Period 1916-1950.* Public Health Monograph No. 32. Washington, D.C.: U.S. Government Printing Office, 1955.

64. Kramer, M., Goldstein, H., Israel, R. H., and Johnson, N. A. "Application of life table methodology to the study of mental hospital populations," *Psychiatric Research Reports,* 5:49-76 (1956).

65. Kramer, M. "A discussion of the concepts of incidence and prevalence as related to epidemiologic studies of mental disorders," *American Journal of Public Health,* 47:826-840 (1957).

66. Kramer, M., and Pollack, E. S. "Problems in the interpretation of trends in the population movement of the public mental hospitals," *American Journal of Public Health,* 48:1003-1019 (1958).

67. Kramer, M., Pollack, E. S., and Redick, R. W. "Studies of the incidence and prevalence of hospitalized mental disorders in the United States: current status and future goals," in *Comparative Epidemiology of the Mental Disorders* (Hoch, P. H. and Zubin, J., eds.). New York: Grune and Stratton, 1961.

68. Kramer, M., Taube, C., and Starr, S. *Patterns of Use of Psychiatric Facilities by the Aged: Current Status, Trends and Implications.* Washington, D.C.: American Psychiatric Association, 1968.

69. Kramer, M. *Applications of Mental Health Statistics.* Geneva: World Health Organization, 1969.

70. Kramer, M. "Cross national study of diagnosis of mental disorders: origin of the problem," *American Journal of Psychiatry,* 125:1-11 (1969).

71. Kreitman, N. "The reliability of psychiatric diagnosis," *Journal of Mental Science,* 107:876-886 (1961).

72. Kreitman, N., et al. "The reliability of psychiatric assessment: an analysis," *Journal of Mental Science,* 107:887-908 (1961).

73. Krupinski, J., and Stroller, A. "A statistical system introduced for the evaluation of the epidemiology of psychiatric disorders in Victoria, Australia," *Health Bulletin,* 27:3 (1962).

74. Lazarus, J., Locke, B. Z., and Thomas, D. S. "Migration differentials in mental disease: state patterns in first admissions to mental hospitals for all disorders and for schizophrenia, New York, Ohio and California as of 1950," *Milbank Memorial Fund Quarterly,* 41:25-42 (1963).

75. Lemkau, P., Tietze, C., and Cooper, M. "Mental hygiene problems in an urban district: I. Description of the study," *Mental Hygiene,* 25:624-646 (1941).

76. Lin, T., and Standley, C. C. "The scope of epidemiology in psychiatry," *Public Health Papers,* no. 16, Geneva: World Health Organization, 1962.

77. Lin, T. "The epidemiological study of mental disorders," *World Health Organization Chronicle,* 21:509 (1967).

78. Lindsay, J. S., et al. "Family size and admission to psychiatric hospitals," *Medical Journal of Australia,* 2:262-264 (1964).

79. Locke, B. Z., et al. "Problems in interpretation of patterns of first admissions to Ohio State public mental hospitals for patients with schizophrenic reactions," *Psychiatric Research Report,* 10:172-196 (1958).

80. Locke, B. Z., Kramer, M., and Pasamanick, B. "Alcoholic psychoses among first admissions to public mental hospitals in Ohio," *Quarterly Journal of Studies on Alcohol,* 21:457-474 (1960).

81. Locke, B. Z., Kramer, M., and Pasamanick, B. "Mental diseases of the senium at mid-century: first admissions to Ohio State pubic mental hospitals," *American Journal of Public Health,* 50:998-1012 (1960).

82. Locke, B. Z., Kramer, M., and Pasamanick, B. "Immigration and insanity," *Public Health Reports,* 75:201-306 (1960).

83. Locke, B. Z. "Hospitalization history of patients with mental diseases of the senium," *Journal of Gerontology,* 17:381-384 (1962).

84. Locke, B. Z. "Outcome of first hospitalization of patients with schizophrenia," *Public Health Reports,* 77:801-805 (1962).

85. Locke, B. Z. "Outcome of first hospitalization of patients with alcoholic psychoses," *Quarterly Journal of Studies on Alcohol,* 23:640-643 (1962).

86. Locke, B. Z., and Duvall, H. J. "Migration and mental illness," *Eugenics Quarterly,* 11:216-221 (1964).

87. Locke, B. Z., and Duvall, H. J. "Alcoholism among first admissions to Ohio public mental hospitals," *Quarterly Journal of Studies on Alcohol,* 25:521-534 (1964).

88. Locke, B. Z. "Notes and comments: alcoholism among admissions to psychiatric facilities," *Quarterly Journal of Studies on Alcohol,* 26:303 (1965).

89. Locke, B. Z., and Duvall, H. J. "Patterns of schizophrenic admissions to Ohio public mental hospitals," *Mental Hygiene,* 49:220-229 (1965).

90. Locke, B. Z. and Duvall, H. J. "First admissions to Ohio mental hospitals for mental diseases of the senium, 1958-1961," *Public Health Reports,* 80:779-789 (1965).

91. MacMahon, B., Pugh, T. F., and Ipsen, J. *Epidemiologic Methods.* Boston: Little, Brown, 1960.

92. MacMahon, B., Johnson, S., and Pugh, T. "Relation of suicide rates to social conditions – evidence from U.S. vital statistics," *Public Health Reports,* vol. 78, no. 4 (1963).

93. MacMahon, B. "Mental illness," in *Preventive Medicine* (Clark, D. W., and MacMahon, B., eds.). London: J. & A. Churchill, 1967, pp. 325-342.

94. Malzberg, B. *Mortality among Patients with Mental Disease.* Utica, N.Y.: State Hospital Press (1934).

95. Malzberg, B. *Social and Biological Aspects of Mental Disease.* Utica, N.Y.: State Hospital Press, 1940.

96. Malzberg, B. *Statistical Data for the Study of Mental Disease in New York State, 1939-1941.* Albany: New York State Department of Mental Hygiene, 1955.

97. Malzberg, B., and Lee, E. S. *Migration and Mental Disease.* New York: Social Science Research Council, 1956.

98. Malzberg, B. *Cohort Studies of Mental Disease in New York State, 1943-1949.* New York: National Association for Mental Health, 1958.

99. McCaffrey, I. *Socioeconomic Environment and First Admissions to Mental Hospitals of Patients with Cerebral Arteriosclerosis and Senile Psychoses, Syracuse City 1935-1941.* New York: Syracuse University Press, 1955.

100. Milbank Memorial Fund. "An approach to the prevention of disability from chronic psychoses: the open mental hospital within the community," *Proceedings of thirty-fourth Annual Conference.* New York: Milbank Memorial Fund, 1957.

101. National Association for Mental Health. *Directory of Facilities for Mentally Ill Children in the United States, 1967.* New York, 1967.

102. National Center for Health Statistics. *Vital Statistics of the United States for 1955 – supplement: Mortality Data, Multiple Causes of Death.* Washington, D.C.: U.S. Government Printing Office, 1965.

103. New York State Department of Mental Hygiene. *Seventy-fourth Annual Report, 1962.* Albany: New York State Department of Mental Hygiene, 1966.

104. Norris, V. "Mental illness in London," *Maudsley Monograph No. 6,* London: Chapman and Hall, 1959.

105. Odegard, O. and Astrup, C. "Continued experiments in psychiatric diagnosis," *Acta Psychiatrica Scandinavica,* 46: 180-210 (1970).

106. Pasamanick, B., Roberts, D. W., Lemkau, P. V., and Krueger, D. E. "A survey of mental disease in an urban population: I. Prevalence by age, sex and severity of impairments," *American Journal of Public Health,* 47:923-929 (1957).

107. Pasamanick, B., Dinitz, S., and Lefton, M. "Psychiatric orientation and its relation to diagnosis and treatment in a mental hospital," *American Journal of Psychiatry,* 116:127-132 (1959).

108. Patton, R. E. "What the tranquilizing drugs are doing to the population in mental hospitals," Proceedings of the Social Statistics Section, American Statistical Association, Washington, D.C. (1958).

109. Plunkett, R. J. and Hayden, A. C. (eds.). *Standard Nomenclature of Diseases and Operations.* Fourth Edition published for the American Medical Association, New York: The Blakiston Company, 1952.

110. Pollack, E. S., et al. *Patterns of Retention, Release and Death of First Admissions to State Mental Hospitals.* Washington, D.C.: U.S. Government Printing Office, 1959.

111. Pollack, E. S., Locke, B. Z., and Kramer, M. "Trends in hospitalization and patterns of care of the aged mentally ill," *Psychopathology of Aging* (Hoch, P. H., and Zubin, J., eds.). New York: Grune & Stratton, 1961.

112. Pollack, E. S., et al., "Socioeconomic and family characteristics of patients admitted to psychiatric services," *American Journal of Public Health,* 54:506-518 (1964).

113. Pollack, E. S. "Use of census matching for study of psychiatric admission rates," *Proceedings of the Social Statistics Section,* American Statistical Association, 107-115 (1965).

114. Pollack, E. S., Redick, R. W., and Taube, C. A. "The application of census socioeconomic and family data to the study of morbidity from mental disorders," *American Journal of Public Health,* 58:83-89 (1968).

115. Pollock, H. M. *Mental Disease and Social Welfare.* Utica, N.Y.: State Hospitals Press, 1941.

116. Powell, E. H. "Occupation, status and suicide: toward a redefinition of anomie" *American Sociological Review,* 23:131-139 (1958).

117. Pugh, T. F., and MacMahon, B. *Epidemiologic Finds in the United States Mental Hospital Data.* Boston: Little, Brown, 1962.

118. Rawnsley, K., et al. "Attitudes of relatives to patients in mental hospitals," *British Journal of Preventive and Social Medicine,* 16:1 (1962).

119. *The Registrar General's Decennial Supplement, England and Wales, 1951.* London: Her Majesty's Stationery Office, 1958.

120. Reid, D. D. "Epidemiological methods in the study of mental disorders," *Public Health Papers,* no. 2, Geneva: World Health Organization, 1960.

121. Richman, A., and Kennedy, P. "Estimating longitudinal changes in the number of patients hospitalized in Canadian psychiatric institutions," *Acta Psychiatrica Scandinavica,* 41:177 (1965).

122. Richman, A. "Long-stay patients in Canadian mental hospitals," *Canadian Medical Association Journal,* 95:337 (1966).

123. Robins, E., Murphy, G. E., et al. "Some clinical considerations in the prevention of suicide based on a study of 134 successful suicides," *American Journal of Public Health,* 49:888-889 (1959).

124. Rosenbaum, M. "Recognition of the suicidal individual," *Symposium on Suicide* (Yochelson, L., ed.). Washington, D.C.: George Washington University, 1967.

125. Roth, W. F. and Luton, F. H. "The mental health program in Tennessee," *American Journal of Psychiatry,* vol. 99, no. 5 (1943).

126. Rutter, M., et al. "A triaxial classification of mental disorders in childhood," *Journal of Child Psychology and Psychiatry,* 10:41-61 (1969).

127. Sainsbury, P. "Suicide in London – an ecological study," *Maudsley Monograph No. 1.* London: Chapman and Hall, 1955.

128. Sainsbury, P. "Suicide in later life," *Gerontologia Clinica,* 4:161-170 (1962).

129. Sandifer, M. G., Jr., Pettus, C., and Quade, D. "A study of psychiatric diagnosis," *Journal of Nervous and Mental Disease,* 139:350-356 (1964).

130. Schmid, C. F. "Suicides in Seattle, 1914-1925: an ecological and behavioristic study," *University of Washington Publication in the Social Sciences,* 5:1-94 (1928).

131. Schmid, C. F., and Van Arsdol, M. D., Jr. "Completed and attempted suicides: a comparative analysis," *American Sociological Review,* 20:273-283 (1955).

132. Schmidt, H. O., and Fonda, C. P. "The reliability of psychiatric diagnosis: a new look," *Journal of Abnormal Social Psychology,* 52:262-267 (1956).

133. Schneidman, E. S., and Farberow, N. S. *The Cry for Help.* New York: McGraw-Hill, 1961.

134. Schneidman, E. S., and Farberow, N. S. "Sociological investigation of suicide," in *Perspectives in Personality Research,* (David, H. P., and Brengelman, J. D., eds.). New York: Basic Books, 1960.

135. Seeman, W. "An investigation of interperson reliability after didactic instruction," *Journal of Nervous and Mental Disease,* 118:541-544 (1953).

136. Shepherd, M., Cooper, B., Brown, A. C., and Kalton, G. W. *Psychiatric Illness in General Practice.* London: Oxford University Press, 1966.

137. Shepherd, M., Brooke, E. M., Cooper, J. E., and Lin, T. "An experimental approach to psychiatric diagnosis," *Acta Psychiatrica et Neurologica Scandinavica,* supp. 201 (1968).

138. Spitzer, R. L., and Endicott, J. "Diagno: a computer program for psychiatric diagnosis utilizing the differential diagnostic procedure," *Archives of General Psychiatry,* 18:746-756 (1968).

139. Srole, L., et al. *Mental Health in the Metropolis: The Midtown Manhattan Study,* vol. 1. New York: McGraw-Hill, 1962.

140. Stengel, E. "Classification of mental disorders," *World Health Organization Bulletin,* 21:601-663 (1959).

141. Svendsen, B. B. "Psychiatric morbidity among civilians in wartime: on trends studies in general and a trends study of Danish psychiatric hospital admissions," *Acta Jutlandica,* 24 supp. A (1952).

142. Taeuber, C., and Hansen, M. H. "A preliminary evaluation of the 1960 censuses of population and housing," *Demography* 1(1):1-14 (1964).

143. Thomas, D. S., and Locke, B. Z. "Marital status, education and occupational differentials in mental disease," *The Milbank Memorial Fund Quarterly,* 41:145-160 (1963).

144. U.S. Department of Commerce, Bureau of the Census. *Patients in Hospitals for Mental Disease, 1923.* Washington, D.C.: U.S. Government Printing Office, 1926.

145. U.S. Department of Commerce, Bureau of the Census. *U.S. Census of Population 1960. Subject Reports – Inmates of Institutions.* Washington, D.C.: U.S. Government Printing Office, 1963.

146. U.S. Department of Health, Education, and Welfare. "Mental health clinic statistics," *Public Health Report,* 69:1008-1011 (1954).

147. U.S. Department of Health, Education, and Welfare, Social Security Administration. *Social Security Bulletin,* 24:12, 1961.

148. U.S. Department of Health, Education, and Welfare. *Patient Movement Data – State and County Mental Hospitals, 1960.* Washington, D.C.: Public Health Service Publication no. 1144, 1962.

149. U.S. Department of Health, Education, and Welfare. *Patients in Mental Institutions 1961 Part II.* Washington, D.C.: U.S. Public Health Service, 1963.

150. U.S. Department of Health, Education, and Welfare. *Patient Movement Data – State and County Mental Hospitals, 1961.* Washington, D.C.: Public Health Service Publication no. 1187, 1964.

151. U.S. Department of Health, Education, and Welfare. *Patient Movement Data – State and County Mental Hospitals, 1962.* Washington, D.C.: Public Health Service Publication no. 1282, 1964.

152. U.S. Department of Interior, Census Office. *Report on the Defective, Dependent, and Delinquent Classes of the Population of the U.S., 1880.* Washington, D.C.: U.S. Government Printing Office, 1888.

153. Ward, C. H., et al. "The psychiatric nomenclature," *Archives of General Psychiatry,* 7:198-205 (1962).

154. Weiss, J. "Suicide: an epidemiologic analysis," *Psychiatric Quarterly,* 1-28 (1954).

155. Wing, J. K., Isaacs, A., and Birley, J. "Reliability of diagnosis in an inpatient population," unpublished paper, Social Psychiatry Research Unit, Maudsley Hospital, London (1965).

156. Wing, L., et al. "The use of psychiatric services in three urban areas: an international case register study," *Social Psychiatry,* 2:158 (1967).

157. World Health Organization. *Manual of the International Statistical Classification of Diseases, Injuries, and Causes of Death.* Geneva, Switzerland, 1948.

158. World Health Organization. *Manual of the International Statistical Classification of Diseases, Injuries, and Causes of Death.* Geneva, Switzerland, 1957.

159. World Health Organization. *Manual of the International Statistical Classification of Diseases, Injuries, and Causes of Death,* vol. 1, Geneva, Switzerland, 1967.

160. World Health Organization. "Psychiatric diagnosis, classification and statistics," Fourth World Health Organization Seminar, Moscow. Geneva, Switzerland (mimeographed Report MH/70.8), 1968.

161. World Health Organization. "Psychiatric diagnosis, classification and statistics," Fifth World Health Organization Seminar, Washington, D.C. Geneva, Switzerland (mimeographed Report MH/70.2), 1969.

162. World Health Organization. World Health Statistical Reports, vol. 26. no. 6, Geneva, Switzerland: World Health Organization Publication, 1968.

163. Yolles, S. F. "The tragedy of suicide in the United States," *Symposium on Suicide* (Yochelson, L., ed.). Washington, D.C.: George Washington University, 1967.

164. Zubin, J. "Classification of the behavior disorders," *Annual Review of Psychology,* 19:373-401 (1967).

165. Zubin, J. "Cross national study of diagnosis of mental disorders: methodology and planning," *American Journal of Psychiatry,* 125:12-20 (1969).

Index

Bei Fragen zur Produktsicherheit wenden Sie sich bitte an:
If you have any questions regarding product safety,
please contact:

Walter de Gruyter GmbH
Genthiner Straße 13
10785 Berlin
productsafety@degruyterbrill.com